Dunmore and Fleischer's

Medical Terminology

Exercises in Etymology

FOURTH EDITION

Dunmore and Fleischer's
Medical Terminology

Exercises in Etymology

FOURTH EDITION

Cheryl Walker-Esbaugh, MA
Instructor
Department of Classics and Letters
University of Oklahoma

Laine H. McCarthy, MLIS
Clinical Associate Professor, Retired
Department of Family & Preventive Medicine
University of Oklahoma Health Sciences Center

Rhonda A. Sparks, MD
Director of Family Medicine
Variety Care

F.A. DAVIS

Philadelphia

F. A. Davis Company
1915 Arch Street
Philadelphia, PA 19103
www.fadavis.com

Printed in the United States of America

Last digit indicates print number: 10 9 8 7 6 5 4 3 2 1

Publisher: T. Quincy McDonald
Director of Content Development: George W. Lang
Developmental Editor: Dean DeChambeau
Content Project Manager: Julie Chase
Art and Design Manager: Carolyn O'Brien

As new scientific information becomes available through basic and clinical research, recommended treatments and drug therapies undergo changes. The author(s) and publisher have done everything possible to make this book accurate, up to date, and in accord with accepted standards at the time of publication. The author(s), editors, and publisher are not responsible for errors or omissions or for consequences from application of the book, and make no warranty, expressed or implied, in regard to the contents of the book. Any practice described in this book should be applied by the reader in accordance with professional standards of care used in regard to the unique circumstances that may apply in each situation. The reader is advised always to check product information (package inserts) for changes and new information regarding dose and contraindications before administering any drug. Caution is especially urged when using new or infrequently ordered drugs.

Library of Congress Control Number: 2022948235

We dedicate this book to the health-care professionals whose courage and dedication has inspired and comforted us in these unprecedented times of the COVID pandemic.

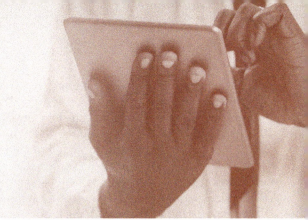

Preface

In 1977, Charles W. Dunmore, an associate professor of classics at New York University, and Rita M. Fleischer, from the Latin/Greek Institute at City University of New York, published a novel approach to teaching the challenging language of medicine. Indeed, medicine does have a language all its own, based largely on a vocabulary drawn from ancient Greek and, to a lesser degree, Latin. This approach involved teaching students to recognize the roots of *medical terminology*, the etymology of the words healthcare professionals use to communicate with each other and with patients. By teaching students the root elements of medical terminology—the prefixes, suffixes, and combining forms from Greek and Latin—Dunmore and Fleischer sought not only to teach students modern medical terminology but also to give them the ability to decipher the evolving language of medicine throughout their careers.

In the fourth edition of this book, we have continued what Dunmore and Fleischer began. This new edition is organized essentially as Dunmore and Fleischer created it, with some important modifications to facilitate ease of use. The text is organized into interrelated units. Unit 1 (Lessons 1 through 7) includes seven lessons based on Greek. Unit 2 (Lessons 8 and 9) is composed of two lessons based on Latin. Unit 3 (Lessons 10 through 15) takes a body systems approach that combines Greek and Latin elements used to describe the digestive system, respiratory system, and so forth. These first 15 lessons comprise the main body of the text. Each lesson builds and expands on the grammar and vocabulary introduced in the previous lessons.

For students who want additional exposure to medical terminology from a body systems perspective, the four lessons in Unit 4 provide just such an opportunity. These lessons include the hematopoietic and lymphatic, musculoskeletal, nervous, and endocrine systems.

Unit 5 stands on its own and provides an overview of *biological nomenclature*, the language used by scientists and physicians to identify the living organisms that exist in our world.

The pronunciation of medical terms follows the same rules that govern the pronunciation of all English words. The consonants *c* and *g* are "soft" before the vowels *e, i,* and *y.* That is, they are pronounced like the *c* and *g* of the words *cement* and *ginger.* Before *a, o,* and *u,* the consonants are "hard" and are pronounced like the *c* and *g* of *cardiac* and *gas.* The consonant *k* is always "hard," as in *leukocyte.* The long vowels *eta* and *omega* of Greek words are marked with the macrons *ē* and *ō;* this indicates that they are pronounced like the *e* and *o* of *hematoma.* Long *i* is pronounced "eye," as in the *-itis* of *appendicitis.* Words are pronounced with a stronger accent (emphasis) on one syllable. The accent falls on the second to last syllable if that syllable is long. To be considered long, a syllable must contain a short vowel followed by two consonants, a diphthong, or a long vowel *(neph-rī'-tis).* If the second to last syllable is short, the accent falls on the third syllable from the end of the word *(gen'-ĕ-sis).*

The appendices include indexes of Latin and Greek suffixes, prefixes, and combining forms, as well as an abbreviated English-to-Greek/Latin glossary and a complete list of terms found in the exercises in Lessons 1 through 15. These appendices provide additional support for students and instructors alike.

The structure of the exercises at the end of each lesson has remained essentially the same as in the third edition. All 15 of the major lessons contain three exercises. The first exercise asks students to analyze 50 terms based on the vocabulary found in that lesson. The second exercise requires students to identify a term based on its definition. The third exercise focuses on the vocabulary found in that lesson and also includes elements from previous lessons. The third exercise can now be used as an alternative to the first exercise.

This approach allows for smooth continuity and ensures that the major body of the text (Lessons 1 through 15) can be covered during a one-semester course. The exercises in Lessons 16 through 19 (Unit 4) are abbreviated and, for the most part, reflect only the material from that specific lesson. This approach allows these lessons to stand alone as additional study material. Lesson 20 (Unit 5), Biological Nomenclature, has also been written as a standalone lesson.

Terms in the lessons and exercises have been checked for currency and accuracy and verified in *Taber's Cyclopedic Medical Dictionary,* 23rd edition (F. A. Davis Company, 2017).

All 20 lessons include etymological notes to give students a historical perspective for medical terminology.

These notes include tales from ancient Greek and Latin writers, mythical stories of gods and goddesses, excerpts from the writings of famous ancient physicians such as Hippocrates and Celsus, and more modern stories of scientists and physicians who struggled to identify and accurately label the phenomena they observed.

This text is a workbook. We encourage you to write in this workbook and to make notes and comments that will help you as you work through the lessons and exercises.

Please note that this is not a medical textbook and should not be used for the diagnosis, treatment, prognosis, or etiology of disease. The medical content of this text, although accurate, is incomplete and is included solely to provide students with a context within which to learn medical terminology.

We hope you enjoy using this text to learn the complex and elegant language of medicine and that the knowledge you gain will benefit you throughout your career.

Cheryl Walker-Esbaugh
Laine H. McCarthy
Rhonda A. Sparks

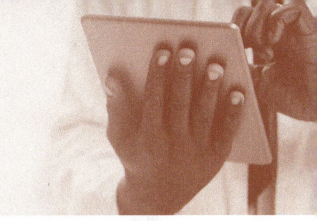

Acknowledgments

We would like to thank F. A. Davis for their generosity in allowing us to use material in *Taber's Cyclopedic Medical Dictionary, 23rd edition*. We also thank the editors at Davis for their advice and support. All of the people involved helped to make this a much better work than we could have made it ourselves. Any errors, of course, are our own.

The fourth edition of this book made it to the finish line because of the kind assistance and guidance from the exceedingly helpful people at Progressive Publishing Services (PPS). Our specials thanks to our Project manager Christine Becker who patiently answered our emails and questions expeditiously. Her kindness and helpfulness cannot be overemphasized. Also, to Carol Lallier, whose suggestions and corrections made it a much better book than it would have been without her expertise.

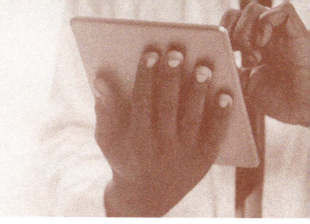

Contents

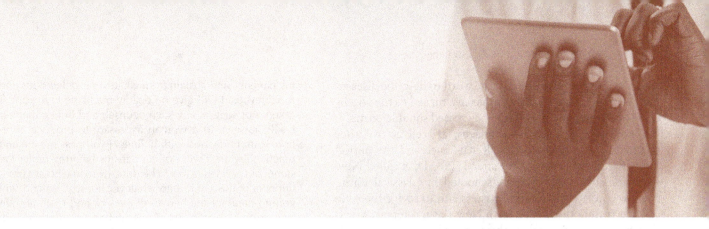

Development of the English Language

In 55 and 54 BC, Julius Caesar invaded Britain. The romanization of Britain, however, did not occur until almost 100 years later, when expeditionary forces were sent out by the Roman emperor Claudius. Although Latin was the official language during the Roman occupation of Britain, Celtic, the native language of the people of Britain, was little affected by it.

The English language began its development as an independent tongue with the migration of Germanic people (Angles, Saxons, and Jutes) from Western Europe (modern-day Denmark and northern Germany) across the English Channel to Britain during the fifth and sixth centuries AD. These Germanic invaders, in contact with the Romans from the first century BC on, brought with them not only their native tongue but also the Latin words they had borrowed from the Romans. Their language, known as Old English or Anglo-Saxon, was a member of the Germanic family of Indo-European languages and gradually superseded the Celtic dialects in most of southern Britain. Many Old English words have survived, with some linguistic change, to form the basic vocabulary of the English language. Words borrowed from other languages—mostly Latin, French, and Greek—have been added to the English language.

During the seventh century AD, after the establishment of the first monastery in 598 AD, the inhabitants of Britain gradually converted to Christianity. Latin, the language of the Western Church, was spoken, written, and read in the churches, schools, and monasteries. This brought many Latin words into the evolving English language, most having to do with religious matters and many derived from Greek.

Beginning in the eighth century AD, as a result of the Viking invasions, additional words of North Germanic origin entered the English language. Living alongside the Anglo-Saxons and eventually assimilated by them, the Norse and Danish invaders and their language had a marked impact on both England and the English language. It is not surprising that, in 1697 AD, writer Daniel Defoe described English as "your Roman-Saxon-Danish-Norman-English."

The Norman invasion in 1066 AD brought a French-speaking aristocracy to England, and for the next 150 years, French was the official spoken and written language of the governing class. In this period, French, with its roots in Latin, existed alongside English but had little effect on it. However, in the 300 years following the expulsion of the Normans from England—from about 1200 to 1500 AD—although English was once again the dominant language, many words were borrowed from French because its vocabulary was far richer. Writers and educated people in England began to look to French as a source of words and concepts lacking in their own language. During these years, the changing English language reached the stage we now know as Middle English.

With the Renaissance (1400–1600 AD) came a revival of classic scholarship. English words began to be formed directly from Latin and Greek and were no longer borrowed through the intermediary of French. Beginning around 1500 AD, for the first time the writings of the ancient Greeks were read in England in their original language. This renewal of interest in Greek and Roman literature and the ideas and concepts expressed in these works created an awareness of the impoverished state of the English language and the difficulty of expressing in English ideas that were easily expressed in Latin or Greek. Words were borrowed extensively from Greek and Latin, both with and without change, and new words were created that combined both Latin and Greek elements. Although most words were borrowed from Latin and Greek, others were borrowed from French and Italian. The English of this period is now known as Modern English.

The extensive borrowing of words from Latin and Greek that began about 1500 AD continued for hundreds of years and continues to this day. As new advances were made in the fields of medicine and science during and after the Renaissance (and continuing up to the present day), words were needed to describe these new discoveries and inventions. Medical scientists turned to the early Greek and Roman physicians, especially Hippocrates, Galen, and Celsus, whom they greatly admired, and borrowed words from their medical treatises. These ancient scientists had an extensive medical vocabulary, which they used to describe their observations and theories. Hippocrates, for example, used the terms *apoplexy, hypochondria, dysentery, ophthalmia, epilepsy,* and *asthma* to describe certain physical features and conditions that he observed. Modern physicians and scientists, who could not find an appropriate word to describe diseases that were unknown to early physicians, turned to the vocabulary of the ancient languages and created suitable terms.

The language used by Linnaeus, as well as by other scientists and scholars of the Renaissance and the period following, that is, the period after 1500 AD, is called New Latin. Scientists and writers, schooled in Classical Latin, tried to emulate the classical writers and to revive the style of Cicero and others. The term New Latin refers to words that have been created in the form of, and on the analogy of, Latin words (e.g., *natrium*, the chemical name for sodium, borrowed from Arabic) or to the use of new meanings applied to extant Latin words (e.g., the word cancer, from *cancer*, crab, or the word bacillus, from *bacillus*, a small rod or staff). New Latin is a rich source of biological terms. *Trichinella spiralis*, the species of *Trichinella* that causes trichinosis, and *Salmonella*, the genus of microorganisms named after the American pathologist Daniel E. Salmon, are two of the many examples of New Latin found in this text.

HIPPOCRATES

Hippocrates, born in 460 BC, was a Greek physician who lived on the Aegean island of Cos. Although he is the most famous of the ancient physicians and is recognized as the father of medicine, very little is actually known about him or his life. The *Hippocratic Corpus*, a work of about 60 medical treatises attributed to Hippocrates, most likely reflects the work of many physicians rather than that of Hippocrates alone. Hippocrates is recognized for separating superstition from medicine. Unlike other physicians of his time, he believed that illness had a rational explanation, rather than being the result of divine anger or possession by evil spirits, and could therefore be treated. Hippocrates based his medical writings on his observation and study of the human body. He was the first to attempt to record his experiences as a physician for future reference. The Hippocratic Oath, although it cannot be directly attributed to him, is said to reflect his philosophy and principles.

THE HIPPOCRATIC OATH

"I swear by Apollo the physician, and Aesculapius, and Hygeia, and Panacea, and all the gods and goddesses, that according to my ability and judgment, I will keep this oath and its stipulation—to reckon him who taught me this art equally dear to me as my parents, to share my substance with him, and to relieve his necessities if required; to look upon his offspring in the same footing as my own brothers, and to teach them this art if they shall wish to learn it, without fee or stipulation, and that by precept, lecture, and every other mode of instruction, I will impart a knowledge of the art to my own sons, and those of my teachers, and to disciples bound by a stipulation and oath according to the law of medicine, but to none other.

"I will follow that system of regimen which, according to my ability and judgment, I consider for the benefit of my patients, and abstain from whatever is deleterious and mischievous. I will give no deadly medicine to anyone if asked, nor suggest any such counsel; and in like manner I will not give to a woman a pessary to produce abortion. With purity and with holiness I will pass my life and practice my art. I will not cut persons laboring under the stone, but will leave this to be done by men who are practitioners of this work. Into whatever houses I enter, I will go into them for the benefit of the sick and I will abstain from every voluntary act of mischief and corruption; and, further, from the seduction of females or males, of freemen and slaves. Whatever, in connection with my professional practice, or not in connection with it, I see or hear, in the life of men, which ought not to be spoken of abroad, I will not divulge, as reckoning that all such should be kept secret.

"While I continue to keep this Oath unviolated, may it be granted to me to enjoy life and the practice of this art, respected by all men, in all times. But, should I trespass and violate this Oath, may the reverse be my lot." (From Venes, D. *Taber's Cyclopedic Medical Dictionary*. 19th ed. F. A. Davis. 2001, pp. 949–950, with permission.)

GALEN

Galen was born in Pergamum, Asia Minor, in 129 AD. After studying medicine at the Asclepium, the famed medical school in his native town, and in Smyrna and Alexandria, he came to Rome in 162 AD, where, except for brief interruptions, he remained until his death, writing philosophical treatises and medical books. His fame and reputation brought him to the attention of the emperor Marcus Aurelius, who appointed him court physician. Galen wrote extensively on anatomy, physiology, and general medicine, relying on his training, the best that was available, and on his dissection of human corpses and experiments on living animals. It was the work of Galen, more than of any other medical writer, that profoundly influenced the physicians of the early Renaissance. His theories on the flow of blood in the human body remained unchallenged until the discovery of the circulation of the blood by William Harvey in the 17th century.

CELSUS

Aulus Cornelius Celsus was a Roman encyclopedist who, under the reign of the emperor Tiberius (14–37 AD), wrote a lengthy work dealing with agriculture, military tactics, medicine, rhetoric, and possibly, philosophy and law. Apart from a few fragments, only his eight books on medicine still exist. It is suggested that Celsus was not a professional physician but rather a layman writing for other laymen. It appears, especially in his treatises on surgery, that he had little firsthand experience in the field of medicine and relied on material selected from other sources. Celsus was highly esteemed during the Renaissance, possibly as a result of his style of writing.

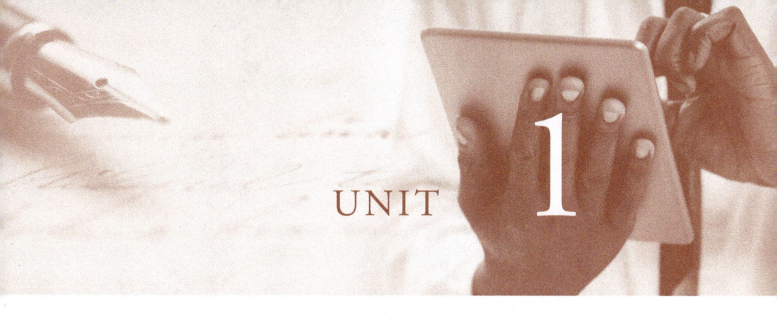

Greek-Derived Medical Terminology

GREEK ALPHABET

Name of Letter	Capital	Lowercase	Transliteration	Name of Letter	Capital	Lowercase	Transliteration
alpha	A	α	a	xi	Ξ	ξ	x
beta	B	ϐ or β	b	omicron	O	ο	o short
gamma	Γ	γ	g	pi	Π	π	p
delta	Δ	δ	d	rho	P	ρ	r
epsilon	E	ε	e short	sigma	Σ	σ or s	s
zeta	Z	ζ	z	tau	T	τ	t
eta	H	η	e long	upsilon	Y	υ	y
theta	Θ	θ	th	phi	Φ	φ or φ	f, ph
iota	I	ι	i	chi	X	x	ch as in
kappa	K	κ	k, c				German
lambda	Λ	λ	l				"echt"
mu	M	μ	m	psi	Ψ	ψ	ps
nu	N	ν	n	omega	Ω	ω	o long

Source: Venes D., ed. *Taber's Cyclopedic Medical Dictionary*. 19th ed. F. A. Davis. 2001, p. 2368.

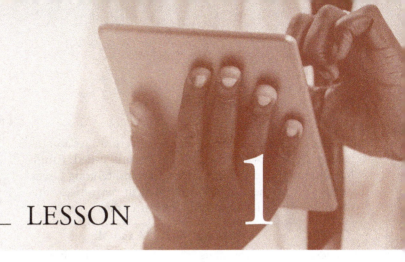
GREEK NOUNS AND ADJECTIVES

A man who is wise should consider health the most valuable of all things to mankind and learn how, by his own intelligence, to help himself in sickness.

[Hippocrates, *Regimen in Health* 9]

In the mid-eighth century BC, the Greeks borrowed the art of writing from the Phoenicians, a Semitic-speaking people of the Levant who inhabited the region in the area of modern Lebanon. The Phoenician system of writing had to be adapted to the Greek language because it contained characters representing sounds in the Semitic language that did not exist in Greek and sounds in Greek for which no characters existed in the Semitic system. In their adaptation of these Phoenician characters, the Greeks began to distinguish between long and short vowels, representing long e by *eta* [H] and short e by *epsilon* [E], and long and short o by *omega* [Ω] and *omicron* [O], respectively. However, the distinction was carried no further, and no differentiation in writing was made between the long and short vowels a, -i, and u. In transliterating Greek words, this text uses a macron (·) to mark the long vowels *ē* and *ō*:

Greek	Meaning	Example
xēros	dry	**xeroderma**
splēn	spleen	**splenomegaly**
phōnē	voice	**phonology**
thōrax	chest cavity	**thoracentesis**

During and after the first century BC, many Greek words were borrowed by the Romans and, in the process of being borrowed, assumed the spelling of Latin words. It has been the practice since then, in the coining of English words from Greek, to use the form and spelling of Latin, even if the word never actually appeared in the Latin language.

The letter *k* was little used in Latin, and Greek *kappa* was transliterated in that language as *c*, which always had the hard sound of *k*. Most English words derived from Greek words containing a *kappa* are spelled with *c*:

Greek	Meaning	Example
kyanos	blue	**cyanotic**
mikros	small	**microscope**
kolon	colon	**colitis**
skleros	hard	**arteriosclerosis**

There are exceptions, and the *kappa* is retained as *k* in some words:

Greek	Meaning	Example
leukos	white	**leukemia**
kinēsis	motion	**dyskinesia**
karyon	kernel	**karyogenesis**
kēlē	swelling	**keloid**

Some words are spelled with either *k* or *c*: **keratocele, ceratocele** (*kerat-*, horn); **cinematics, kinematics** (*kinēma*, motion).

In Latin, the letter *k* is rarely used and is found only in the following:

- *Kalendae*, the Calends, the first day of the month, and its derivatives *Kalendalis, Kalendaris, Kalendarium,* and *Kalendarius*
- *Karthago*, Carthage, the Phoenician city in North Africa

- *kalo* (archaic), call
- *koppa* (archaic), Greek symbol for 90

Greek words beginning with *rho* [r] were always accompanied by a strong expulsion of breath called **rough breathing** (also called aspiration). In transliterating Greek words and in the formation of English derivatives, this rough breathing is indicated by an *h* after the *r*:

Greek	Meaning	Example
rhombos	rhombus	**rhombencephalon**
rhodon	rose	**rhodopsin**
rhiza	root	**rhizoid**
rhythmos	rhythm	**rhythmic**

There are exceptions: **rhachis, rachis** (*rhachis*, spine). Words beginning with *rho* [r] usually double the *r* when following a prefix or another word element, and the **rough breathing** [h] follows the second *r* (note: the following words are from Greek verbs):

Greek	Meaning	Example
rhe-	flow	**diarrhea**
rhag-	burst forth	**hemorrhage**
rhaph-	sew	**cystorrhaphy**

When Greek words containing diphthongs were borrowed and used in Latin, the diphthongs *ai*, *ei*, *oi*, and *ou* were changed to the Latin spelling of these sounds, but these Latin diphthongs usually undergo a further change in English:

Greek	Latin	English	Greek Example	Meaning	English Example
ai	*ae*	*e*	*haima*	blood	**hematology***
			aitia	cause	**etiology***
ei	*ei*	*ei* or *i*	*cheir*	hand	**cheirospasm, dyschiria**
			leios	smooth	**leiomyofibroma**
			meiōn	less	**miotic**
oi	*oe*	*e*	*oidēma*	swelling	**edema***
			oistros	desire	**estrogen***
ou	*u*	*u*	*gloutos*	buttock	**gluteal**

*British spelling usually retains the Latin diphthongs *ae* and *oe*: haematology, aetiology, oedema, oestrogen.

In the Greek language, words beginning with the sound of the rough breathing [h] often lost their aspiration when another word element preceded the aspirated word (except after the prefixes *anti-*, *apo-*, *epi-*, *hypo-*, *kata-*, and *meta-*). However, the spelling of English derivatives of such words varies, and the aspiration is often retained:

Greek	Meaning	Example
hidros	sweat	**chromidrosis**
		hyperhidrosis

Greek is an **inflected** language—that is, words have different endings to indicate their grammatical function in a sentence. The inflection of nouns, pronouns, and adjectives is called **declension.** Greek nouns are declined in five grammatical cases in both singular and plural: nominative, genitive, dative, accusative, and vocative. There are three declensions of Greek nouns, each having its own set of endings for the cases. Nouns are cited in dictionaries and vocabularies in the form of the nominative singular, often called the **dictionary form.**

Nouns of the first declension, mostly feminine, end in *-ē* or *-ā* and sometimes in short *-a*. Second declension nouns, mostly masculine or neuter, end in *-os* if masculine and in *-on* if neuter. Third declension nouns are discussed in Lesson 2.

The base of nouns of the first and second declensions is found by dropping the ending of the nominative case, resulting in the **combining form,** to which suffixes and other combining forms are added to form words:

Greek	Meaning	Example
nephros	kidney	**nephr**-itis
neuron	nerve	**neur**-otic
psōra	sore	**psor**-iasis
psychē	mind	**psych**-osis

Rarely, the entire word is used as the combining form: **colonoscopy** (*kolon*, colon), **neuronitis** (*neuron*, nerve).

If a suffix or a combining form that begins with a consonant is attached to a combining form that ends in a consonant, then a vowel, called the **connecting vowel,** usually **o** and sometimes **i** or **u** (especially with words derived from Latin), is inserted between the two forms.†

leuk-**o**-cyte
neur-**o**-blast
psych-**o**-neurosis
calc-**i**-pexis
vir-**u**-lent

---

†Medical dictionaries and English dictionaries usually give the connecting vowel as part of the combining form, as in leuko-, neuro-, psycho-, and so forth.

Exceptions occur when suffixes beginning with *s* or *t* follow an element ending with *p* or *c*:

eclamp-sia
apoplec-tic
epilep-tic

Adjectives agree in gender, number, and case with the noun they modify. They are cited in dictionaries and vocabularies in the form of the nominative singular masculine. The dictionary form of most Greek adjectives ends in *-os*, and the combining form is found by dropping this ending. Some adjectives end in *-ys*, and the combining form of these is found by dropping the *-s* or, rarely, the *-ys*:

Greek	Meaning	Example
leukos	white	**leuk**-emia
kyanos	blue	**cyan**-osis
tachys	swift	**tachy**-gastria
glykys	sweet	**glyc**-emia

When Greek nouns are used in English, they usually appear in one of four ways:

1. In the original vocabulary form:
kolon	**colon**
mania	**mania**
omphalos	**exomphalos**
psyche	**psyche**

2. With the ending changed to the Latin form:
aortē	**aorta**
bronchos	**bronchus**
kranion	**cranium**
tetanos	**tetanus**

3. With the ending changed to silent *-e*:
gangraina	**gangrene**
kyklos	**cycle**
tonos	**tone**
zōnē	**zone**

4. With the ending dropped:
organon	**organ**
orgasmos	**orgasm**
spasmos	**spasm**
stomachos	**stomach**

PREFIXES

Prefixes modify or qualify in some way the meaning of the word to which they are affixed. It is often difficult to assign a single specific meaning to each prefix, and it is often necessary to adapt a meaning that fits the particular use of a word. A complete list of prefixes is found in Appendix B.

---

a- (**an-** before a vowel or *h*): not, without, lacking, deficient:

a-biogenesis	**an**-algesia
a-sthenia	**an**-hydrous
encephal-**a**-trophy	**an**-hidrosis

anti- (**ant-** often before a vowel or *h*; hyphenated before *i*): against, opposed to, preventing, relieving:

anti-biotic	**anti**-retroviral
anti-histamine	**anti**-septic
anti-toxin	**ant**-acid

di- (rarely **dis-**): two, twice, double:

di-otic	**di**-oxide
di-plegia	**dis**-mutase

dys-: difficult, painful, defective, abnormal:

dys-menorrhea	**dys**-pepsia
dys-pnea	**dys**-genesis
dys-ostosis	**dys**-trophy

ec- (**ex-** before a vowel): out of, away from:

ec-tasis	**ex**-encephalia
ec-topic	**ex**-cision

The prefix **ex-** in most words is derived from Latin: **excrete, exhale, extensor, exudate,** and so forth.

ecto- (**ect-** often before a vowel): outside of:

ecto-derm	**ecto**-plasm
ecto-cervix	**ect**-ostosis

en- (**em-** before *b*, *m*, and *p*): in, into, within:

en-cephalitis	**em**-metropia
em-bolism	**em**-physema

endo-, ento- (**end-, ent-** before a vowel): within:

endo-genous	**ento**-cele
endo-metritis	**end**-odontics
endo-cardium	**ent**-optic

epi- (**ep-** before a vowel or *h*): upon, over, above:

epi-cardium	**epi**-demic
epi-dermis	**ep**-onychium

exo-: outside, from the outside, toward the outside:

exo-cardia	**exo**-genous
exo-crine	**exo**-thermal

hemi-: half, partial; (often) one side of the body:

hemi-crania	**hemi**-paralysis
hemi-plegia	**hemi**-gastrectomy

hyper-: over, above, excessive, beyond normal:

hyper-hidrosis	**hyper**-lipemia
hyper-glycemia	**hyper**-parathyroidism

hypo- (hyp- before a vowel or *h*): under, deficient, below normal:

hypo-chondria	**hyp-**algesia
hypo-dermic	**hyp-**oxia

mono- (mon- before a vowel or *h*): one, single:

mono-blast	**mono-**chromatic
mon-ocular	**mono-**neuritis

peri-: around, surrounding:

peri-aortic	**peri-**gastric
peri-cardium	**peri-**neuritis

syn- (sym- before *b*, *p*, and *m*; the *n* assimilates or is dropped before *s*): together, with, joined:

syn-apse	**sym-**pathy
syn-thetic	**sym-**metry
sym-biosis	**sy-**stolic

Note that words can have more than one prefix and that a prefix can follow a combining form:

exo-anti-gen	cardi-**ec-**tomy
tachy-**a-**rrhythmia	**dys-dia-**dochokinesia

SUFFIXES

Suffixes are elements that are added to combining forms. Suffixes form nouns, adjectives, and verbs or adverbs. Most of these nouns are abstract; that is, they indicate a state, quality, condition, procedure, or process. In medical terminology, most conditions indicated by these suffixes are pathological or abnormal: **psoriasis, hepatitis, pneumonia, myopia, astigmatism,** and so forth. Some nouns indicating procedures or processes are **amniocentesis, appendectomy, gastroscopy,** and **gastropexy.** A complete list of suffixes is found in Appendix C.

-a: abstract noun-forming suffix: state, condition:

dyspne-**a**	anasarc-**a**
erythroderm-**a**	rhinorrhe-**a**

-ac (rare): adjective-forming suffix: pertaining to, located in:

cardi-**ac**	ile-**ac**
celi-**ac**	myocardi-**ac**

-ia: abstract noun-forming suffix: state, condition:

anem-**ia**	hyposm-**ia**
pneumon-**ia**	vagoton-**ia**

-iac (rare): noun-forming suffix: person afflicted with:

hemophil-**iac**	insomn-**iac**
hypochondr-**iac**	amnes-**iac**

-iasis: abstract noun-forming suffix: disease, abnormal condition, abnormal presence of; often used with the name of a parasitic organism to indicate infestation of the body by that organism. When used with **lith-** [Gr. *lithos*, stone]: formation and/or presence of calculi in the body:

elephant-**iasis**	ancylostom-**iasis**
nephrolith-**iasis**	schistosom-**iasis**

-ic: adjective-forming suffix: pertaining to, located in; words ending in **-ic** can be used as both adjectives and nouns and, as nouns, often indicate a drug or agent:

analges-**ic**	hypoderm-**ic**
gastr-**ic**	tox-**ic**

Words ending in **-ic** can refer to a person suffering from a certain disability or condition:

parapleg-**ic**	anorex-**ic**

-in, -ine: noun-forming suffix: form names of substances:

diox-**in**	chlor-**ine**
antitox-**in**	epinephr-**ine**

-ist: noun-forming suffix: a person interested in:

cardiolog-**ist**	hematolog-**ist**
dermatolog-**ist**	orthodont-**ist**

-itic: adjective-forming suffix: pertaining to; pertaining to inflammation; words ending in **-itic** can be used as both adjectives and nouns and, as nouns, often indicate a drug or agent:

antineur-**itic**	arthr-**itic** (Fig. 1-1)
laryng-**itic**	nephr-**itic**

-itis: noun-forming suffix: indicating an inflamed condition; inflammation:

gastr-**itis**	laryng-**itis**
hepat-**itis**	periton-**itis**

-itides is the plural form for nouns ending in **-itis**:

arthr-**itides**	dermat-**itides**

-ium (rarely **-eum**): noun-forming suffix: membrane, connective tissue:

endometr-**ium**	pericard-**ium**
epicran-**ium**	periton-**eum**

In a few words, **-ium** names a region of the body:

epigastr-**ium**	hypogastr-**ium**
hypochondr-**ium**	splen-**ium**

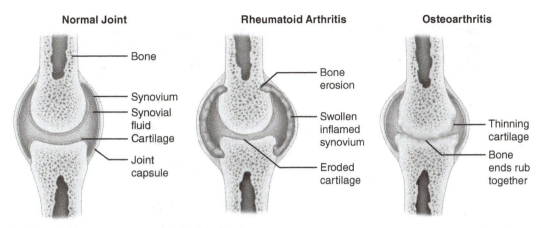

Figure 1-1. Rheumatoid arthritis. (From Hull, M., *Medical Language: Terminology in Context*, F. A. Davis, 2013.)

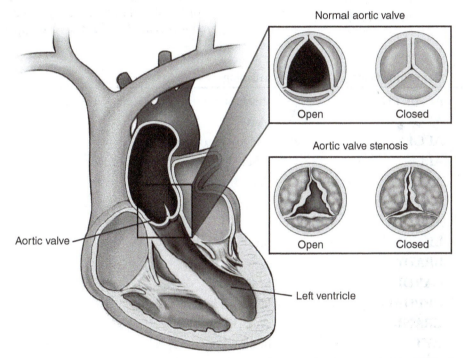

Figure 1-2. Stenosis. (From Gylys, B., and Masters, R., *Medical Terminology Simplified: A Programmed Learning Approach by Body System*, 6th ed., F. A. Davis, 2019.)

-ma: noun-forming suffix: (often) abnormal or diseased condition. The combining form for nouns ending in **-ma** is **-mat-.** Sometimes the final **-a** drops off the noun:

ede-**ma**	ede-**mat**-ogenic
trau-**ma**	trau-**mat**-ic
phleg-**m**	phleg-**mat**-ic
sper-**m**	sper-**mat**-ic

-osis*: noun-forming suffix: abnormal or diseased condition:

nephr-**osis**	scler-**osis**
neur-**osis**	sten-**osis** (Fig. 1-2)

---

*(See the Etymological Notes in this lesson for other uses of **-osis.**)

-otic: adjective-forming suffix from nouns ending in **-osis:** pertaining to:

nephr-**otic**	scler-**otic**
neur-**otic**	sten-**otic**

-sia: abstract noun-forming suffix: state, condition:

amne-**sia**	dyspha-**sia**
ecta-**sia**	eclamp-**sia**

-sis: abstract noun-forming suffix: state, condition, quality, process, procedure:

antisep-**sis**	cente-**sis**
eme-**sis**	prophylaxis (prophylac-**sis**)

-tic: adjective-forming suffix from nouns ending in **-sis:** pertaining to; words ending in **-tic** can be used as both adjectives and nouns and, as nouns, often indicate a drug or agent:

    antisep-**tic**   paraly-**tic**

    eme-**tic**   prophylac-**tic**

Words ending in **-itic** or **-tic** can form nouns referring to a person suffering from a certain disability or condition and, as such, **-itic** and **-tic** are noun-forming suffixes:

    neuro-**tic**   arthr-**itic**

-y: abstract noun-forming suffix: state, condition, quality, process, procedure:

    hypertroph-**y**   microcephal-**y**

    symmetr-**y**   neuroton-**y**

Words can have more than one suffix. Sometimes the suffix **-iac** or **-ic** is affixed to the noun-forming suffix **-sia** or **-sis.** When this occurs, the only vestige left of the noun-forming suffix is the **-s:**

    amne-**sia**   amne-**s-ic,** amne-**s-iac**

A suffix can appear in the middle of a word affixed to a combining form:

    hyperinsul-**in**-emia   hepat-**ic**-o-enterostomy

VOCABULARY

The following is a list of combining forms derived from Greek. (When the meaning of the original Greek word differs from its modern meaning, the original meaning of the word is placed in brackets.) For a complete list of combining forms used in this text, see Appendix A.

Greek	Combining Form	Meaning	Example
akantha	**ACANTH-**	thorn, spine	**acanth**-ocytosis
algos	**ALG-**	pain	my-**alg**-ia
algēsis	**ALGES-**	sensitivity to pain	an-**alges**-ia
allos	**ALL-**	other, divergence, difference from	**all**-ostery
angeion	**ANGI-**	(blood) vessel, duct	**angi**-ography
arteria	**ARTERI-**	[air passage] artery (Fig. 1-3)	**arteri**-ogram
arthron	**ARTHR-**	joint	**arthr**-itis
bios	**BI-**	life	**bi**-ology
bradys	**BRADY-**	slow	**brady**-rhythmia
kardia	**CARDI-**	heart	**cardi**-ograph
kephalē	**CEPHAL-**	head	**cephal**-algia
kranion	**CRANI-**	skull (Fig. 1-4)	epi-**crani**-um
kytos	**CYT-**	[hollow container] cell	leuko-**cyt**-e
enkephalon	**ENCEPHAL-**	brain (a combination of *en*, in, and *kephalē*, head)	**encephal**-itis
erythros	**ERYTHR-**	red, red blood cell	**erythr**-ocyte
leptos	**LEPT-**	thin, fine, slight	**lept**-omeninges
leukos	**LEUK-**	white, white blood cell	**leuk**-emia
lithos	**LITH-**	stone, calculus	micro-**lith**
logos	**LOG-**	word, study	bio-**log**-y
malakos	**MALAC-**	soft	**malac**-oplakia
mesos	**MES-**	middle, secondary, partial, mesentery	**mes**-oderm
metron	**-METER, METR-**	measure, measuring device (Words ending in **-meter** indicate instruments for measuring.)	bio-**metr**-y, cyto-**meter**
nephros	**NEPHR-**	kidney	**nephr**-ectomy

Greek	Combining Form	Meaning	Example
neuron	**NEUR-**	[tendon] nerve, nervous system	**neur-**ology
osteon	**OSTE-**	bone	**oste-**oporosis
praxis	**PRAX-**	act, action	echo-**prax-**ia
prōtos	**PROT-**	first, primitive, early	**prot-**opathic
skleros	**SCLER-**	hard	**scler-**oderma
stenos	**STEN-**	narrow	**sten-**otic
stereos	**STERE-**	solid, having three dimensions	**stere-**otropism
tachys	**TACHY-**	rapid	**tachy-**cardia
toxon	**TOX(I)-**	poison	**tox-**in

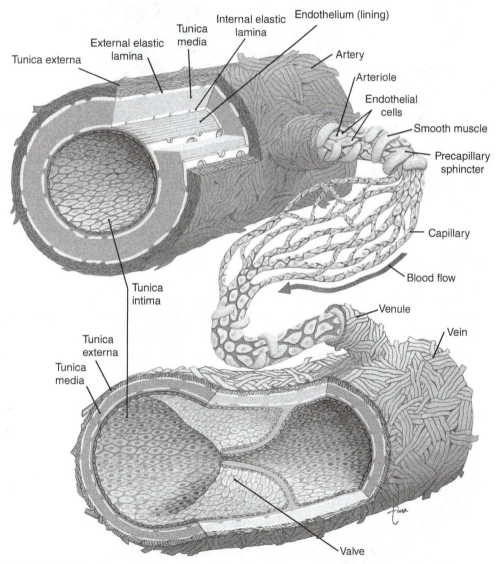

Figure 1-3. Structure of an artery. (From Scanlon, V. C., and Sanders, T., *Essentials of Anatomy and Physiology*, 8th ed., F. A. Davis, 2020.)

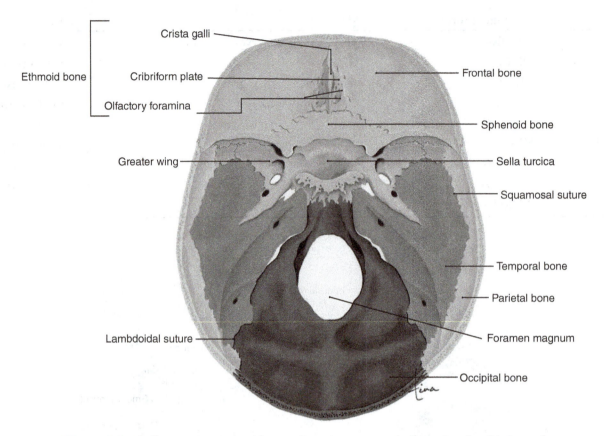

Figure 1-4. Skull. Superior view with top of cranium removed. (From Scanlon, V. C., and Sanders, T., *Essentials of Anatomy and Physiology*, 8th ed., F. A. Davis, 2020.)

SUFFIX FORMS

Many combining forms are used with certain suffixes so commonly that this combination can be called a **suffix form**. Some common suffix forms include the following:

Combining Form	Suffix Form	Meaning	Example
LOG-	**-logy**	study, science, the study or science of	cardio-**logy**
	-logist	one who specializes in a certain study or science	neuro-**logist**
MALAC-	**-malacia**	the softening (of tissues) of	osteo-**malacia**
SCLER-	**-sclerosis**	the hardening (of tissues) of	arterio-**sclerosis**
STEN-	**-stenosis**	the narrowing (of a part of the body)	cranio-**stenosis**
TOX-	**-toxic**	poisonous (to an organ)	cyto-**toxic**
	-toxin	a substance poisonous to (a part of the body)	neuro-**toxin**

ETYMOLOGICAL NOTES

Throughout its history, the English language has been enriched by borrowing words from other languages, particularly Latin, Greek, and French. Borrowing from French began as early as the period of the Norman conquest of England and reached its high point during and immediately after the Renaissance. Because French is based largely on Latin and because many Latin words are derived from Greek, various French words have Greek origins. One such word is **migraine,** a severe form of headache, usually unilateral. The French word *migraine*, the British word *megrim*, and the Italian word *emicránia* are derived from the Latin word *hemicrania*, which was borrowed from the Greek word *hemikrania*, meaning "pain on one side of the head," from the prefix *hemi* (half) and *kranion* (skull).

The ancient Greeks used to smear poison on their arrowheads for use in hunting, and this poison was called *toxicon pharmakon* (*toxon*, bow, archery; *pharmakon*, drug), thus providing the modern word **toxic.** A **toxicologist** is a specialist in the field of poisons and toxins, whereas a **toxophilite** is a lover (*philos*) of archery. **Toxicity** means the extent, quality, or degree of being poisonous; toxicity is also used to describe specific poisonous effects as in **neurotoxicity,** the capability of harming nerve cells or tissues.

The suffix **-osis** indicates an abnormal condition: **neurosis, psychosis** (*psychē*, mind). When affixed to a combining form indicating an organ or a part of the body, it usually indicates a noninflammatory diseased condition: **nephrosis, endometriosis** (*endo*, within, *mētra*, uterus). Following the combining form **cyt-** (cell) it means an abnormal increase in number of the type of cell indicated: **leukocytosis, erythrocytosis.** Following the combining form for an adjective, it indicates the abnormality characterized by the meaning of the adjective: **stenosis,** narrowing of a passage; **sclerosis,** hardening of tissues; **cyanosis** (*kyanos*, blue), bluish discoloration of a part.

A few words ending in **-osis** have special meanings:

anastomosis: a surgical or pathological connection between two passages
exostosis: a bony growth arising from the surface of a bone
aponeurosis: a sheet of tissue connecting muscles to bones
symbiosis: the living together in close association of two organisms of different species
antibiosis: the association between two organisms in which one is harmful to the other

The adjectival form for words ending in **-osis** is **-otic: neurosis, neurotic; psychosis, psychotic; nephrosis, nephrotic; symbiosis, symbiotic.**

The word **etiology** is from the Greek noun *aitia* (cause, origin) with the suffix form **-logy.** The etiology of a disease or an abnormal condition is its cause or origin. In medical dictionaries, it is usually abbreviated **etiol.**

Exercise 1:   Analyze and Define

Analyze and define each of the following words. In this and in succeeding exercises, analysis should consist of separating the words into prefixes (if any), combining forms, and suffixes or suffix forms (if any) and giving the meaning of each. Be certain to differentiate between nouns and adjectives in your definitions. Consult a medical dictionary for the current meanings of these words. Use a separate paper if you need more room for an answer.

1. acanthocytosis _____

2. acephalia _____

3. allostery _____

4. alogia _____

5. analgesic _____

6. angiology _____

7. antibiosis _____

8. anticytotoxin _____

9. apraxia _____

10. arthritides _____

11. arthritis _____

12. arthrology _____

13. arthrosclerosis _____

14. biologist _____

15. bradycardia _____

16. cardioangiology _____

17. dysostosis _____

18. ectostosis _____

19. encephalolith _____

20. endarteritis _____

21. endosteum _____

22. endotoxin _____

23. epinephrine _____

24. episcleritis _____

25. erythrocyte _____

26. erythroleukemia _____

27. erythrosis _____

28. exocardia _____

29. exotoxin _____

30. hemicrania _____

31. hypalgesia _____

32. hyperalgesia _____

33. hyperostosis _____

34. leukotoxin _____

35. lithiasis _____

36. mesocardia _____

37. nephrolithiasis _____

38. nephrosclerosis _____

39. neuritis _____

40. osteometry _____

41. osteosclerosis _____

42. ostosis _____

43. pericyte _____

44. perinephric _____

45. scleromalacia _____

46. sclerosis _____

47. stenotic _____

48. stereology _____

49. synosteology _____

50. tachycardiac _____

Exercise 2:   Word Derivation

Give the word derived from Greek elements that matches each of the following. It is not necessary to give combining terms for words in parentheses. Verify your answer in a medical dictionary. **Note that the wording of the dictionary definition may vary from the wording used here.**

1. Inflammation of the kidney _____

2. The science (and technology) of measurement _____

3. (Mesodermal) bone-forming cell _____

4. Having a medium-sized head _____

5. Absence of life _____

6. White blood cell _____

7. Membrane that lines (the chambers of) the heart _____

8. Increased heart rate alternating with slow rate _____

9. Instrument for counting and measuring cells _____

10. Measurement of a solid body _____

11. Substance toxic to kidney (tissue) _____

12. Softening of the heart (muscle) _____

13. Deep-seated head pain _____

14. Hardening of the arteries _____

15. The science dealing with calculi _____

16. Narrowing of a passage or orifice _____

17. Pain occurring along a nerve _____

18. Increased rate (of contractions) of the stomach _____

19. Inflammation of the white matter of the brain _____

20. Living together of two organisms _____

Exercise 3:   Drill and Review

Analyze and define each of the following words. Analysis should consist of separating the words into prefixes (if any), combining forms, and suffixes or suffix forms (if any), and give the meaning of each. Be certain to differentiate between nouns and adjectives in your definitions. Using the elements in the word determine its meaning. Consult a medical dictionary for the current meanings of these words. Use a separate paper if you need more room for an answer.

1. abiotic _____

2. acanthocyte _____

3. angiitis _____

4. antiarthritic _____

5. antibiotic _____

6. antilithic _____

7. antineuritic _____

8. antitoxin _____

9. arteritis _____

10. arthritic _____

11. arthrosis _____

12. biologic _____

13. biometry _____

14. biotoxin _____

15. cardionephric _____

16. cephalalgia _____

17. craniomalacia _____

18. craniosclerosis _____

19. cytobiology _____

20. cytotoxin _____

21. dysarthrosis _____

22. encephalic _____

23. encephalomalacia _____

24. endangiitis _____

25. endocranium _____

26. endoneurium _____

27. erythrocytosis _____

28. exencephalia _____

29. exocardia _____

30. exocytosis _____

31. exoerythrocytic _____

32. hemianalgesia _____

33. hyperalgia _____

34. hyperleukocytosis _____

35. hypostosis _____

36. mesencephalic _____

37. mesonephric _____

38. monocyte _____

39. mononeuritis _____

40. neurotoxin _____

41. osteomalacia _____

42. periarteritis _____

43. periarthritis _____

44. pericarditis _____

45. stenosis _____

46. symmetry _____

47. synostosis _____

48. tachycardia _____

49. toxicology _____

50. toxin _____

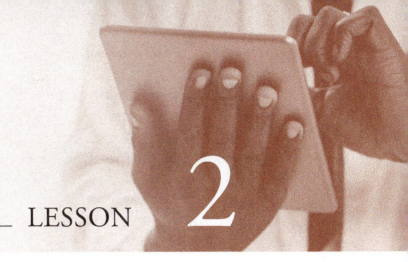

NOUNS OF THE THIRD DECLENSION

The learning of medicine can be compared to the growth of plants in the earth. Our inherent ability is the soil. The precepts of our teachers are the seeds. Learning from childhood is like the seeds falling into the plowed land at the proper season. The place of learning is like the nourishment that arises from the surrounding air to the seeds that are planted. Love of work is the labor. Time strengthens all of these things so that their nurture is completed.

[Hippocrates, *Law* 3]

Nouns of the third declension are somewhat different from those of the first and second declensions in that this class of nouns usually has two combining forms: one formed from the nominative singular, the dictionary form, and the other from a case other than the nominative. For this reason, Greek dictionaries and vocabularies cite the genitive singular, which usually ends in -*os*, along with the nominative case of these nouns. The combining form is found by dropping the ending -*os*. Sometimes the base of the genitive case is the same as the nominative case: *cheir, cheiros* (hand), and there is only one combining form. But usually they differ:

derma, dermatos	skin	**derm**-oid
		hypo-**derm**-ic
		dermat-ology
		dermat-itis
gastēr, gastros	stomach	**gastr**-ic
		gastr-itis
		epi-**gaster**

Sometimes the nominative singular, the dictionary form of a noun, is itself a word without a prefix or suffix:

derma	the skin
hepar	the liver
meninx	one of the coverings of the brain and spinal cord
soma	the body

PREFIXES

amphi-, ampho-: on both sides, around, both:
    amphi-bious   **ampho**-philic

ana-: up, back, against:
    ana-tomy   **ana**-gen

apo-: away from:
    apo-crine   **apo**-ptosis

cata- (**cat-** before a vowel or *h*): downward, disordered:

cata-bolism	**cat**-hode

dia- (**di-** before a vowel): through, across, apart:

dia-lysis	**di**-opter

eso-: within, inner, inward:

eso-gastritis	**eso**-tropia
eso-phoria	**eso**-sphenoiditis

eu-: good, normal, healthy:

eu-thyroid	**eu**-phoria
eu-pepsia	**eu**-thanasia

heter-, hetero-: different, other, relationship to another:

hetero-chromia	**heter**-odont
hetero-sexual	**hetero**-cephalus

homo-, homeo-: same, likeness:

homo-topic	**homo**-genize
homeo-stasis	**homeo**-pathic

meta- (**met-** before a vowel or *h*): change, transformation, after, behind:

meta-bolism	**met**-encephalon
meta-morphopsia	**met**-hemoglobin

para- (often **par-** before a vowel): alongside, around, abnormal, beyond:

para-thyroid	**par**-enteral
para-metrium	**par**-onychia

pro-: before:

pro-dromal	**pro**-gnosis
pro-gnathous	**pro**-phylaxis

pros-, prosth-: in place of:

pros-thesis	**prosth**-odontics

SUFFIXES

-al: adjective-forming suffix (from Latin): pertaining to, located in:

bronchi-**al**	parenter-**al**
epiderm-**al**	psychologic-**al**

-ase: noun-forming suffix: forms names of enzymes:

sucr-**ase**	lip-**ase**
lact-**ase**	malt-**ase**

-asia, -asis (rare): abstract noun–forming suffix: state, condition:

metachrom-**asia**	achal-**asia**
phlegm-**asia**	blepharochal-**asis**

-ema: abstract noun–forming suffix: state, condition. The combining form of nouns ending in **-ema** is **-emat-**:

emphys-**ema**	emphys-**emat**-ous
eryth-**ema**	eryth-**emat**-ous

-esis: abstract noun–forming suffix: state, condition, procedure:

amniocent-**esis**	diur-**esis**
diaphor-**esis**	hematopoi-**esis**

-etic: adjective-forming suffix, often from nouns ending in **-esis**: pertaining to:

diaphor-**etic**	gen-**etic**
diur-**etic**	sympath-**etic**

-ics: noun-forming suffix indicating a particular science or study: science or study of:

geriatr-**ics**	endodont-**ics**
pediatr-**ics**	biometr-**ics**

-ism: abstract noun–forming suffix: state, condition, quality:

astigmat-**ism**	phototrop-**ism**
hypothyroid-**ism**	asynchron-**ism**

-ismus: abstract noun–forming suffix: state, condition; muscular spasm:

esophag-**ismus**	strab-**ismus**
laryng-**ismus**	vagin-**ismus**

-oid, (rarely) **-ode, -id**: both noun- and adjective-forming suffix indicating a particular shape, form, or resemblance: like, resembling:

aden-**oid**	nemat-**ode**
arachn-**oid**	lip-**id**

-oma: abstract noun–forming suffix: usually tumor; occasionally disease. The combining form of nouns ending in **-oma** is **-omat-**; the plural often is **-omata**:

carcin-**oma**	carcin-**omat**-osis
xanth-**oma**	xanth-**omata**

-ose: adjective-forming suffix (from Latin); full of, resembling an noun-forming suffix used to form names of chemical substances:

angin-**ose**	fruct-**ose**
varic-**ose**	gluc-**ose**

-ous: adjective-forming suffix (from Latin): pertaining to, characterized by, full of:

bili-**ous**	atrich-**ous**
ven-**ous**	venom-**ous**

-tics: noun-forming suffix indicating a particular science or study: science or study of:

ortho-**tics**	therapeu-**tics**
gene-**tics**	acous-**tics**

-us: a Latin noun-forming ending: condition, person (sometimes a malformed fetus):

hypothalam-**us**	microphthalm-**us**
hydrocephal-**us**	tetan-**us**

Verb-Forming Suffix

-ize: a commonly used Greek-derived verb-forming suffix that means "to make, become, cause to be, subject to, engage in."

hypnot-**ize**	internal-**ize**

CHEMICAL SUBSTANCES

There are many noun-forming suffixes used to form names of chemical substances. Some of these are:

-ate	(chlor-**ate**)
-ide	(brom-**ide**)
-ite	(nitr-**ite**)
-one	(testoster-**one**)

PRECEDING HYPHENS

Combining forms preceded by a hyphen (e.g., **-em-**) are found only following a prefix or another combining form: anemia, leukemia, and so forth.

COLI-, CYSTI-, CHOLECYST-

Words beginning with or containing **coli-** usually refer to the colon bacillus, *Escherichia coli*.

Words containing **cyst(i)-** usually refer to the urinary bladder.

Words containing **cholecyst-** refer to the gallbladder.

VOCABULARY

Greek	Combining Form	Meaning	Example
akron	ACR-	[highest point] extremities (particularly the hands and feet)	**acr**-odermatitis
amblys	AMBLY-	dull, faint	**ambly**-opia
karkinos	CARCIN-	[crab] (Fig 2-1) carcinoma, cancer	**carcin**-oma
kēlē	-CEL-*	hernia, tumor, swelling	hydro-**cel**-e
cheir	CHEIR-, CHIR-	hand	**cheir**-ospasm
cholē	CHOL(E)-	bile, gall	**chol**-olith
kolon	COL(I)-, COLON-	colon	**colon**-oscope
kyanos	CYAN-	blue	**cyan**-otic
kystis	CYST(I)-, -CYSTIS	bladder, cyst	**cyst**-itis
diploos	DIPLO-	double, twin	**diplo**-coccus
enteron	ENTER-	(small) intestine	**enter**-algia
ergon	ERG-	action, work	**erg**-ometer
gastēr, gastros	GASTR-	stomach	**gastr**-ectomy
haima, haimatos	HEM-, HEMAT-, -EM-	blood	**hem**-orrhage
hēpar, hēpatos	HEPAR-, HEPAT-	liver	**hepat**-itis
lipos	LIP-	fat	**lip**-osuction
makros	MACR-	(abnormally) large or long	**macr**-oglossia

*See the Etymological Notes in this lesson for uses of **-CEL-**.

Greek	Combining Form	Meaning	Example
*megas, megalou**	**MEGA-, MEGAL-**	(abnormally) large or long	**mega**-colon
melas, melanos	**MELAN-**	dark, black	**melan**-in
mikros	**MICR-**	(abnormally) small	**micr**-obe
nyx, nyctos	**NYCT-**	night	**nyct**-amblyopia
odynē	**ODYN-**	pain	**odyn**-ophagia
onkos	**ONC-**	tumor	**onc**-ologist
pachys	**PACHY-**	thick	**pachy**-derma
pseudēs	**PSEUD-**	false	**pseud**-oxanthoma
pyon	**PY-**	pus	**py**-emia
sarx, sarcos	**SARC-**	flesh, soft tissue	**sarc**-openia
spasmos	**SPASM-**	spasm, involuntary muscular contraction	neuro-**spasm**
splēn	**SPLEN-**	spleen	**splen**-omegaly
stoma, stomatos	**STOM-, STOMAT-**	mouth, opening	**stomat**-ogastric

*The forms of this adjective are irregular.

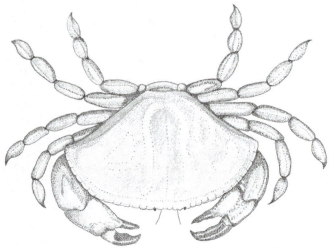

Figure 2-1. Coral crab. The Greek word *karkinos*, as well as the Latin word *cancer*, meant crab. The Greek and Roman medical writers used these words to name any spreading, ulcerous growth on the body. Hippocrates also used the word *karkinoma* (carcinoma) to refer to a growth of this sort. (Drawing by Laine McCarthy.)

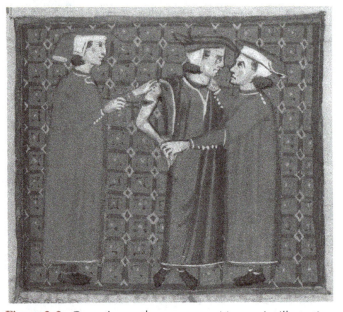

Figure 2-2. Operating on the upper arm. Manuscript illustration for *Chirurgia* by Theodoric of Cervia, 13th century AD. (From Special Collections, University of Leiden, Netherlands: Leiden, University Library, ms. Voss. Lat. F. 3, fol. 43r. with permission.)

ETYMOLOGICAL NOTES

The word **surgeon** came into English indirectly from two Greek words: *cheir* (hand) and *ergon* (action, work) (Fig. 2-2). The Greek verb *cheirourgoun*, meaning to work with the hands, and the noun *cheirourgos*, one who works with his hands, were applied to the surgeon. The words came into Latin as *chīrurgus*. Celsus, the Roman writer of the first century AD, had this to say about the surgeon:

> A surgeon (chirurgus) should be a young man, or certainly one not long out of youth. He should have a strong and steady hand, one which never trembles, and he should be able to use both the right and left hand equally well. He must have a sharp and keen eye and be of a firm spirit, feeling a sense of pity deep enough that he wishes to cure his patient, but not so sensitive as to be so influenced by his cries of pain that he acts in haste or cuts less than necessary;

on the contrary, he should go about everything just as if he were not at all affected by the moans that he hears.

[*De Medicina*, Preface 4]

The Latin word *chirurgus* came into Old French as *cirurgien* and was used in English as early as the 13th century in the form *sorgien*. Among the subsequent forms of the word in English were *surgeyn, surgyen, surgien*, and ultimately *surgeon*. However, a collateral form of the word also developed, giving rise to the spelling *chirurgeon*. In 1760, Samuel Johnson wrote to Boswell concerning a friend, "I am glad that the chirurgeon at Coventry gives him so much hope." The modern French word for surgeon is *chirurgien*, and the Italian word is *chirúrgo*.

The Greek noun *ergon* has given rise to the words **synergy** and **synergism**. *Taber's Cyclopedic Medical Dictionary* (2017) defines synergy, synergism as "an action of two or more agents, muscles, or organs working with each other, cooperatively." From the same root come the words **synergia, synergic, synergetic,** and **synergist.**

The Greek word *stoma* (mouth, opening) has a specialized use in medical terminology. In surgical procedures, an **anastomosis** (*ana-*, up, back) is the surgical or pathological connection of two tubular structures. An **arteriovenous anastomosis** is an opening between an artery and a vein. Words ending in **-stomy** indicate such surgical procedures. An **enteroenterostomy** is the creation of a communication between two noncontiguous segments of the intestine. A **colostomy** is the opening of a portion of the colon to the skin surface of the abdomen. This opening is known as a **stoma.** The plural of **stoma** is **stomata** or **stomas.**

The suffix **-oma** often indicates an abnormal or diseased condition, such as **trachoma,** a chronic contagious form of bacterial conjunctivitis, or **glaucoma,** a destructive disease of the eye caused by increased intraocular pressure. However, it usually denotes an abnormal growth of tissue (neoplasm) or a tumor (Latin *tumor,* swelling). *Taber's Cyclopedic Medical Dictionary* (2017) defines tumor as "1. A swelling or enlargement; one of the four classic signs of inflammation. 2. An abnormal mass. Growth or proliferation that is independent of neighboring tissue is characteristic of all tumors, benign and malignant." Tumors are generally benign, but there are exceptions. **Sarcoma** is a malignant tumor originating in mesenchymal tissue such as muscle (**myosarcoma;** Greek *mys,* muscle) or bone (**osteosarcoma).** If the tumor arises in the muscular tissue of a blood vessel, it is called **angiosarcoma** or **hemangiosarcoma.** A sarcoma containing nerve cells is called **neurosarcoma.**

The word element to which the suffix **-oma** is affixed indicates either the location of the growth or its nature: **hepatoma,** tumor of the liver; **nephroma,** tumor of a kidney; **cholangioma,** a tumor of the bile ducts; **hemangioma,** a tumor of the blood vessels—that is, the swelling consists of dilated blood vessels; **hematoma,** a swelling comprising a mass of blood, which occurs when ruptured blood vessels flood the nearby tissues. **Melanoma** is a malignant tumor composed of darkly pigmented cells **(melanocytes). Melanomatosis** is the formation of numerous melanomas on or beneath the skin.

The Greek noun *onkos* meant bulk, mass. This word has given rise to the combining form indicating a swelling or tumor: **oncogenesis,** tumor formation and development. **Oncology** is the branch of medicine that addresses cancer care, diagnostics, therapeutics and research.

Another combining form indicating an abnormal swelling comes from the noun *kēlē*. The form **-cele,** which is generally used as a suffixed element of a word, usually means hernia, the protrusion of an organ or part of an organ through the wall of the cavity that normally contains it: **cystocele,** hernia of the bladder; **rectocele,** hernia of the rectum into the vagina. Sometimes a word ending in **-cele** indicates a swelling caused by an abnormal accumulation of fluid, as in **hydrocele,** an accumulation of serous fluid in a saclike structure such as the scrotum in a newborn male child. A **keloid** is a scarlike growth of tissue on the skin **(kel-** is an alternate form of **cel-,** from Greek *kēlē*).

The term **cyst** refers to either a cyst or the urinary bladder (Fig. 2-3). *Taber's Cyclopedic Medical Dictionary* (2017)

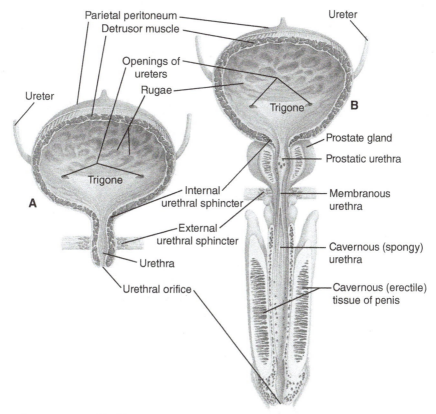

Figure 2-3. Urinary bladder. (From Venes, D., *Taber's Cyclopedic Medical Dictionary,* 21st ed. F. A. Davis, 2009.)

defines cyst as "a closed sac or pouch, with a definite wall, containing fluid, semifluid, or solid material. It is usually an abnormal structure resulting from developmental anomalies, obstruction of ducts, or parasitic infection." There are many types of cysts, including the following: **dermoid cyst,** a cyst containing elements of hair, teeth, or skin; **ovarian cyst,** a sac that develops in the ovary. **Cystalgia** is pain in the bladder, and **cholecystitis** is inflammation of the gallbladder wall. Words containing **cholecyst-** refer to the gallbladder. In ophthalmology the **dacryocyst** is the lacrimal sac. Some words containing **cyst-** refer to the growth called a cyst: **cystoid.**

Words beginning with, ending in, or containing **coli-** refer to the colon bacillus *Escherichia coli,* named after the German physician Theodor Escherich (1857–1911). **Colinephritis** is inflammation of the kidney caused by the presence of *Escherichia coli* (usually abbreviated *E. coli*).

Exercise 1:   Analyze and Define

Analyze and define each of the following words. In this and in succeeding exercises, analysis should consist of separating the words into prefixes (if any), combining forms, and suffixes or suffix forms (if any) and giving the meaning of each. Be certain to differentiate between nouns and adjectives in your definitions. Consult a medical dictionary for the current meanings of these words. Use a separate paper if you need more room for an answer.

1. acrocephaly _____

2. allodynia _____

3. amphibious _____

4. analogy _____

5. anastomosis _____

6. anatoxin _____

7. anemic _____

8. antilipemic _____

9. asynergy _____

10. carcinoma _____

11. cheirospasm _____

12. chiromegaly _____

13. cholangioma _____

14. cholelithiasis _____

15. colicystitis _____

16. colonocyte _____

17. diploid _____

18. dyschiria _____

19. endostoma _____

20. enterocystocele _____

21. enterostenosis _____

22. epigastrium _____

23. esogastritis _____

24. eubiotics _____

25. gastroenteric _____

26. hematoma _____

27. hemopericardium _____

28. heparin _____

29. hepatosplenomegaly _____

30. heterocephalus _____

31. homology _____

32. hyperemia _____

33. lipocyte _____

34. lipoid _____

35. macrocythemia _____

36. megalocephaly _____

37. melanoma _____

38. metabiosis _____

39. microbe* _____

40. microstomia _____

41. pachymeter _____

42. parabiosis _____

43. paraneural _____

44. parenteral _____

45. pseudoanemia _____

46. pyonephrosis _____

47. sarcomatoid _____

48. splenomegaly _____

49. stomatocyte _____

50. symbiosis _____

---

*The *b* in *microbe* is the only surviving part of the Greek noun *bios*. The final *-e* is an English noun-forming suffix.

Exercise 2:   Word Derivation

Give the word derived from Greek elements that matches each of the following. It is not necessary to give combining forms for words in parentheses. Verify your answer in a medical dictionary. **Note that the wording of the dictionary definition may vary from the wording used here.**

1. Lack of energy _____

2. Bladder cancer arising from (mesenchymal) tissue _____

3. Drug that relieves pain _____

4. Inflammation of the (mucous membrane of) the small and large intestines _____

5. Blue (gray, slate, or dark purple) discoloration of the skin _____

6. Growth containing cysts _____

7. Spasm of the hand (muscle) _____

8. Unusual amount of blood (in a part) _____

9. Inflammation of the mouth _____

10. Surrounding the liver _____

11. (Abnormal amount of) fat in the blood _____

12. Apparatus for measuring the amount of work done _____

13. (Purple or) blue discoloration of the extremities _____

14. Pain in the bladder _____

15. Enlargement of the liver _____

16. Inflammation (of tissues) surrounding a bile duct _____

17. Pertaining to the stomach and liver _____

18. Any blood cell _____

19. (Unusual) smallness of the stomach _____

20. Pertaining to the spleen and colon _____

Exercise 3: Drill and Review

Analyze and define each of the following words. Analysis should consist of separating the words into prefixes (if any), combining forms, and suffixes or suffix forms (if any), and give the meaning of each. Be certain to differentiate between nouns and adjectives in your definitions. Using the elements in the word determine its meaning. Consult a medical dictionary for the current meanings of these words. Use a separate paper if you need more room for an answer.

1. acromegaly _____

2. acromicria _____

3. antianemic _____

4. biotics _____

5. cephalocele _____

6. cholecystogastrostomy _____

7. cholecystolithiasis _____

8. colonic _____

9. colostomy _____

10. cystic _____

11. cystocele _____

12. cystolith _____

13. dyscephaly _____

14. endocystitis _____

15. enteralgia _____

16. enterocholecystostomy _____

17. enterodynia _____

18. erythrism _____

19. erythrocytometer _____

20. gastroenteritis _____

21. hemangioma _____

22. hemangiosarcoma _____

23. hemarthrosis _____

24. hemocytometer _____

25. heparin _____

26. hepatologist _____

27. hypogastrium _____

28. hypomelanosis _____

29. leukocytic _____

30. liposarcoma _____

31. macrocephalous _____

32. macrocranial _____

33. megacolon _____

34. melanomatosis _____

35. mesogastrium _____

36. microlithiasis _____

37. microcephaly _____

38. oncology _____

39. osteocarcinoma _____

40. pachymetry _____

41. periarterial _____

42. perichondrium _____

43. periostosis _____

44. pseudoarthrosis _____

45. pseudocyst _____

46. pyemic _____

47. splenocyte _____

48. splenohepatomegaly _____

49. symbiotic _____

50. toxemia _____

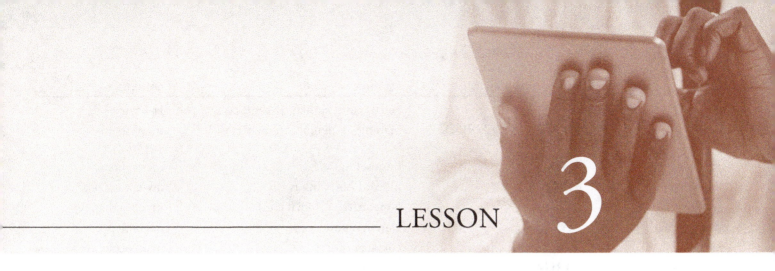

BUILDING GREEK VOCABULARY I: NOUNS AND ADJECTIVES

For those who have a fever, if jaundice occurs on the seventh, the ninth, the eleventh, or the fourteenth day, it is a good sign, provided the right hypochondrium does not become rigid. Otherwise it is a bad sign.

[Hippocrates, *Aphorisms* 4.64]

VOCABULARY

Greek	Combining Form	Meaning	Example
arachnē	**ARACHN-**	spider, web; arachnoid membrane	**arachn-**ophobia
chlōros	**CHLOR-**	green	**chlor-**ine
chondros	**CHONDR-**	cartilage	costo-**chondr-**al
daktylos	**DACTYL-**	finger, toe	poly-**dactyl-**y
derma, dermatos	**DERM(AT)-, -DERMA**	skin (Fig. 3-1)	**dermat-**ology
helkos	**(H)ELC-**	ulcer	kerato-**helc-**osis
hidrōs, hidrōtos	**HIDR(OT)-, -IDR-**	sweat	**hidr-**adenoma
histos	**HIST(I)-***	[web] tissue	**hist-**oblast
hydor, hydatos	**HYDR-†**	water, fluid	**hydr-**olysis
hypnos	**HYPN-**	sleep	**hypn-**osis
ikteros	**ICTER-**	jaundice	**icter-**ogenic
inos	**IN-, INOS-**	fiber, muscle	**in-**otropic

*The combining form HISTI- is from the diminutive noun *histion*.
†This combining form is slightly irregular.

Greek	Combining Form	Meaning	Example
isos	**IS-**	equal, same, similar, alike	**is**-ocytosis
mēninx, mēningos (plural, *mēninges*)	**MENING-, -MENINX**	meningeal membrane, meninges	**mening**-itis
mys, myos	**MY(S)-**	[mouse] muscle	**my**-olipoma
mykēs, mykētos	**MYC(ET)-**	[mushroom] fungus	**mycet**-omata
myelos	**MYEL-**	bone marrow, spinal cord	**myel**-orrhaphy
narkē	**NARC-**	stupor, numbness	**narc**-olepsy
nekros	**NECR-**	corpse; dead	**necr**-opsy
oligos	**OLIG-**	few, deficient	**olig**-ospermia
onyx, onychos	**ONYCH-**	fingernail, toenail	**onych**-omycosis
pous, podos	**POD-**	foot	**pod**-iatrist
polios	**POLI-**	[gray] gray matter of the brain and spinal cord	**poli**-ovirus
polys	**POLY-**	many, excessive	**poly**-morphic
poros	**POR-**	passage, opening, duct, pore, cavity	osteo-**por**-osis
psychē	**PSYCH-**	[soul] mind	**psych**-iatric
sōma, somatōs	**SOM(AT)-, -SOMA**	body	**somat**-ization
sthenos	**STHEN-**	strength	a-**sthen**-ia
trachēlos	**TRACHEL-**	neck, cervix	**trachel**-odynia
xanthos	**XANTH-**	yellow	**xanth**-ochromia

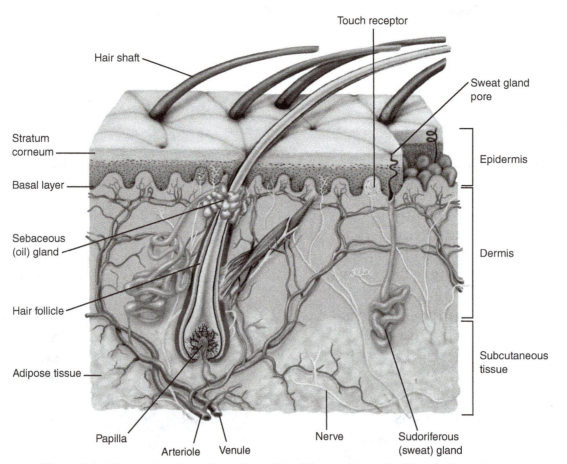

Figure 3-1. Skin section. (From Gylys, B., and Wedding, M. E., *Medical Terminology Systems: A Body Systems Approach*, 8th ed., F. A. Davis, 2017.)

ETYMOLOGICAL NOTES

Arachne, in Greek mythology, was a young girl of Maeonia, a land of Asia Minor, who became so skilled in the art of weaving that she challenged Athena, a goddess unequaled at the loom, to a contest (Fig. 3-2). Ovid, the first century BC Roman poet, tells us the story in the *Metamorphoses*, a poem that deals with mythological metamorphoses.

Athena took up the challenge, and the two, goddess and girl of humble origins, began to weave their tapestries. The goddess began by depicting the Acropolis in Athens with the twelve Olympian gods seated on their lofty thrones in serene majesty, with Jove [Zeus] in their midst. Then, so that Arachne might know what reward she could expect for her mad presumption, she wove in the four corners scenes showing punishments meted out to mortals who had dared to challenge the gods.

Arachne, in her tapestry, wove pictures of the gods in various disguises seducing mortal women. Athena could find no flaw in Arachne's work but, indignant at her success, tore the tapestry showing the celestial crimes, and with her shuttle struck Arachne again and again. The wretched girl could bear the punishment no longer and bound a noose around her neck and hanged herself. Ovid tells us that as Arachne hung there, Athena felt pity and lifted her, saying:

> Live, wicked girl, but hang forever; and so that you may never feel secure in time to come, let this same punishment fall upon all your generations, even to remote posterity.
>
> And as the goddess turned to leave, she sprinkled Arachne with the juices from Hecate's herb, and the girl's hair, touched by the poison, fell off, and her nose and ears fell off, and her head became shrunken, and her whole body was tiny. There was nothing left but belly and slender fingers clinging to her side as legs. And as a spider she still spins and practices her ancient art.

[Ovid, *Metamorphoses* 6.136–145]

The arachnoid membrane, or **arachnoidea,** is a thin, delicate membrane, the intermediate of the three that enclose the brain and spinal cord. The outer, tough, fibrous membrane is the dura mater (Latin, hard mother), sometimes called simply the dura. The innermost of the three meninges is the pia mater (devout mother). The arachnoidea is separated from the dura by the subdural (Latin *sub*, under) space, and from the pia by the subarachnoid space. **Subdural hematoma** is caused by venous blood occupying the subdural space of the brain. It is usually the result of trauma, and even a comparatively trivial injury can result in severe and steady headaches and sometimes coma. Symptoms of subdural hematoma may not be apparent for a period of several days or even several weeks after the initial injury.

Meningitis is inflammation of the meninges of the brain or spinal cord, and there are several types, the most severe of which is acute bacterial meningitis. This may be caused by one of several bacteria; however, regardless of the causative organism, the resulting disorders are similar. Classic symptoms are headache, fever, stiff neck, and lethargy. Unfortunately, typical manifestations of the disease are not seen in infants ages 3 months to 2 years, and, although antibiotics have reduced the mortality rate to less than 10 percent for cases recognized early, undiagnosed meningitis remains a lethal disease, with the prognosis for life progressively bleaker the younger the patient.

The combining form MYEL- refers to either bone marrow or the spinal cord. A **myeloma** is a tumor originating in the bone marrow. **Multiple myeloma** is a neoplastic disease characterized by the infiltration of bone and bone marrow by myeloma cells forming multiple tumor masses that lead to pathological fractures.

Poliomyelitis, inflammation of the gray matter of the spinal cord, is also known as infantile paralysis, or simply polio. As recently as 1988, the World Health Organization (WHO), the agency within the United Nations charged with directing international health, reported 350,000 cases of polio worldwide; in 2018, WHO reported only 33 cases worldwide. The dramatic decline in this highly communicable and debilitating disease seen mostly in children is due to the work of two renowned scientists: Dr. Jonas E. Salk (1914–1995), who developed the first polio vaccine, the Salk vaccine, and Dr. Albert B. Sabin (1906–1993), who later developed a second polio vaccine, the Sabin vaccine. Though cases of polio are extremely rare today, WHO continues to monitor polio outbreaks and stated, "As long as a single child remains infected, children of all countries are at risk for contracting polio. Failure to eradicate polio from these last remaining strongholds could result in as many as 200,000 new cases every year, within 10 years, all over the world."* **Postpolio syndrome** (PPS) is the development of motor and respiratory weakness, limb muscle atrophy, and fatigue 15 to 25 years after an acute episode of paralytic poliomyelitis.

Jaundice is a condition that manifests itself externally by a yellow staining of the skin caused by the deposition of bile pigments. The word jaundice is from the French *jaunisse*, which is from the Latin *galbinus* meaning yellowish green in color. Another term for jaundice is **icterus,**

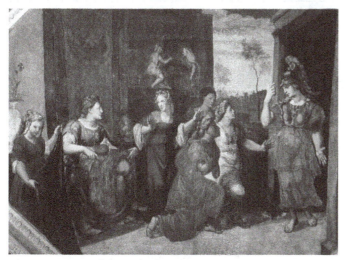

Figure 3-2. Arachne and Athena.

---

*World Health Organization, Poliomyelitis, July 22, 2019, https://www.who.int/news-room/fact-sheets/detail/poliomyelitis

from the Greek *ikteros* (jaundice). Pliny the Elder, the first century AD Roman writer whose 37-volume *Natural History* provides us with an encyclopedia of geography, botany, zoology, and other information, writes on jaundice, which was called the royal disease *(rēgius morbus):*

> There are certain remedies for jaundice: a dram of dirt from the ears and teats of sheep mixed with a pinch of myrrh and two cups of wine; the ashes of the head of a dog mixed with honey wine; a millipede in a half-cup of wine; earthworms in vinegar mixed with myrrh; wine in which a hen's feet have been rinsed—but the feet must be yellow and be washed in water first; a partridge's or an eagle's brain in three cups of wine; the ashes of a pigeon in honey wine; the intestines of a pigeon in wine; the ashes of sparrows in honey wine and water.
>
> There is a bird that is called icterus because of its color. People say that if one with jaundice looks at this bird the disease leaves him. But the bird dies. I think that this bird is the one that in Latin is called galgulus (the golden oriole).

[Pliny, *Natural History* 30.28]

The phrase "scleral icterus" is used to describe the yellow staining of the sclera (the white part of the eye) often associated with jaundice.

The **hypochondrium** is the soft part of the abdomen beneath the cartilage of the lower ribs, the upper central region of the abdomen over the pit of the stomach and located on either side of the **epigastrium.** This area, in which are situated the gallbladder, liver, and spleen, was thought of as the seat of melancholy. The form **hypochondria,** properly the plural of hypochondrium, entered the English language in the 17th century as an abstract noun meaning a melancholy state for which there is no apparent cause.

Exercise 1:   Analyze and Define

Analyze and define each of the following words. In this and in succeeding exercises, analysis should consist of separating the words into prefixes (if any), combining forms, and suffixes or suffix forms (if any) and giving the meaning of each. Be certain to differentiate between nouns and adjectives in your definitions. Consult a medical dictionary for the current meanings of these words. Use a separate paper if you need more room for an answer.

1. achlorhydria _____

2. amyosthenia _____

3. anhydrous _____

4. antinarcotic _____

5. antipsychotic _____

6. arachnodactyly _____

7. chloroleukemia _____

8. chondrolipoma _____

9. dermatitis _____

10. dermatomyositis _____

11. histiocyte _____

12. histiocytosis _____

13. hydrocephalus _____

14. hydronephrosis _____

15. hyperchlorhydria _____

16. hyperhidrosis _____

17. hypnotize _____

18. inosemia _____

19. isocytosis _____

20. macrosomia _____

21. melanonychia _____

22. meningomyelocele _____

23. mesoderm _____

24. micropsychotic _____

25. myasthenia _____

26. mycology _____

27. myeloid _____

28. myonecrosis _____

29. narcotism _____

30. narcotize _____

31. necrobiosis _____

32. neurasthenia _____

33. neurohistology _____

34. oligoarthritis _____

35. onychoid _____

36. osteochondroma _____

37. pachymeningitis _____

38. pachyonychia _____

39. podocyte _____

40. poliomyelitis _____

41. polyostotic _____

42. psychometry _____

43. psychosomatic _____

44. sthenia _____

45. syndactyly _____

46. toxicoderma _____

47. trachelismus _____

48. trachelocele _____

49. xanthoma _____

50. xanthomatosis _____

Exercise 2:   Word Derivation

Give the word derived from Greek elements that matches each of the following. It is not necessary to give combining terms for words in parentheses. Verify your answer in a medical dictionary. **Note that the wording of the dictionary definition may vary from the wording used here.**

1. Muscle (tissue) cell _____

2. (Unusual) thickness of the skin _____

3. Full of pores _____

4. Pertaining to the body _____

5. Fusion of the lower extremities _____

6. Fungal infection of the nails _____

7. Condition of (excessive) inequality in the size of cells _____

8. Agent that prevents or inhibits sleep _____

9. Lack or loss of strength _____

10. Pain in or around a cartilage _____

11. Pertaining to muscle and nerve _____

12. Excessive sweating _____

13. Pertaining to or causing sleep _____

14. Having fingers and toes of equal length _____

15. Inflammation of cartilage _____

16. Pain in the neck _____

17. Science of the skin and its diseases _____

18. Inflammation of bone and marrow _____

19. (Unconsciousness or) stupor produced by drugs _____

20. Excess of (red) blood cells _____

Exercise 3:   Drill and Review

Analyze and define each of the following words. Analysis should consist of separating the words into prefixes (if any), combining forms, and suffixes or suffix forms (if any) and giving the meaning of each. Be certain to differentiate between nouns and adjectives in your definitions. Using the elements in the word determine its meaning. Consult a medical dictionary for the current meanings of these words. Use a separate paper if you need more room for an answer.

1. achondrogenesis _____

2. acrodermatitis _____

3. amyosthenic _____

4. anonychia _____

5. antihidrotic _____

6. arachnoid _____

7. chloronychia _____

8. chlorosis _____

9. chondrocranium _____

10. chondrocyte _____

11. dermatomycosis _____

12. dermatomyositis _____

13. dermic _____

14. dyshidrosis _____

15. epidermoid _____

16. epidermomycosis _____

17. hematomyelia _____

18. histiocytoma _____

19. hypochloremia _____

20. icteroid _____

21. isocytotoxin _____

22. isodiametric _____

23. lipodermatosclerosis _____

24. melanoderma _____

25. meningitis _____

26. meningocele _____

27. mycetoma _____

28. myelocystocele _____

29. myelography _____

30. myospasm _____

31. necrosis _____

32. neuroectoderm _____

33. oligogenic _____

34. osteoporosis _____

35. paronychia _____

36. podocyte _____

37. polioencephalomyelitis _____

38. polydactyly _____

39. polymyositis _____

40. polyneuritis _____

41. polyp _____

42. psychoneurotic _____

43. psychosis _____

44. scleroderma _____

45. somatogenic _____

46. synchondrosis _____

47. trachelitis _____

48. trachelology _____

49. xanthomatous _____

50. xanthous _____

GREEK VERBS

In the winter eat as much as possible and drink as little as possible. The drink should be undiluted wine, and the food should be bread and roasted meat. Eat as few vegetables as possible during this season. In this way the body will be most dry and hot.

[Hippocrates, *Regimen in Health* 1]

For those who have a fever (pyretos), if deafness occurs, if blood flows from the nose, or if the bowels become disordered, the disease will be cured.

[Hippocrates, *Aphorisms* 4.40]

Greek verbs are **conjugated.** This means that there are different endings for person and number, and sometimes for tense, mood, and voice. A Greek verb normally has six different forms, called principal parts, on which the various tenses are built. Many verbs lack one or more of the principal parts, and verbs are often irregular. Thus, knowing the dictionary form of a verb does not always allow one to predict the other forms.

Greek dictionaries and grammar texts cite verbs in the first person singular. English and medical dictionaries, however, usually cite verbs in the form of the present infinitive, and they are given in this form in this manual. The present infinitive of most verbs ends in *-ein*, but there are other infinitival endings such as *-ai, -an, -oun,* and *-sthai.* Not all of the principal parts of a verb are used in forming English derivatives, and in this manual only the combining forms of principal parts that have produced English derivatives are given.

Often the entry form of a verb has not yielded any English derivatives. For example, the principal parts of the verb *gignesthai* (come into being) are:

gignomai, genēsomai, egenomēn, gegenēmai, gegona, egenēthēn

The third principal part, which supplies one of the past tenses (the aorist), furnishes the combining form GEN-, as in the words **pathogenic, genesis, carcinogen,** and so forth. Greek grammar texts often cite the verb *lyein* (loosen, destroy) as an example of a model verb:

lyō, lysō, elysa, lelyka, lelymai, elythēn

The combining form of *lyein* is LY(S)-, as in **analysis** or **hemolysin.**

VOCABULARY

Greek	Combining Form	Meaning	Example
autos	AUT-	self	**aut**-ism
krinein	CRIN-	[separate] secrete, secretion	endo-**crin**-ology
aisthēsis	ESTHE(S)-	sensation, sensitivity, sense	**esthe**-tics
gignesthai	GEN(E)-, -GEN	come into being; produce	**gene**-tics
gramma	GRAM-	[something written] a record	echocardio-**gram**
graphein	GRAPH-	write, record	**graph**-ology
iatros	IATR-	healer, physician; treatment	**iatr**-ogenic
idios	IDI-	of one's self	**idi**-opathic
kinein	KINE-	move	**kine**-tics
kinēsis	KINES(I)-	movement, motion	**kines**-iology
lyein	LY(S)-	destroy, break down	hemo-**lys**-is
myxa	MYX-	mucus	**myx**-ofibroma
orthos	ORTH-	straight, erect; normal	**orth**-odontia
ous, ōtos	OT-	ear	**ot**-algia
pathos	PATH-	[suffering] disease	**path**-ogen
philein	PHIL-	love; have an affinity for	hemo-**phil**-iac
piptein	PT-	fall, sag, drop, prolapse	entero-**pt**-osis
pyr, pyros	PYR-	[fire] fever, burning	**pyr**-osis
pyretos	PYRET-	fever	anti-**pyret**-ic
pyressein	PYREX-	be feverish	**pyrex**-ia
rhein	RHE-	[run] flow, secrete	diar-**rhe**-a
rhēgnynai	RHAG-	[burst forth] flow profusely,	menor-**rhag**-ia
rhēxis	RHEX-	hemorrhage rupture	**rhex**-is
rhis, rhīnos	RHIN-	nose	**rhin**-oplasty
skopein	SCOP-	look at, examine	oto-**scop**-y
sēpein	SEP-	[be putrid] be infected	**sep**-sis
tasis	TA-	stretching	ec-**ta**-sis
telos	TEL-	end, completion	**tel**-encephalia
tenōn, tenontos	TEN-, TENON(T)-	tendon	**ten**-odesis
therapeuein	THERAP(EU)-	treat medically, heal	**therapeu**-tics
tomē	TOM-	a cutting, slice, incision	**tom**-ography
tonos	TON-	[a stretching] (muscular) tone, tension	**ton**-icity

COMPOUND SUFFIX FORMS

Some combining forms of verbs, usually with the addition of a suffix and/or prefix, have become so commonly used in a certain form and meaning as to remain fixed as **compound suffix forms:**

Compound Suffix Form	Meaning	Example
-ectasia, -ectasis	dilation, enlargement	cardi-**ectasia**, esophag-**ectasis**
-ectomy	surgical excision; removal of all (total excision) or part (partial excision) of an organ	gastr-**ectomy**, nephr-**ectomy**
-gen*	substance that produces (something)	antitoxino-**gen**, carcino-**gen**
-genesis	formation, origin	lipo-**genesis**, patho-**genesis**
-genic, -genous	causing, producing, caused by, produced by or in	carcino-**genic**, hepato-**genous**†
-gram	a record of the activity of an organ (often an x-ray)	echocardio-**gram**, angio-**gram**
-graph	an instrument for recording the activity of an organ	poly-**graph**, cardio-**graph**
-graphy	(1) the recording of the activity of an organ (usually by x-ray examination) (2) a descriptive treatise (on a subject)	cholangio-**graphy**, cysto-**graphy** phlebo-**graphy**, mammo-**graphy**
-lysis	dissolution, reduction, decomposition, disintegration	hemo-**lysis**, bacterio-**lysis**
-lytic	pertaining to dissolution or decomposition, disintegration (forms adjectives from words ending in -lysis)	hemo-**lytic**, bacterio-**lytic**
-pathy	disease	neuro-**pathy**, cardio-**pathy**
-ptosis	dropping, sagging, prolapse (of an organ or part)	glosso-**ptosis**, colo-**ptosis**
-rrhagia‡	profuse discharge, hemorrhage	leuko-**rrhagia**, meno-**rrhagia**
-rrhea	profuse discharge, excessive secretion	rhino-**rrhea**, dia-**rrhea**
-rrhexis	bursting (of tissues), rupture	kerato-**rrhexis**, entero-**rrhexis**
-scope	an instrument for examining	rhino-**scope**, colpo-**scope**
-scopy	examination	endo-**scopy**, cysto-**scopy**
-tome	a surgical instrument for cutting	myo-**tome**, derma-**tome**
-tomy	surgical incision	cholecysto-**tomy**, laparo-**tomy**

*Strictly speaking, -gen, -gram, and -graph are not suffix forms because there is no suffix on the combining form. It seemed desirable, however, that -gen, -genesis, -genic, and -genous as well as -gram, -graph, and -graphy should be listed together as suffix forms in order to show the relationship between words using these forms.

†Because these suffix forms can mean either producing or produced by, the meaning of some words is ambiguous: urogenous means either producing urine or originating in urine.

‡Words beginning with the letter r- [Greek rho] usually double this letter when following another element. Craniorhachischisis is an exception.

ETYMOLOGICAL NOTES

There is no disease more grievous or severe than that which, by a certain stiffness of the nerves, now draws the head back toward the shoulder blades, now draws the chin down toward the chest, and now holds the neck stretched out immobile. The Greeks call the first *opisthotonos*, the second *emprosthotonos*, and the third *tetanus*.

[Celsus, *De Medicina* 4.6]

The name of the disease **tetanus** (Greek *tetanos*) is related linguistically to the nouns *tasis* (stretching), and *tonos* (tension); this acute disease was known to ancient physicians. Hippocrates wrote, "Spasm or tetanus following severe burns is a bad sign" [*Aphorisms* 7.13]. Signs of tetanus are stiffness of the muscles of the jaw, esophagus, and neck.

For this reason, the disease is often called lockjaw. In the advanced stage, these and other muscles become fixed in a rigid position. If the body is stretched backward in a tetanic spasm, the position is called **opisthotonos** (Greek *opisthen*, in back) (Fig. 4-1); if stretched forward, it is called **emprosthotonos** (*emprosthen*, in front); if stretched to the side, **pleurothotonos** (*pleurothen*, on the side); and if the body is held rigidly stretched in a straight line, the condition is called **orthotonos** (*orthos*, straight, upright).

Tetanus is a life-threatening illness caused by the toxin **tetanospasmin**, produced in infected wounds by the bacillus *Clostridium tetani*, which takes its name from *klōstēr* (spindle), after the rodlike shape of these bacilli. The suffix -*id* indicates a member of a genus, and -*ium* is a Latin diminutive ending, from the Greek -*ion*. The word *klōstēr*

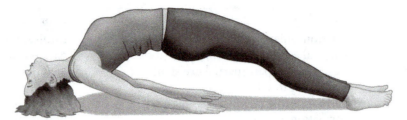

Figure 4-1. Opisthotonos. (From Venes, D., *Taber's Cyclopedic Medical Dictionary*, 24th ed., F. A. Davis, 2021, with permission.)

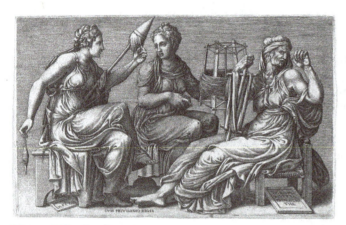

Figure 4-2. The Three Fates.

is derived from the verb *klōthein* (spin). Clotho, the Spinner, is one of the three sisters, the Fates (in Greek *Moirai*, in Latin *Parcae*), who spins the thread of life for each of us. Her sister Lachesis, the Apportioner, determines the length of the thread, and the third sister, Atropos, Irreversible, cuts it (Fig. 4-2).

The adjective *idios* meant of one's self, pertaining to one's own interest. Galen, the second-century AD Roman physician, used the term *idiopatheia* to refer to an ailment having a local origin—that is, originating within the body. We speak of an **idiopathic** disease as one with an uncertain or undetermined cause. There was a noun *idiōma*, meaning a peculiarity or particular feature of something. Our word idiom is ultimately derived from this noun. An *idiōtēs* was a person in private life, as opposed to one holding public office. It came to mean one who was unlearned or unskilled. The word idiot entered the English language early in the 14th century in the sense of a person who was so lacking in mental ability as to be incapable of acting in a rational way: an idiot. In the 16th century, the term "an idiot" mistakenly came to be "a nidiot," and then, through the influence of the pronunciation of the term, the spelling was changed to nidget or nigit. Thomas Heywood, the 17th-century English dramatist, wrote in *The Wise Woman of Hogsdon* (1638), "I think he saith we are a company of fooles and nigits."

The **parotid** gland, which runs alongside the ear, is one of the glands that supply saliva to the mouth. Inflammation of this gland is called **parotitis.** Mumps is a contagious form of parotitis caused by the **paramyxovirus.** Mumps can lead to inflammation of the parotid gland and other organs. In about 10% of cases, involvement of other organs

can result in deafness, pancreatitis, and meningitis. Like mumps, measles is one of the world's most contagious diseases. It is spread by coughing, sneezing, and close personal contact with infected nose or throat secretions. Before routine vaccination for measles began in 1963, the annual mortality rate worldwide from the virus was reported to be 2.6 million deaths, mostly children under the age of 5 years. In 1971, a combination vaccine for measles, mumps, and rubella (MMR vaccine) became widely available. The World Health Organization (WHO) reported that the MMR vaccine prevented 23.2 million deaths between 2000 and 2018. 140,000 deaths from measles were reported for 2018, a decrease of 76% from 2000. Sporadic outbreaks of the highly infectious measles virus continue to occur, especially in undernourished children and "in countries with low per capita incomes and weak health infrastructures."*

The Roman physician Celsus knew of mumps, although there was no Latin name for it:

Parotid swellings (parotides) are likely to occur below the ears, sometimes in periods of health when inflammation occurs here, and sometimes after long fevers when the force of the disease has turned in that direction.

[*De Medicina* 6.16]

As a remedy for these swellings, he recommended a mixture of pumice, liquid pine resin, frankincense, soda scum, iris, wax, and oil. Pliny the Elder, the Roman author, philosopher, and encyclopedist, recommended a mixture of foxes' testicles and bull's blood, dried and pounded together and mixed with the urine of a she-goat, all of this to be poured drop by drop into the ear and followed by an external application of she-goat's dung mixed with axle grease [*Natural History* 28.49].

Rheum, a watery discharge, is from *rheuma, rheumatos,* a word related to the verb *rhein* and meaning "that which flows." The ancient Greek writers used the word to refer to the current of a river, the eruption of lava from a volcano, or to anything that flowed. Hippocrates used it in the sense of a discharge of liquid from the body:

Those of us with a cold in the head and a discharge (rheuma) from the nostrils generally find that this discharge is more acrid than that which formerly accumulated there and daily passed from the nostrils.

[*Ancient Medicine* 18]

---

*World Health Organization, Measles Fact Sheet, December 2019, https://www.who.int/news-room/fact-sheets/detail/measles

Rheumatism *(rheumatismos)* was thought to be caused by a flowing of the humors in the body, and was thus named.

The ancient Greeks were unaware of the existence of capillaries in the human body simply because they did not have the optical devices with which to see these microscopic vessels. It was not until the 17th century that their existence was demonstrated by the Italian anatomist Marcello Malpighi as a result of his discovery of capillary anastomosis in the lungs. The word **capillary** is from Latin *capillāris*, pertaining to hair *(capillus)*. But many terms for abnormal conditions of the capillaries have been formed from the Greek elements *tel-* (end) and *angi-* (vessel), as both the arterial and the venous systems terminate in capillaries. **Telangiectasia** is a vascular lesion formed by dilation of a group of small blood vessels. It can appear as a birthmark or be caused by long-term exposure to the sun.

Exercise 1:   Analyze and Define

Analyze and define each of the following words. In this and in succeeding exercises, analysis should consist of separating the words into prefixes (if any), combining forms, and suffixes or suffix forms (if any) and giving the meaning of each. Be certain to differentiate between nouns and adjectives in your definitions. Consult a medical dictionary for the current meanings of these words. Use a separate paper if you need more room for an answer.

1. abiogenesis _____

2. akinesia _____

3. anesthesia _____

4. antibiogram _____

5. antihemorrhagic _____

6. arachnolysin _____

7. atelencephalia _____

8. autism _____

9. autoantitoxin _____

10. biokinetics _____

11. carcinogenesis _____

12. cholecystectomy _____

13. cystorrhexis _____

14. dermatoscopy _____

15. dysgraphia _____

16. endocrinology _____

17. endocrinopathy _____

18. esthesiometer _____

19. gastroscope _____

20. genetics _____

21. graphology _____

22. hemophiliac _____

23. hepatocarcinogen _____

24. iatrology _____

25. idiogram _____

26. idiolysin _____

27. kinesimeter _____

28. lipophile _____

29. myxoid _____

30. myxolipoma _____

31. nephroscope _____

32. orthokinetics _____

33. orthopsychiatry _____

34. otitis _____

35. otorhinology _____

36. pathologist _____

37. podiatrist _____

38. pyrexia _____

39. pyrogenic _____

40. rhinocephaly _____

41. rhinorrhea _____

42. sclerotome _____

43. sepsis _____

44. septicemia _____

45. telangiectasis _____

46. tenocyte _____

47. tenolysis _____

48. therapeutics _____

49. therapist _____

50. toxigenic _____

Exercise 2:   Word Derivations

Give the word derived from Greek elements that matches each of the following. It is not necessary to give combining terms for words in parentheses. Verify your answer in a medical dictionary. **Note that the wording of the dictionary definition may vary from the wording used here.**

1. Any substance or agent that produces cancer _____

2. Instrument used for cutting muscles _____

3. Incision of the heart _____

4. Defect in the ability to perform voluntary movement _____

5. Originating in the liver _____

6. Increased tension _____

7. Injury or illness that occurs because of medical care _____

8. (Extreme) slowness of movement _____

9. Disease of the brain and spinal cord _____

10. Excision of (a portion of) a muscle _____

11. Pertaining to, caused by, or originating in dead matter _____

12. Infection of the ear caused by fungus _____

13. Renal incision for removal of kidney stones _____

14. Prolapse of the heart _____

15. Agent that causes fever _____

16. Dropping or drooping of an organ or part _____

17. Pertaining to the arrest of spasms _____

18. Lack of sensation in (one or more of) the extremities _____

19. Nasal stone _____

20. Mucous tumor with fatty tissue elements _____

Exercise 3:   Drill and Review

Analyze and define each of the following words. Analysis should consist of separating the words into prefixes (if any), combining forms, and suffixes or suffix forms (if any), and give the meaning of each. Be certain to differentiate between nouns and adjectives in your definitions. Using the elements in the word determine its meaning. Consult a medical dictionary for the current meanings of these words. Use a separate paper if you need more room for an answer.

1. amyotonia _____

2. anesthesiology _____

3. angiogram _____

4. antiangiogenesis _____

5. atelia _____

6. autohemolysis _____

7. autosepticemia _____

8. catagenesis _____

9. chondromyxosarcoma _____

10. cystoscopy _____

11. dermatopathology _____

12. dyspraxia _____

13. endotoscope _____

14. epiotic _____

15. erythrocytorrhexis _____

16. exocrine _____

17. exogenous _____

18. gastrectomy _____

19. hepaticotomy _____

20. histolysis _____

21. hyperesthesia _____

22. idioisolysin _____

23. isotonia _____

24. leukorrhea _____

25. lithogenesis _____

26. macrotia _____

27. metakinesis _____

28. mycosis _____

29. myopathy _____

30. myotonia _____

31. myxoid _____

32. myxoma _____

33. nephrectomy _____

34. oncotherapy _____

35. orthosis _____

36. orthotics _____

37. osteitis _____

38. osteoarthropathy _____

39. osteogeny _____

40. ototoxic _____

41. paracrine _____

42. pathogenetic _____

43. pathology _____

44. rhinogenous _____

45. rhinoscleroma _____

46. rhinoscopy _____

47. septicemic _____

48. telogen _____

49. therapy _____

50. tomography _____

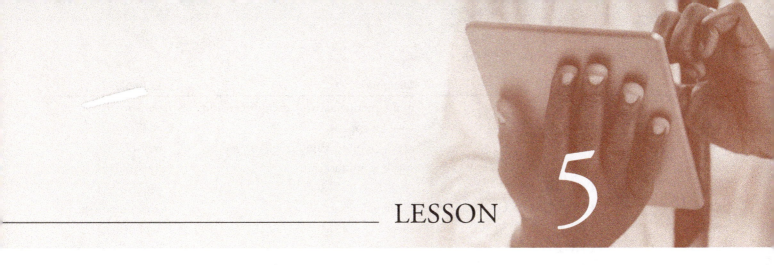

BUILDING GREEK VOCABULARY II

γνῶθι σαυτόν. Know thyself.

> [Thales, sixth-century BC philosopher, as quoted by Diogenes Laertius (third century AD), *Lives of the Philosophers*]

VOCABULARY

Greek	Combining Form	Meaning	Example
akouein	ACOU(S)-, ACU(S)-	hear	**acous**-tics
amnion	AMNI-	fetal membrane, amniotic sac, amnion	**amni**-ocentesis
*askitēs**	ASC-, ASCIT-	[leather bag] bladder, sac, bag	**ascit**-es
baros	BAR-	weight, pressure	**bar**-iatrics
kentein	CENTE-	pierce	cardio-**cente**-sis
chrōma, chrōmatos	CHROM-, CHROMA-, CHROMAT-	color, pigment	**chromat**-ography
dipsa	DIPS-	thirst	poly-**dips**-ia
ēkhō	ECHO-	reverberating sound, echo	**echo**-cardiogram
oidēma, oidēmatos	EDEMA, EDEMAT-	swelling	**edemat**-ogenic
emein	EME-	vomit	**eme**-sis
gignōskein	GNO(S)-	know	dia-**gno**-sis
lalein	LAL-	talk	echo-**lal**-ia
lapara	LAPAR-	abdomen, abdominal wall	**lapar**-oscope
legein	LEX-	read	dys-**lex**-ia
mimnēskein	MNE-	remember	**mne**-monics
neos	NE-	new	**ne**-onatal

*See the Etymological Notes in this lesson.

Greek	Combining Form	Meaning	Example
nous	**NO-**	mind, mental activity, comprehension	para-**no**-ia
oregein	**OREC-, OREX-**	have an appetite	an-**orex**-ia
oxys	**OX(Y)-**	acute, pointed; rapid; acid; oxygen	**oxy**-chloride
phēnai	**PHA-**	speak, communicate	dys-**pha**-sia
phagein	**PHAG-**	swallow, eat	**phag**-ocyte
pharmakon	**PHARMAC(EU)-***	medicine, drug	**pharmaceu**-tics
phēmē	**PHEM-**	speech	a-**phem**-ia
phobos	**PHOB-**	(abnormal) fear	hydro-**phob**-ia
phonē	**PHON-**	voice, sound	**phon**-ograph
phrazein	**PHRAS-**	speak	poly-**phras**-ia
phrēn	**PHREN-**	mind; diaphragm	**phren**-ic
phylattein	**PHYLAC-**	protection (against disease)	pro-**phylax**-is†
physis	**PHYS(I)-**	nature, appearance	**physi**-ology
phyton	**PHYT-**	plant (organism), growth	**phyt**-otoxin
poiein	**POIE-**	produce, make	leuko-**poie**-sis
prosopon	**PROSOP-**	face	**prosop**-agnosia
sapros	**SAPR-**	rotten, putrid, decaying	**sapr**-ophyte
stear, steatos	**STEAR-, STEAT-**	fat, sebum, sebaceous glands	**steat**-onecrosis

*The combining form PHARMACEU- is from the Greek adjective *pharmakeutikos* (concerning drugs).
†Words ending in -phylaxis are from PHYLAC- and -sis.

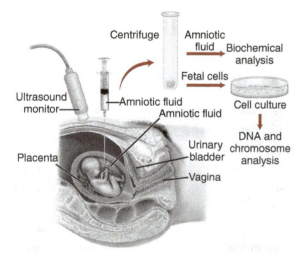

Figure 5-1. Amniocentesis. (From Gylys, B. A., and Wedding, M. E., *Medical Terminology Systems: A Body Systems Approach*, 8th ed., F. A. Davis, 2017.)

OX-

The combining form **OX-** indicates the presence of oxygen: anoxia, hypoxia, hypoxemia, and so forth. In a few words, **OXY-** means rapid: oxytocin, oxytocic. In some words, **OXY-** has the meaning of acid: oxyphil.

ETYMOLOGICAL NOTES

On August 1, 1774, Joseph Priestley, the British clergyman and chemist, focused the rays of the sun through a magnifying glass onto red oxide of mercury and produced a vapor that he named dephlogisticated air. Scientists of that time commonly believed that all matter contained a substance called phlogiston (Greek *phlogistos*, inflammable), which was released during burning. Priestley, after discovering that his lungs felt particularly light and easy for some time after breathing the vapor, asked, "Who can tell but that, in time, this pure air may become a fashionable article in luxury? Hitherto, only two mice and myself have had the privilege of breathing it."‡

Priestley journeyed to Paris in the fall of 1774 and described his experiment to the French scientist Antoine Lavoisier, who renamed the newly discovered vapor oxygen, meaning acid producing.

Oedipus, the tragic hero of Sophocles' *Oedipus the King*, owes his name to the verb *oidein*, meaning to become swollen. An oracle had told Laius, king of Thebes, that if his wife bore him a son, this child would eventually kill him. When a son was born to the queen, Laius pierced the infant's feet and tied them together and gave him to a shepherd to expose on the mountainside. But instead, the child was given to the childless king of Corinth, who brought him up as his own son, naming him *Oidipous* (swollen foot). As is well known, Oedipus (to give his name the Latin spelling) did eventually

‡Copyright 1974 by the New York Times Company. Reprinted by permission.

kill his father and, furthermore, marry Jocasta, his own mother; hence the Freudian term Oedipus complex.

The Greek noun *oidēma* (swelling), from the verb *oidein* (become swollen), has given us the word **edema,** meaning a swelling caused by an accumulation of fluid in tissue. If the condition is generalized over large areas of the body, it is sometimes called **hydrops** (Greek *hydrōps,* from *hydōr,* water) or **hydropsy.**

The Greek noun *askos* meant skin or hide but more commonly referred to a bag or sack made of skin, especially a wineskin. Homer tells us that when Odysseus and his men departed from the island of Aeolia, where Aeolus, the Keeper of the Winds, had entertained them for a full month, Aeolus gave Odysseus a bag *(askos)* made of the hide of a 9-year-old ox in which he bound the blustering winds, allowing only the breath of the west wind to blow, thus affording Odysseus and his men a sure passage across the sea [*Odyssey* 10.19ff].

The ancient Greeks knew of the condition that we call **ascites,** and named it *ascitēs,* the baggy disease, from the baggy aspect of the human body resulting from the accumulation of serous fluid in the peritoneal cavity.

In Greek mythology, Mnemosyne (Memory) was a Titaness, one of the children of Sky and Earth. The eighth-century BC poet Hesiod tells us of the union of Mnemosyne and Zeus:

> For nine nights did all-wise Zeus lie with her, entering her holy bed far away from the immortals. And when a year had passed and the seasons turned as the months waned, and many days were fulfilled, she bore nine daughters, all of like mind, whose hearts are turned to song and whose spirits are free from care, a little way from the highest peak of snow-clad Olympus.

[*Theogony* 56 ff]

These daughters were the nine Muses: Clio, Euterpe, Thalia, Melpomene, Erato, Terpsichore, Polyhymnia, Urania, and Calliope, patron goddesses of the arts.

There was a Greek verb *mimnēskein* (remember), related to the name of the goddess of memory, Mnemosyne, and from it we get such words as **amnesia, amnesty, mnemonic,** and so forth. The Latin nouns *memotia* and *mēns, mentis* (mind), are related to this Greek verb and have given us the words **memory** and **mental.**

The Greek word *amnos* (lamb) had a diminutive form, *amnion,* meaning the innermost of the membranes surrounding the human fetus, and this is the modern meaning of the word. The **amnion** is a thin, transparent sac in which the fetus is suspended, surrounded by the amniotic fluid, or **liquor amnii,** which protects the fetus from injury. The Greek diminutive form *amnion* (little lamb) was probably so named because this membrane resembles the extremely thin and delicate skin of the newborn lamb. **Amniocentesis** (Fig. 5-1) is the puncturing of the abdomen with a long, thin, hollow needle and the removal of a small amount of the amniotic fluid surrounding the fetus. This fluid contains some fetal cells that are grown in a laboratory, then examined microscopically to determine if there is any abnormality in the chromosome number or structure. Each human somatic cell contains 23 pairs of chromosomes, the genetic and hereditary determinants of human beings. Abnormalities in the number of chromosomes in the cells can indicate genetic defects in the unborn fetus.

The often fatal disease **hydrophobia,** which, literally translated, means fear of water, is characterized by excruciating spasms of the throat muscles whenever the victim attempts to drink, even though the victim is at the point of death from dehydration. The incubation period of this disease varies from 10 days to 3 months. If the carrier of the virus, often a dog, squirrel, or bat, is identified, treatment may begin immediately and recovery is normal. The Latin word *rabiēs,* which is commonly used for this disease, means simply madness. Celsus wrote about hydrophobia and its cure:

> Certain physicians, after the bite of a rabid dog, send the victims directly to the bath, and there allow them to sweat as long as their strength permits, with the wound kept exposed so that the poison may readily drip from it. Then much undiluted wine is drunk, as this is an antidote to all poisons. After three days of this treatment, the patient is thought to be out of danger. But if the wound is not sufficiently treated there arises a fear of water which the Greeks call *hydrophobia,* an exceedingly distressing disease in which the sufferer is tormented simultaneously by thirst and dread of water. There is little hope for those who are in this state. However, there remains one last remedy: throw the patient unexpectedly into a pool of water when he is not looking. If he cannot swim, allow him to sink and drink the water and then raise him up; but if he can swim, keep pushing him under so that he becomes filled with water, although unwillingly. In this way both his thirst and his fear of water are removed at the same time.

[*De Medicina* 5.27.2]

The ancients believed that the midriff was the seat of the emotions, and thus the word *phrēn* was applied to this area as a physical part of the body and also as the center of the emotions, the heart, or the mind. Homer tells us in the *Odyssey* that Odysseus, after the Cyclops Polyphemus (Fig. 5-2) had

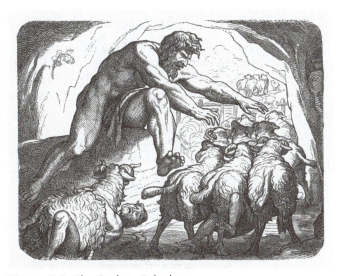

Figure 5-2. The Cyclops Polyphemus.

made a meal of two of his companions, pondered how to deal with this monster:

> And I formed a plan to steal near to him and, drawing my sharp sword from beside my thigh, to strike him in the breast, at the point where the midriff (*phrēn*) holds the liver (*hēpar*).

> [*Odyssey* 9.299–301]

Later in the poem, Odysseus becomes enraged when one of his companions speaks slightingly of him.

> So he spoke, and I pondered in my mind (*phrēn*) whether or not to draw my long sword from beside my thigh and strike off his head and bring it to the ground, even though he was a kinsman of mine by marriage.

> [*Odyssey* 10.438–441]

Thus, derivative words of *phrēn* in medical terminology refer to either the diaphragm or the mind or the mental processes. The adjective **phrenic** can mean pertaining to the diaphragm or mind. The right and left phrenic nerves provide motor innervation and control of the diaphragm. Irritation of the phrenic nerves is one cause of hiccups. The Greek verb *gignōskein* meant to know or to understand; a secondary meaning was to examine, form an opinion, or determine. From this verb were derived the nouns *gnōsis* (knowledge), *diagnōsis* (means of discerning, opinion, diagnosis), and *gnōmōn* (one who knows, judge).

The verb *phyein* meant to grow according to the laws of nature. From this verb was derived a noun, *physis*, meaning natural growth, the outward form or appearance of anything. The word *physiognōmia* meant the study of one's appearance, a judgment of character from an individual's appearance. Our word is **physiognomy,** the human countenance. From *gnōsis* and *diagnōsis* we get **serodiagnosis,** diagnosis based on tests of serum including immunological tests, and **immunodiagnosis,** the use

of immunocytochemistry, detection of lymphocyte markers, and other strategies to diagnose autoimmune diseases and disorders. Other derivatives of the noun *physis* include **physic, physics, physical,** and **physician.**

The Greek nouns *phyton* (plant, growth) has given us **phytochemistry,** the study of plant chemistry; **phytotoxin,** a poison derived from plants; **dermatophyte,** a fungal (that is, plant) parasite growing in or on the skin; and **osteophyte,** a bony outgrowth.

> In cases where there are swellings (*phymata*) and pains in the joints following fevers, those afflicted are eating too much food.

> [Hippocrates, *Aphorisms* 7.45]

Horace, the Roman poet of the first century BC, mentions in two of his poems a girl whom he calls Lalage. She is otherwise unknown. Horace may have made up the name from the Greek verb *lalein* (talk) because his Lalage seems to be fond of chattering.

> *pone me pigris ubi nulla campis*
> *arbor aestiva recreatur aura,*
> *quod latus mundi nebulae malusque*
> *iuppiter urget;*
>
> *pone sub curru nimium propinqui*
> *solis in terra domibus negata:*
> *dulce ridentem Lalagen amabo,*
> *dulce loquentem.*

> [*Odes* 1.22.17–24]

Place me on a barren plain
where no tree grows in the summer breeze,
a land overhung by mists and gloomy skies;

place me in a land too close to the chariot
of the sun, a land barren of homes.
I will love my sweetly laughing,
sweetly chattering Lalage.

Exercise 1:   Analyze and Define

Analyze and define each of the following words. In this and in succeeding exercises, analysis should consist of separating the words into prefixes (if any), combining forms, and suffixes or suffix forms (if any) and giving the meaning of each. Be certain to differentiate between nouns and adjectives in your definitions. Consult a medical dictionary for the current meanings of these words. Use a separate paper if you need more room for an answer.

1. achromatolysis _____

2. acousmatamnesia _____

3. agnostic _____

4. alexia _____

5. amniocentesis _____

6. amnioscope _____

7. anamnesis _____

8. anaphylaxis _____

9. anorexia _____

10. aphemia _____

11. aphonia _____

12. bariatrics _____

13. bradyphrenia _____

14. chromesthesia _____

15. diagnosis _____

16. dysphagia _____

17. echolalia _____

18. echopraxia _____

19. edema _____

20. emesis _____

21. histophysiology _____

22. hyperemesis _____

23. laparoscope _____

24. leukopoiesis _____

25. monochromatic _____

26. monophasia _____

27. myelopoiesis _____

28. neogenesis _____

29. neophobia _____

30. oxygenase _____

31. paracentesis _____

32. paranoid _____

33. paraphasia _____

34. phagocyte _____

35. pharmacotherapy _____

36. phoniatrics _____

37. phonocardiogram _____

38. phrenic _____

39. physiologist _____

40. phytotherapy _____

41. phytotoxin _____

42. polydipsia _____

43. prognosis _____

44. prosopagnosia _____

45. psychodiagnosis _____

46. psychokinesis _____

47. saprobe _____

48. somatoparaphrenia _____

49. steatohepatitis _____

50. xanthochromia _____

Exercise 2: Word Derivation

Give the word derived from Greek elements that matches each of the following. It is not necessary to give combining terms for words in parentheses. Verify your answer in a medical dictionary. **Note that the wording of the dictionary definition may vary from the wording used here.**

1. Without color _____

2. Formation of the amnion _____

3. Abnormal sensitivity to sound _____

4. Loss of memory _____

5. Condition of having a normal (clear) voice _____

6. Puncture (of a cavity) _____

7. Sense or perception of pressure _____

8. Absence of oxygen _____

9. Surgical opening of the abdomen _____

10. Difficulty reading _____

11. Agent that promotes vomiting _____

12. Organism living on decaying or dead organic matter _____

13. Person affected with aphasia _____

14. Newly invented word _____

15. Use of (colored) light to treat disease _____

16. Capable of producing echoes _____

17. Formation of red blood cells _____

18. Study of drugs (and their origin) _____

19. Fungal parasite that grows in or on the skin _____

20. Science of sound _____

Exercise 3:   Drill and Review

Analyze and define each of the following words. Analysis should consist of separating the words into prefixes (if any), combining forms, and suffixes or suffix forms (if any), and give the meaning of each. Be certain to differentiate between nouns and adjectives in your definitions. Using the elements in the word determine its meaning. Consult a medical dictionary for the current meanings of these words. Use a separate paper if you need more room for an answer.

1. achromatosis _____

2. acoustic _____

3. agnosia _____

4. amniotomy _____

5. anamniotic _____

6. antiemetic _____

7. antiphagocytic _____

8. aphemia _____

9. barognosis _____

10. chromatogram _____

11. chromidrosis _____

12. dysphasia _____

13. echoendoscope _____

14. echopathy _____

15. ectophyte _____

16. edematogenic _____

17. enterocentesis _____

18. erythrophage _____

19. hematophagous _____

20. hematopoiesis _____

21. homophobe _____

22. hypophonia _____

23. hypoxia _____

24. isochromatic _____

25. laparocele _____

26. laparoscopy _____

27. leptochromatic _____

28. leukoedema _____

29. monochromatism _____

30. necrophagous _____

31. neostomy _____

32. odynophagia _____

33. orexigen _____

34. osteophyte _____

35. oxygenic _____

36. paranoia _____

37. phagocytize _____

38. pharmaceutics _____

39. phonophobia _____

40. physical _____

41. physiotherapy _____

42. polyphagia _____

43. prophylactic _____

44. psychodiagnostics _____

45. psychophysical _____

46. pyemia _____

47. stearin _____

48. steatonecrosis _____

49. steatorrhea _____

50. tachyphylaxis _____

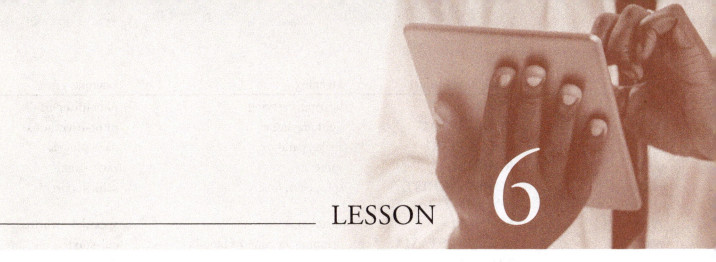

BUILDING GREEK VOCABULARY III

ΝΙΨΟΝΑΝΟΜΗΜΑΤΑΜΗΜΟΝΑΝΟΨΙΝ: Νίψον ἀνομήματα, μὴ μόναν ὄψιν.

Wash your sins, not only your face.

[A palindromic inscription on the sacred font in the courtyard of Hagia Sophia in Istanbul]

VOCABULARY

Greek	Combining Form(s)	Meaning	Example
anēr, andros	**ANDR-**	man, male	**andr-**ogynous
ankylos	**ANKYL-, ANCYL-**	fused, stiffened; hooked, crooked	**ankyl-**odactylia
Aphrodisios	**APHRODIS(I)-**	[of or pertaining to Aphrodite, Greek goddess of love] sexual desire	**aphrodis-**iac
brachys	**BRACHY-**	short	**brachy-**cephalous
kryptos	**CRYPT-**	hidden, latent	**crypt-**ic
dēmos	**DEM-**	people, population	epi-**dem-**ic
dolichos	**DOLICH-**	long, narrow, slender	**dolich-**omorphic
dromos	**DROM-**	a running	**drom-**otropic
Erōs, Erōtos	**ER-, EROT-**	[Eros, son of Aphrodite, Greek goddess of love] sexual desire	**erot-**ic
gynē, gynaikos	**GYN(EC)-**	woman, female	**gynec-**ologic
helmins, helminthos	**HELMINT(H)-**	(intestinal) worm	**helminth-**iasis
nēma, nēmatos	**NEMAT-**	thread (worm)	**nemat-**ode
nosos	**NOS-**	disease, illness	**nos-**ophyte
odous, odontos	**ODONT-**	tooth	orth-**odont-**ist
palin	**PALI(N)-**	back, again	**palin-**dromic
pas, pantos	**PAN(T)-**	all, entire, every	**pan-**carditis

Greek	Combining Form(s)	Meaning	Example
phoros	**PHOR-**	bearing, carrying	phos-**phor**-us
phōs, phōtos	**PHOS-, PHOT-**	light, daylight	**phot**-osynthesis
plēssein	**PLEC-, PLEG-**	strike, paralyze	para-**pleg**-ia
rhachis	**R(H)ACHI-**	spine	**rachi**-tome
schizein	**SCHIZ-, SCHIST, -SCHISIS**	split, cleft, fissure	**schiz**-ophrenia
spondylos	**SPONDYL-**	vertebra	**spondyl**-arthritis
staxis	**-STAXIS, -STAXIA**	dripping, oozing (of blood)	epi-**staxis**
thanatos	**THAN(AT)-**	death	**thanat**-ology
tithenai	**THE-**	place, put	syn-**the**-sis
thrix, trichos	**TRICH-**	hair	**trich**-algia
trophē	**TROPH-**	nourishment	a-**troph**-y

ETYMOLOGICAL NOTES

Trichinosis (Greek *trichinos*, of hair), also called Trichinellosis, is a disease caused by ingesting the larvae of the parasitic worm *Trichinella spiralis* by eating raw or insufficiently cooked pork or wild game meat (Fig. 6-1). The larvae penetrate the mucous lining of the intestinal tract and, in a few days, mature and mate, after which the males die. The females begin to discharge their young larvae after about a week, a process that continues for up to 6 weeks. These tiny larvae enter the bloodstream of the host and are carried to the tissues and organs of the body, where they lodge in muscle tissue, causing, among other symptoms, pain, nausea, diarrhea, edema, fever, chills, and general weakness. Most people afflicted with trichinosis recover, although involvement of the respiratory muscles can lead to death. In the United States, 90 cases of trichinosis were reported between 2008 and 2012. Worldwide, the Centers for Disease Control and Prevention (CDC) estimates the incidence of trichinosis to be approximately 10,000 new cases annually.*

The name *Trichinella spiralis* is New Latin. The term New Latin is applied to words and names that have been coined in modern times in the form of, and on the analogy of, Latin words. In some instances, New Latin has been used for new meanings applied to extant Latin words. In the name *Trichinella spiralis*, *-ella* is a Latin diminutive suffix added to the stem of the Greek adjective *trichinos*, and *spiralis* is a modern adjectival formation of the Latin noun *spīra* (coil or spiral), borrowed from the Greek noun *speira*, meaning anything that is coiled or twisted. In the binomial system of biological nomenclature, the generic name is indicated by a capitalized noun; the species is indicated by an adjective agreeing with this noun in gender and number.†

The Greek word *trophē* (nourishment) has given us such words as **trophic,** meaning concerned with nourishment. Most of the words in medical terminology that use the form TROPH- have to do with nourishment that is carried to the cells of the body by circulating blood. Any impediment to the flow of blood to a part will result in **hypotrophy** and eventually **atrophy.** Hypotrophy is the gradual degeneration and loss of function of tissue—usually muscle tissue—resulting from a decrease in the flow of blood to that part. Atrophy is a decrease in size of a part resulting from lack of cell nourishment, as in muscle atrophy, which occurs with long periods of nonuse of muscles in bedridden individuals. **Hypertrophy** is an increase in the size of an organ or part as a consequence of increased absorption of nutrients. This is usually caused by an increase in functional activity, as in **cardiac hypertrophy,** an increase in the size of

HELMINTHS

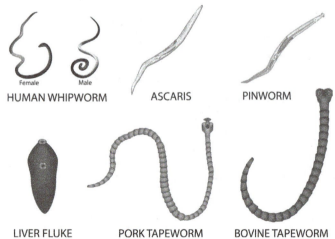

Figure 6-1. Representative helminths. (From Getty Images, iStock: Timoninalryna)

---

*Morbidity & Mortality Weekly Report, Centers for Disease Control and Prevention, January 16, 2015.
†See Unit 5, Lesson 20, Biological Nomenclature.

the heart resulting from overgrowth of the tissues of the heart muscle. This condition is caused by continued stress beyond normal limits, such as occurs in long-standing hypertension with resultant stress on the heart. One of the four signs of the tetralogy of Fallot (a congenital disorder caused by a defect in the heart that allows blood to pass from the left ventricle to the right) is hypertrophy of the right ventricle. This is caused by the extra stress placed on this part of the heart muscle by the burden of pumping the additional blood that accumulates there.

Amyotrophy is muscular atrophy. **Dystrophy** is the name given to any disorder of the body caused by defective nutrition, such as **muscular dystrophy,** a familial disease characterized by progressive atrophy of muscles.

The words **euphoria** and **dysphoria** are formed from the Greek compound nouns *euphoria*, a sense of well-being or comfort, and *dysphoria*, a sense of discomfort.

The Greek adjective *ankylos* meant crooked or curved, and the noun *ankylē* meant a joint that was bent and stiffened by disease; both words are derivatives of the noun *ankos* (bend or hollow). **Ankylosis** is abnormal immobility of a joint caused by some pathological changes in the joint or its surrounding tissue. The combining form ANKYL- means a fusion of parts normally separate, as in **ankylodactylia** (*daktylos*, finger, toe) and **ankylotia** (*ous*, *ōtos*, ear). **Ankylosing spondylitis** is a progressive condition in which inflammatory changes and new bone formation occur at the site of attachment of tendons and ligaments to bone. This most commonly affects the spine and leads to chronic pain and debilitation.

The Greek word *Aphrodisia* meant sexual pleasures, things connected with Aphrodite, the goddess of love (Fig. 6-2). There was an adjective *Aphrodisiakos*, from which we get the word **aphrodisiac.** Aphrodite did not confine her amorous attentions to Hephaestus, her husband and god of the forge, but had numerous affairs with immortals and mortals alike. One such relationship, with Hermes, a Greek god of many functions, resulted in the birth of a son who grew to be a handsome young man resembling both his mother and his father. His name was Hermaphroditus. Ovid, the first-century BC Roman poet, tells us an anecdote about this young man.

As the story goes, there was once a naiad, a water nymph, named Salmacis, who dwelled in a pool in Caria, a land of Asia Minor. One day, 15-year-old Hermaphroditus came to the place and Salmacis fell in love with him on sight. A shy young man, he refused her advances. But she waited until he went bathing in the pool and, casting off all her garments, dived in, crying, "I win, he is mine!"

Hermaphroditus resists and denies the nymph the pleasures she has hoped for, but she clings to him, pressing her whole body to him as if they were grown together. *Struggle as hard as you wish, you wicked boy, she says, but you will not escape. May the gods grant me this, that no day ever come that will take him from me.* The gods heard her. Their two bodies were joined together, one face and one form for both. Just as one grafts a twig onto a branch and sees them join and grow together, so were these two

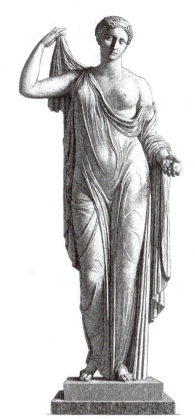

Figure 6-2. Aphrodite. (From Getty Images, clu: DigitalVision Vectors)

bodies joined in close embrace, no longer two beings, yet no longer either man or woman, but neither, and yet both.

[*Metamorphoses* 4.368ff]

Thus, **hermaphrodite** came to mean a person with the genital organs of both sexes. Hesiod, a Greek poet of the mid-eighth century BC, tells us in his *Theogony* (Origin of the Gods) that in the beginning of Creation, Chaos first came into being; then Earth, dark Tartarus in the depths of Earth; and then Eros, "fairest among the deathless gods, who unnerves the limbs and overcomes the counsels of a prudent mind of all gods and men" (*Theogony* 120–123). But in the sense in which he is usually conceived, that of the Latin Cupid, Eros is the creation of later Greek poets. Far from remaining the primeval deity of Hesiod, he grows younger. From the handsome youth of the sixth to fifth centuries BC, Eros becomes a wanton, lascivious boy in the Alexandrian period (third to first centuries), whose arrows kindle passion in the heart. The parentage of the second Eros is in some dispute, but the most commonly held belief makes Aphrodite his mother and either Hermes or Ares, the god of war, his father. Cicero holds to the latter view (*On the Nature of the Gods* 3.23). Eros's Latin name, Cupid (*cupīdō*, desire), gives us the word **cupidity;** his Greek name gives us **erotic** and **eroticism.**

To the ancient Greeks, Thanatos was the god of death. Thanatos appears as a character on the stage in the opening scene of Euripides' tragedy *Alcestis*, when he comes to claim Alcestis, the lovely young wife of King Admetus, for whom she has offered to die. Admetus had offended the goddess Artemis, and she decreed that he must die on a certain date—unless someone would voluntarily die for him. When Admetus could find no one to make this sacrifice, Alcestis agreed to take his place. But this was a tragedy with a happy ending, for the great hero Heracles went to the underworld and succeeded in taking Alcestis away from Thanatos, and the drama ends with Heracles leading Alcestis back to her husband.

Homer, in the *Iliad* (16.666 ff), tells us that when Zeus's son, Sarpedon, was killed in the fighting before the walls of Troy, the god ordered Apollo to remove Sarpedon's body from the field of battle and entrust it to Sleep (Hypnos) and his twin brother Death (Thanatos), who would return it to Sarpedon's home in Lycia. This legend is the subject of the painting on a famous ancient Greek vase, the Euphronios Krater (vase), now in the Metropolitan Museum of Art in New York City (Fig. 6-3). Sleep and Death are depicted lifting the body of Sarpedon while Apollo looks on.

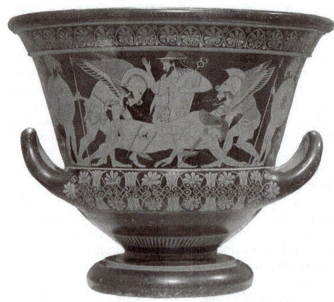

Figure 6-3. Euphronios Krater (vase). (Metropolitan Museum of Art, New York City)

Exercise 1:   Analyze and Define

Analyze and define each of the following words. In this and in succeeding exercises, analysis should consist of separating the words into prefixes (if any), combining forms, and suffixes or suffix forms (if any) and giving the meaning of each. Be certain to differentiate between nouns and adjectives in your definitions. Consult a medical dictionary for the current meanings of these words. Use a separate paper if you need more room for an answer.

1. abiotrophy _____

2. acrobrachycephaly _____

3. amyotrophia _____

4. android _____

5. ankylotia _____

6. anthelmintic _____

7. aphrodisiac _____

8. apoplectic _____

9. atrichia _____

10. atrophy _____

11. autoerotism _____

12. brachytherapy _____

13. cataplexy _____

14. chromatophore _____

15. cryptography _____

16. demographics _____

17. diaphoresis _____

18. diplegia _____

19. dolichoectasia _____

20. dysondontiasis _____

21. dystrophoneurosis _____

22. endemoepidemic _____

23. endodontics _____

24. epidemiologist _____

25. epistaxis _____

26. erogenous _____

27. euphoria _____

28. euthanasia _____

29. gynecology _____

30. helminthology _____

31. hemiatrophy _____

32. homoerotic _____

33. nematology _____

34. nosophyte _____

35. odontocele _____

36. odontogenesis _____

37. osteosynthesis _____

38. palindromic _____

39. pandemic _____

40. panencephalitis _____

41. paraplegia _____

42. photosynthesis _____

43. prodromal _____

44. rachiometer _____

45. rachischisis _____

46. schistocyte _____

47. schizencephaly _____

48. spondylopathy _____

49. thanatology _____

50. trichonosis _____

Exercise 2:   Word Derivation

Give the word derived from Greek elements that matches each of the following. It is not necessary to give combining terms for words in parentheses. Verify your answer in a medical dictionary. **Note that the wording of the dictionary definition may vary from the wording used here.**

1. Fusion of two or more fingers or toes _____

2. Abnormal deficiency of hair _____

3. Toothache _____

4. Found in a specific population _____

5. Inflammation of (all the structures of) the heart _____

6. Device for measuring (the intensity of) light _____

7. (Congenital) fissure (that remains open in the wall) of the abdomen _____

8. Exposure to sunlight for therapeutic purposes _____

9. Infestation with worms _____

10. Inflammation of the joints of the vertebrae _____

11. Science (of the description or classification) of diseases _____

12. Pertaining to nutrients carried in the blood _____

13. Having a short (broad) head _____

14. Abnormal fear of hair _____

15. Pertaining to nourishment _____

16. Fissure of a tooth _____

17. Inflammation of the spine _____

18. Hidden _____

19. (Scientific) study of men's health _____

20. Pertaining to (or stimulating) sexual desire _____

 ## Exercise 3:   Drill and Review

Analyze and define each of the following words. Analysis should consist of separating the words into prefixes (if any), combining forms, and suffixes or suffix forms (if any), and give the meaning of each. Be certain to differentiate between nouns and adjectives in your definitions. Using the elements in the word determine its meaning. Consult a medical dictionary for the current meanings of these words. Use a separate paper if you need more room for an answer.

1. androgynous _____

2. ankylosis _____

3. apoplexy _____

4. brachialgia _____

5. brachycephalic _____

6. cataphoresis _____

7. chondrodystrophy _____

8. chromophore _____

9. craniorachischisis _____

10. cryptogenic _____

11. demography _____

12. diaphoretic _____

13. dolichocephalic _____

14. dystrophy _____

15. endodontist _____

16. epidemic _____

17. eroticism _____

18. exodontia _____

19. gynecologist _____

20. helminthic _____

21. hemiplegia _____

22. hypertrichosis _____

23. hypertrophy _____

24. melanophore _____

25. metachromasia _____

26. microphotograph _____

27. nematocyst _____

28. nosode _____

29. odontography _____

30. oligodontia _____

31. onychodystrophy _____

32. panarteritis _____

33. panendoscope _____

34. periodontal _____

35. peritrichous _____

36. phosphorolysis _____

37. photobiology _____

38. photogenic _____

39. prosthesis _____

40. prosthodontics _____

41. protopathic _____

42. rachitome _____

43. rhachialgia _____

44. schistocytosis _____

45. spondyloptosis _____

46. spondylosis _____

47. synthetic _____

48. tomosynthesis _____

49. trichotoxin _____

50. trophedema _____

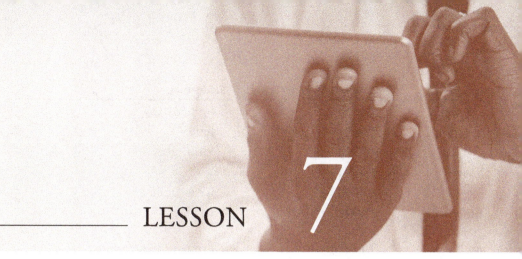

LESSON

7

BUILDING GREEK VOCABULARY IV

The art of medicine would never have been discovered, nor would there have been any medical research—for there would have been no need for medicine—if sick men had benefited by the same manner of living and by the same food and drink of men in health.

[Hippocrates, *Ancient Medicine* 3]

VOCABULARY

Greek	Combining Form(s)	Meaning	Example
adēn	**ADEN-**	gland	**aden-**oids
aēr	**AER-**	air, gas	**aer-**obe
blennos	**BLENN-**	mucus	**blenn-**orrhea
koilia	**CEL(I)-**	abdomen	**celi-**ocentesis
cheilos	**CH(E)IL-**	lip	**cheil-**oschisis
chronos	**CHRON-**	time, timing	**chron-**ic
klān	**CLA(S)-, -CLAST**	break (up), destroy	osteo-**clas-**tic
desis	**-DESIS**	binding	syn-**desis**
desmos	**DESM-**	[binding] ligament, connective tissue	**desm-**oplasia
dynamis	**DYNAM-**	force, power, energy	**dynam-**ic
gēras	**GER-**	old age	**ger-**iatrics
gnathos	**GNATH-**	(lower) jaw	pro-**gnath-**ous
ischein	**ISCH-, -SCHE-**	suppress, check	**isch-**emia
kleptein	**KLEPT-**	steal	**klept-**omania
leios	**LEI-**	smooth	**lei-**omyoma
lēpsis	**LEP-**	attack, seizure	epi-**lep-**tic

Greek	Combining Form(s)	Meaning	Example
mainesthai	**MAN-**	be mad	**man**-ic
melos	**MEL-**	limb	**mel**-algia
morphē	**MORPH-**	form, shape	**morph**-ology
nomos	**NOM-**	law	**nom**-ogram
omphalos	**OMPHAL-**	navel, umbilicus	**omphal**-ocele
pais, paidos	**PED-**	child	**ped**-iatrics (British: paediatrics)
penia	**PEN-**	decrease, deficiency	leuko-**pen**-ia
pexis	**-PEX-**	fixing, (surgical) attachment	gastro-**pex**-y
plassein	**PLAS(T)-**	form, develop	a-**plas**-ia
presbys	**PRESBY-**	old, old age	**presby**-opia
prostatēs	**PROSTAT-**	[one who stands before] prostate gland	**prostat**-itis
ptyein	**PTY-**	spit	hemo-**pty**-sis
ptyalon	**PTYAL-**	saliva	**ptyal**-in
rhaptein	**-RRHAPH-**	suture	cardio-**rrhaph**-y
sitos	**SIT-**	food	**sit**-osterol
histanai	**STA(T)-**	stand, stop	**sta**-sis
taxis	**TAX-**	(muscular) coordination	a-**tax**-ia
thermē	**THERM-**	heat, (body) temperature (Table 7-1)	**therm**-ometer
tropē	**TROP-**	turning	**trop**-ism

-PLASTY, -TROPISM

Words ending in **-plasty** (molding, surgically forming) refer to plastic or restorative surgery: rhino-**plasty**, angio-**plasty** (Fig. 7-1).

Words ending in **-tropism** refer to the turning of living organisms toward (positive tropism) or away from (negative tropism) an external stimulus: photo-**tropism**, stereo-**tropism**.

INSTRUMENTS

Words ending in **-clast** indicate an instrument or device for breaking or crushing: litho-**clast**.

Words ending in **-stat** indicate a device or agent for stopping the flow of something: hemo-**stat**.

Words ending in **-meter** (Lesson 1) indicate an instrument for measuring: cephalo-**meter**.

Words ending in **-tome** (Lesson 4) indicate a device for cutting or excising: myo-**tome**.

Table 7-1. Comparative Thermometric Scale

	Celsius*	Fahrenheit
Boiling point of water	100°	212°
	90	194
	80	176
	70	158
	60	140
	50	122
	40	104
Body temperature	37°	98.6°
	30	86
	20	68
	10	50
Freezing point of water	0°	32°
	−10	14
	−20	−4

*Also called *centigrade*.
Source: From *Taber's Cyclopedic Medical Dictionary*, 23rd ed., F. A. Davis, 2017, p. 2335, with permission.

ETYMOLOGICAL NOTES

The verb *mainesthai* (to be mad) is one of several words in both Greek and Latin that have the root MN-, all having to do with mental processes: Greek, *mimnēskein* (remember) (cf. *Mnemosyne* [Memory], *manteia* [prophetic power], *manthanein* [learn], *ma[n]thematikos* [mathematical], *mantis* [prophet or prophetic]); and Latin, *mēns, mentis* (mind),

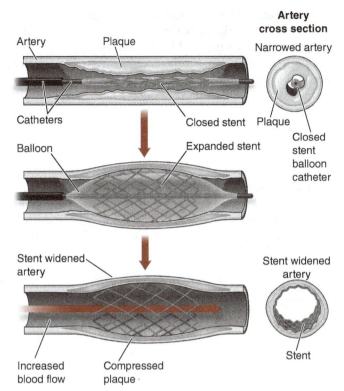

Figure 7-1. Arterial balloon angioplasty. (From Capriotti, T., *Pathophysiology: Introductory Concepts and Clinical Perspectives*, 2nd ed., F. A. Davis, 2020.)

Morpheus is the cleverest of all of Sleep's sons in imitating the form of humans:

> No other is more skilled than he in simulating the gait, the countenance, and the speech of mortals, or in assuming their clothing and the words that each is accustomed to use.

[*Metamorphoses* 11.635–638]

The *Metamorphoses*, Ovid's greatest work, was written before he was banished to Tomis on the Black Sea by the emperor Augustus in AD 8. A long poem (11,990 lines), the *Metamorphoses* tells stories from Greek mythology and Near Eastern legend, all involving a change in shape or form. The poem begins with the creation of the universe and ends with the transformation of Julius Caesar into a star after his death. The poet declares his intentions at the opening of the work:

> My purpose is to tell of bodies changed to new forms.
> Gods—for it is you who made the changes—
> give me inspiration for this poem
> that runs from the beginning
> of the world down to our own days.

The verb *ptyein* and its derivative noun *ptyalon*, both meaning spit, are examples of onomatopoeia (*onoma, onomatos*, name, *poiein*, make), the formation of words in imitation of sounds. One of the best-known examples of this from antiquity is found in a fragment of the *Annales* by

mentiō, mentiōnis (mention), *mentīrī* (lie, cheat). In the beginning of the *Iliad*, Apollo rains his arrows upon the Greek camp. Agamemnon, the leader of the Greek army, refuses to return the girl, whom he has taken captive, to her father, a priest of Apollo. Achilles rises in the assembly and speaks:

> Come, let us consult some seer *(mantis)* or priest, or some interpreter of dreams—for dreams are sent by Zeus—who can tell us why Phoebus Apollo has conceived such anger.

[*Iliad* 1.62–64]

Tiresias, the famous blind prophet of Thebes, had a daughter, Manto, who also became a famous seer. Manto is also the name of an Italian nymph who had the gift of prophecy and who founded the city of Mantua in Lombardy, the birthplace of Virgil.

Theocritus, the third-century BC Greek bucolic poet, called the orthopterous insect *Mantis religiosa* (praying mantis) the prophetic grasshopper *(mantis kalamaia)*. Perhaps this insect was given its Latin name because of its posture, holding its forelegs in a position that suggests hands folded in prayer (Fig. 7-2) [*Idylls* 10.18].

The narcotic drug morphine takes its name from Morpheus, the Greco-Roman god of dreams (Greek *morphē*, form, shape). Morpheus was one of the thousand sons of Sleep. Morphine takes its name from Morpheus because of the dreams induced by it, especially by opium, from which morphine is derived. The Roman poet Ovid tells us that

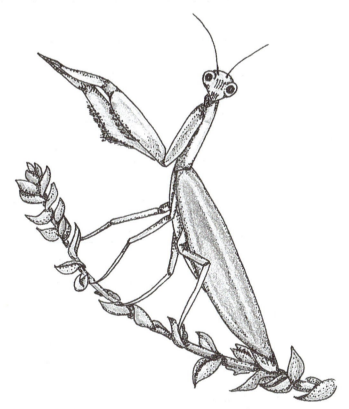

Figure 7-2. Praying mantis. (Drawing by Laine McCarthy, 2000.)

the second-century BC Roman poet Ennius, whose works are mostly lost:

At tuba terribili sonitu taratantara dixit.

But the trumpet, with a terrible sound, went *taratantara*.

The prostate gland was called *prostatēs* (*pro-*, in front of, *histanai*, stand) by the early Greek physicians because of its location in front of the bladder and urethra.

The term "stat" used in hospitals is from Latin *statim*, meaning immediately.

Exercise 1:   Analyze and Define

Analyze and define each of the following words. In this and in succeeding exercises, analysis should consist of separating the words into prefixes (if any), combining forms, and suffixes or suffix forms (if any) and giving the meaning of each. Be certain to differentiate between nouns and adjectives in your definitions. Consult a medical dictionary for the current meanings of these words. Use a separate paper if you need more room for an answer.

1. adenoidectomy _____

2. adenotome _____

3. aerobe _____

4. aerometer _____

5. alloplasty _____

6. aplasia _____

7. arthroclasia _____

8. arthrodesis _____

9. ataxiaphasia _____

10. blennorrhea _____

11. celiomyositis _____

12. cheiloschisis _____

13. cholestasia _____

14. chronological _____

15. chronophobia _____

16. cystopexy _____

17. desmoplasia _____

18. dynamometry _____

19. enteropexy _____

20. epileptic _____

21. erythromelalgia _____

22. erythropenia _____

23. exomphalos _____

24. geriatrician _____

25. hemiataxia _____

26. hemodynamics _____

27. hepatorrhaphy _____

28. hypoplasia _____

29. ischemia _____

30. kleptomania _____

31. leiomyosarcoma _____

32. leukopenia _____

33. melalgia _____

34. micrognathia _____

35. morphogen _____

36. narcolepsy _____

37. nomography _____

38. omphalotomy _____

39. parasitemia _____

40. parasitologist _____

41. pediatrics _____

42. polymorphism _____

43. presbycardia _____

44. prognathous _____

45. prostatodynia _____

46. ptyalism _____

47. rhinoplasty _____

48. somatotropic _____

49. thermodynamics _____

50. thermometry _____

Exercise 2:   Word Derivation

Give the word derived from Greek elements that matches each of the following. It is not necessary to give combining terms for words in parentheses. Verify your answer in a medical dictionary. **Note that the wording of the dictionary meaning may vary from the wording used here.**

1. Looking like a gland _____

2. Swallowing of air _____

3. Puncture of the abdomen _____

4. Pertaining to a body type that is long and slender _____

5. Difficulty standing _____

6. Condition of being bound together _____

7. Deficiency in the number of red blood cells (in the body) _____

8. Any disease of the abdomen _____

9. Inflammation (or chapping) of the lips _____

10. Branch of health care concerned with (the care of) the aged _____

11. (Congenital) hernia of the umbilicus _____

12. Production of heat _____

13. Destruction of cells _____

14. Suppression of perspiration _____

15. (Benign) tumor consisting principally of smooth muscle (and fibrous connective) tissue _____

16. Condition marked by possession of the same form _____

17. Measurement of the shape or form of an object _____

18. Device for fracturing bones (for therapeutic purposes) _____

19. Abnormal size of a lip _____

20. Reduction in all cellular elements of the blood _____

Exercise 3:   Drill and Review

Analyze and define each of the following words. Analysis should consist of separating the words into prefixes (if any), combining forms, and suffixes or suffix forms (if any), and give the meaning of each. Be certain to differentiate between nouns and adjectives in your definitions. Using the elements in the word determine its meaning. Consult a medical dictionary for the current meanings of these words. Use a separate paper if you need more room for an answer.

1. adenoiditis _____

2. aerotitis _____

3. aptyalism _____

4. ataxia _____

5. biodynamics _____

6. celiac _____

7. celiorrhaphy _____

8. cheilectomy _____

9. cholecystopexy _____

10. chronobiology _____

11. chronophobia _____

12. desmoplastic _____

13. dynamic _____

14. dynanometer _____

15. endoparasite _____

16. enterorrhaphy _____

17. erotomania _____

18. erythromelia _____

19. gastropexy _____

20. geriatric _____

21. hemopexin _____

22. hemoptysis _____

23. hemostasis _____

24. hidradenitis _____

25. homeostasis _____

26. homeotherm _____

27. hydropenia _____

28. ischemic _____

29. kleptomaniac _____

30. leiomyomata _____

31. leptomeninges _____

32. lithoclast _____

33. logopenia _____

34. maniacal _____

35. morphography _____

36. nomogram _____

37. odontoclasis _____

38. omphalitis _____

39. parasitize _____

40. pediatrician _____

41. phototropism _____

42. presbyacusia _____

43. prognathic _____

44. prostatectomy _____

45. pytalin _____

46. sitotoxism _____

47. stasis _____

48. stereotropism _____

49. syndesmopexy _____

50. tenodesis _____

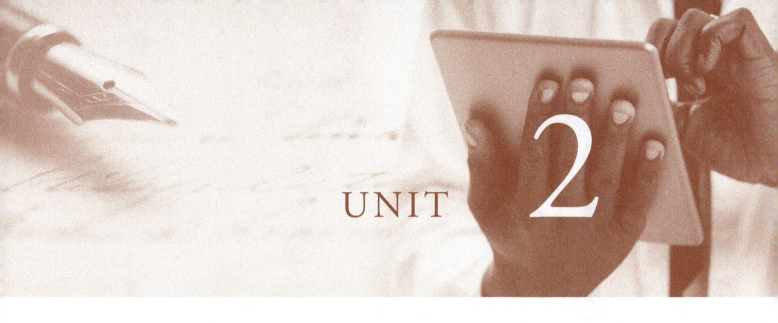

Latin-Derived Medical Terminology

Latin Nouns and Adjectives
Latin Verbs

Roman Numerals

A line placed over a letter increases its value one thousand times.

1	I	6	VI	11	XI	40	XL	90	XC	5000	$\overline{\text{V}}$
2	II	7	VII	12	XII	50	L	100	C	10,000	$\overline{\text{X}}$
3	III	8	VIII	15	XV	60	LX	500	D	100,000	$\overline{\text{C}}$
4	IV	9	IX	20	XX	70	LXX	1000	M	1,000,000	$\overline{\text{M}}$
5	V	10	X	30	XXX	80	LXXX	2000	MM		

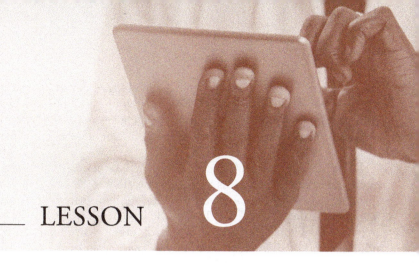

LESSON 8

LATIN NOUNS AND ADJECTIVES

Just as agriculture promises nourishment to healthy bodies, so does the practice of medicine promise health to the sick.

[Celsus, *De Medicina*, Prœmium 1]

Latin, like Greek, is an **inflected** language. Nouns, pronouns, and adjectives have different endings to indicate their grammatical function in a sentence. Latin nouns are divided into five classifications, or groups, called **declensions.** In each of these declensions, the endings of the various grammatical cases are substantially different in both singular and plural. The first three declensions produce most of the English derivatives.

Nouns of the first declension, mostly feminine, have the ending *-a* in the nominative singular, the vocabulary form of the noun. The combining form of these nouns is found by dropping the final *-a*. Latin nouns of the first declension appear in English in either their vocabulary form or with the final *-a* dropped or changed to a silent *-e*.

Latin Noun	Meaning	English Derivative
fistula	pipe	**fistula**
vāgīna	sheath	**vagina**
tībia	shin bone	**tibia**
axilla	armpit	**axilla**
larva	ghost	**larva**
lympha	clear water	**lymph**
forma	shape	**form**
palma	palm	**palm**
tunica	garment	**tunic**
membrāna	skin	**membrane**
ūrīna	urine	**urine**
sūtūra	seam	**suture**
tuba	trumpet	**tube**
valva	folding door	**valve**

The nominative plural of first declension nouns is *-ae*: *antenna, antennae; larva, larvae; vertēbra, vertēbrae.* The genitive singular of first declension nouns ends in *-ae*. This form is sometimes found in descriptive terminology and can be translated by the word *of*: **os coxae** (*os*, bone; *coxa*, hip), bone of the hip; **cervix vesicae** (*cervix*, neck; *vēsīca*, bladder), neck of the bladder.

Nouns of the second declension are either masculine or neuter. Masculine nouns in the nominative end in *-us* and neuter nouns end in *-um*. The combining form of these nouns is found by dropping this ending. Second declension nouns are usually found in the vocabulary form, but sometimes the ending is dropped or changed to silent *-e*.

Latin Noun	Meaning	English Derivative
bacillus	small staff	**bacillus**
cuneus	wedge	**cuneus**
fungus	mushroom	**fungus**
humerus	upper arm	**humerus**
globus	sphere	**globe**
digitus	finger	**digit**
ileum	groin	**ileum**
ōvum	egg	**ovum**
cerebrum	brain	**cerebrum**
palātum	palate	**palate**
intestīnum	intestine	**intestine**

The nominative plural of second declension masculine nouns is *-ī*: *bacillus, bacillī; fungus, fungī.* The plural of neuter nouns is *-a*: *cilium, cilia; ovum, ova.* The genitive singular of second declension nouns ends in *-ī*. This form

81

is sometimes found in descriptive terminology: **cervix uteri** (*cervix*, neck; *uterus*, womb), neck of the uterus. The genitive plural of these nouns ends in -*ōrum*: **icterus neonatorum** (Greek *neos*, new, Latin *nātus*, born), jaundice of newborns.

Latin nouns of the third declension are like Greek third declension nouns in that it is not always possible to determine the base of these nouns by knowing the nominative singular, the dictionary form. To find the base, it is usually necessary to know the form of some case other than the nominative. For this reason, dictionaries and vocabularies cite the nominative case along with the genitive singular, which ends in -*is*. The base is found by dropping this ending. In forming English words, often the nominative case is used alone, and sometimes suffixes are added directly to it. More often, however, the base of these nouns is used to form compound words.

Third declension nouns can be masculine, feminine, or neuter. (In this manual, if the base of a noun is the same as the dictionary form, or if the genitive case is the same as the nominative case, the genitive case is not given in the vocabularies.)

Latin Noun	Combining Form	Meaning	English Derivative
auris (auris)	*AUR-*	ear	**auris, auricle**
latus, lateris	*LATER-*	side	**latus, lateral**
os, ossis	*OSS-*	bone	**os coxae, ossify**
rādix, rādīcis	*RADIC-*	root	**radix, radical**
sopor (sopōris)	*SOPOR-*	sleep	**sopor, soporific**
vās (vāsis)	*VAS-*	vessel	**vas deferens, vascular**

LATIN GENITIVE ENDINGS

	Genitive Ending	Example	Meaning
First Declension			
Singular	-*ae*	**vesicae**	of the bladder
Second Declension			
Singular	-*ī*	**uteri**	of the uterus
Plural	-*ōrum*	**neonatorum**	of newborns
Third Declension			
Singular	-*is*	**dentis**	of the tooth

GENITIVE SINGULAR

The genitive singular of nouns of the first, second, and third declensions is sometimes found in descriptive terminology and can be translated by the word *of*: **corona dentis** (*corōna*, crown, *dens, dentis*, tooth), crown of the tooth.

The nominative plural of third declension masculine and feminine nouns ends in -*ēs*: *cervix, cervīcis* (neck): **cervix** (plural, **cervices**); *nāris, nāris* (nostril): **naris** (plural, **nares**); *rēn, rēnis* (kidney): **ren** (plural, **renes**). The plural of neuter nouns ends in *a*: *corpus, corporis* (body): **corpus** (plural, **corpora**); *genus, generis* (kind): **genus** (plural, **genera**); *viscus, visceris* (internal organ): **viscus** (plural, **viscera**).

There are a few nouns of the fourth and fifth declensions in medical terminology. Most fourth declension nouns are masculine and end in -*us* in the nominative singular, with the plural ending in -*ūs*: *meātus* (passage): **meatus** (plural, **meatus**), **meatoplasty, meatotomy**; *plexus* (a braid): **plexus** (plural, **plexus** or **plexuses**). Neuter nouns of the fourth declension end in *ū* in the nominative singular: *genū* (knee): **genupectoral**, pertaining to the knees and chest (*pectus, pectoris*, chest). The nominative plural of fourth declension neuter nouns ends in -*ua*: *cornū* (horn): **cornu** (plural, **cornua**). The nominative singular of fifth declension nouns ends in -*ēs*: *cariēs* (decay); *rabiēs* (madness); *scabiēs** (itch). Most fifth declension nouns are feminine; the plural is identical to the singular in the nominative case.

---

*Most fifth declension nouns end in -*iēs* in the nominative singular and plural.

LATIN NOMINATIVE SINGULAR AND PLURAL ENDINGS

	Singular	Example	Plural	Example
First and Second Declensions				
Masculine	*-us*	**fungus**	*ī*	**fungi**
Feminine	*-a*	**larva**	*-ae*	**larvae**
Neuter	*-um*	**ovum**	*-a*	**ova**
Third Declension				
Masculine/Feminine	*s**	**cervix**	*-ēs*	**cervices†**
Neuter	***	**viscus**	*-(i)a*	**viscera‡**
Fourth Declension				
Masculine	*-us*	**meatus**	*-ūs*	**meatus**
Neuter	*-u*	**genu**	*-ua*	**genua**
Fifth Declension				
Feminine	*-ēs*	**rabies**	*-ēs*	**rabies**

*Third declension nouns have a variety of endings in the nominative singular.
†Latin *cervix, cervicis*.
‡Latin *viscus, visceris*.

LATIN ADJECTIVES

There are two classes of Latin adjectives: they are either of the first and second declension, with endings like those of masculine, feminine, and neuter nouns of the first and second declensions, or of the third declension. Latin dictionaries and grammar texts cite first- and second declension adjectives by using the masculine singular, ending in *-us*, as the entry form, and following it with the feminine and neuter endings *-a* and *-um; bonus, -a, -um* (good); *magnus, -a, -um* (large); *medius, -a, -um* (middle). In this manual, adjectives of this class are cited only in the form of the masculine nominative singular, ending in *-us*, the dictionary form. There are some adjectives of the first and second declension with masculine forms ending in *-er*; but with the feminine and neuter forms ending in *-a* and *-um*, respectively: *asper, aspera, asperum* (rough); *tener, tenera, tenerum* (tender). Some adjectives ending in *-er* drop the *-e-* in the feminine and neuter: *integer, integra, integrum* (whole); *ruber, rubra, rubrum* (red).

Third declension adjectives usually have two terminations: *-is* for the masculine and feminine and *-e* for the neuter: *gravis, -e* (severe); *fortis, -e* (strong); *levis, -e* (light). There are some adjectives of the third declension with masculine forms ending in *-er*; these have *-ris* in the feminine and *-re* in the neuter: [*ācer, ācris, ācre* (sharp)]; *salūber, salūbris, salūbre* (healthful). Some adjectives of the third declension have one form for the masculine, feminine, and neuter genders: *ātrox*, genitive *ātrōcis* (fierce), *praegnāns*, genitive *praegnantis* (pregnant); *sapiēns*, genitive *sapientis* (knowing, wise). There are no adjectives of the fourth and fifth declensions.

Latin adjectives usually follow the nouns they modify and agree with them in gender and number:

myasthenia **gravis**

genu **recurvatum**

vena **cava**

LATIN PREFIXES

Latin prefixes, like Greek prefixes, modify or qualify the meaning of the word to which they are affixed. It is difficult to assign a single specific meaning to each prefix. Often, it is necessary to adapt a meaning that fits the particular use of a word. A word may have more than one prefix. In compound words, a prefix may follow a combining form. Latin prefixes (and suffixes) are frequently used with Greek combining forms.

---

ab- (**a-** rarely before certain consonants; **abs-** before *c* and *t*): away from:

ab-ductor	**abs**-cess
ab-lation	**abs**-tract
ab-ortion	**a**-vulsion

---

ad- (**ac-** before *c*; **af-** before *f*; **ag-** before *g*; **al-** before *l*; **an-** before *n*; **ap-** before *p*; **as-** before *s*; **a-** before *sp*; **at-** before *t*): to, toward:

ad-aptation	**al**-literation
ad-renaline	**an**-nectent
ac-cessory	**ap**-pendix
af-fection	**as**-sisted
af-ferent	**a**-spirate
ag-glomerate	**at**-traction

---

ambi-: both:

ambi-dextrous	**ambi**-sexual
ambi-lateral	**ambi**-valence

ante-: before, forward:

ante-flexion	**ante**-natal
ante-mortem	**ante**-version

bi- (bin-, bis-): two, twice, double, both:

bi-parous	**bin**-aural
bi-furcate	**bin**-ocular
bi-lateral	**bis**-iliac

circum-: around:

circum-corneal	**circum**-nuclear
circum-duction	**circum**-ocular

con- (co- before *h;* **col-** before *l;* **com-** before *e, m,* and *p;* **cor-** before *r*): together, with; thoroughly, very:

con-genital	**com**-mensal
co-hesion	**com**-press
col-lapse	**cor**-rosive
com-edo	**co**-hesion

contra-: against, opposite:

contra-ception	**contra**-indication
contra-fissura	**contra**-lateral

de-: down, away from, absent:

de-generation	**de**-saturation
de-hydration	**de**-sensitize

dis- (di- before *g, v,* and usually before *l;* **dif-** before *f*): apart, away:

dis-infect	**di**-gest
dif-fusate	**di**-lation
dif-fuse	**di**-vergent

ex- (e- before certain consonants; **ef-** before *f*): out of, away from:

ex-halation	**ef**-ferent
ex-pectoration	**e**-visceration

extra- (rarely **extro-**): on the outside, beyond:

extra-sensory	**extro**-version
extra-vasation	**extro**-vert

(1) in- (il- before *l;* **im-** before *b, m,* and *p;* **ir-** before *r*): in, into:

in-cubation	**im**-bibition
in-farct	**im**-mersion
in-gestion	**im**-pregnate
il-lumination	**ir**-radiate

(2) in- not:

in-continence	**im**-balance
in-firm	**im**-mune
in-nominate	**im**-potent
il-legal	**ir**-reducible

(3) in-: very, thoroughly:

in-duration	**in**-flammation
in-ebriation	**in**-toxication

infra-: beneath, below:

infra-mammary	**infra**-renal
infra-psychic	**infra**-sonic

inter-: between:

inter-cerebral	**inter**-dental
inter-costal	**inter**-renal

intra- (rarely **intro-**): within:

intra-gastric	**intra**-venous
intra-muscular	**intro**-version

mult- (often **multi-**): many, much, affecting many parts:

mult-angular	**multi**-gravida
multi-cuspid	**multi**-parous

non-: not:*

non-conductor	**non**-toxic
non-protein	**non**-viable

ob- (oc- before *c;* **op-** before *p*): against, toward; very, thoroughly:

ob-session	**oc**-cult
oc-clusion	**op**-position

per- (pel- before *l*): through; very, thoroughly:

per-manent	**per**-spiration
per-meable	**pel**-lucid

post-: after, following, behind:

post-mortem	**post**-partum
post-nasal	**post**-uterine

pre-: before, in front of:

pre-digestion	**pre**-tibial
pre-gnant	**pre**-tracheal

pro-: forward, in front:

pro-cedure	**pro**-jection
pro-cess	**pro**-tection

---

*Non is not a prefix in Latin, but an adverb. Because it is used as a prefix in English, it is included here with prefixes.

re-: back, again:

re-cess	**re**-sonance
re-fraction	**re**-suscitation

retro-: backward, in back, behind:

retro-grade	**retro**-peritoneal
retro-nasal	**retro**-pharyngeal

se-: apart, away from:

se-crete	**se**-gregation
se-duce	**se**-paration

semi-: half:

semi-conscious	**semi**-permeable
semi-flexion	**semi**-prone

sub- (**suf-** before *f;* **sup-** before *p*): under:

sub-costal	**suf**-fusion
sub-dural	**sup**-purate

super- (often **supra-**): over, above; excess:

super-ficial	**supra**-costal
super-virulent	**supra**-renal

trans-: across, through:

trans-parent	**trans**-thoracotomy
trans-plant	**trans**-vaginal

ultra-: beyond, excess:

ultra-microtome	**ultra**-sound
ultra-sonic	**ultra**-violet

Numeric Combining Forms and Prefixes

Combining Form/Prefix	Meaning	Example
uni-	one	**uni**-form
bi-, bin-, bis-	two, twice, double, both	**bi**-modal, **bin**-aural, **bis**-iliac
tri-*	three	**tri**-cuspid
quadr-	four	**quadr**-iplegia, **quadr**-uped
quint-	five, fifth	**quint**-ipara, **quint**-uplet
sex-, sext-	six, sixth	**sex**-digital, **sext**-uplet, **sext**-igravida
sept-	seven	**sept**-ivalent, **sept**-uplet
oct-, octa-	eight	**oct**-ane, **octa**-hedron, **oct**-ogenarian, **oct**-ipara
non-	nine, ninth	**non**-igravida, **non**-ose
dec-, deca-	ten, one-tenth	**dec**-igram, **deca**-meter

*Derived from Greek.

LATIN SUFFIXES

Suffixes are elements that are added to the combining forms of nouns, adjectives, and verbs to form new words. Nouns are either abstract or concrete. Abstract nouns indicate a state, quality, condition, procedure, or process; concrete nouns give names to objects and agents. Adjectives impart qualities or characteristics to nouns. The Latin language was rich in suffixes, but only those that are in common use in modern medical terminology are presented here.

Most of the abstract noun-forming suffixes that were used in Latin were affixed to verbal stems and are presented in Lesson 9. The suffixes given here are attached to the combining forms of adjectives or nouns. In most instances, Latin suffixes have come into English in a form slightly changed from their original as a result of their transition through French. The following list gives their English form. Note that when the base of a noun or adjective ends in a consonant and the suffix begins with a consonant, a **connecting vowel,** usually **i,** but sometimes **o** or **u,** is inserted.

The Latin language was particularly rich in adjective-forming suffixes. Only those suffixes that are frequently found are listed here; the less common ones will be identified as they occur. As with the noun-forming suffixes, adjective-forming suffixes usually come into English in a form slightly changed from their original. The following list gives their English form. Many Latin adjectives end in *-eus*, *-ea*, or *-eum*, which explains the presence of -e- in many English words: **esophageal, sanguineous, cesarean,** and so forth.

-al: adjective-forming suffix: pertaining to:

dors-**al**	ren-**al**

-an: adjective-forming suffix: pertaining to, located in:

medi-**an**	ovari-**an**

-ar: adjective-forming suffix: pertaining to, located in:

ocul-**ar**	vascul-**ar**

-arium: noun-forming suffix: denotes a place for something:

aqu-**arium**	herb-**arium**

-ary: noun-forming suffix: denotes a place for something:

libr-**ary**	mortu-**ary**

-ary: adjective-forming suffix: pertaining to:

saliv-**ary**	axill-**ary**

-ate: adjective-forming suffix: having the form of, possessing:

cord-**ate**	caud-**ate**

-ia: abstract noun-forming suffix: state, quality, condition:

inert-**ia**	insomn-**ia**

-ian: noun-forming suffix: indicates an expert in a certain field:

librar-**ian**	mortic-**ian**

-ic: adjective-forming suffix: pertaining to:

pelv-**ic**	rhythm-**ic**

-id*: adjective-forming suffix: pertaining to:

morb-**id**	rab-**id**

-ile: adjective-forming suffix: pertaining to, capable of:

sen-**ile**	febr-**ile**

-ine: adjective-forming suffix: pertaining to, located in:

uter-**ine**	amygdal-**ine**
sangu-**ine**	femin-**ine**

-ive: adjective-forming suffix: pertaining to:

tuss-**ive**	palliat-**ive**

-lent: adjective-forming suffix: full of:

somno-**lent**	puru-**lent**

-ose: adjective-forming suffix: full of:

adip-**ose**	varic-**ose**

-ous: adjective-forming suffix: full of:

bili-**ous**	sanguine-**ous**

-ty: abstract noun-forming suffix: state, quality, condition:

gravi-**ty**	morbidi-**ty**

-y: abstract noun-forming suffix: state, quality, condition:

memor-**y**	remed-**y**

---

*Note that there is a Greek-derived suffix *-id*, an alternative form of *-oid*, meaning, "having the form of": hominid (*homo, hominis*, man).

-AD

The English adverb-forming suffix **-ad** forms adverbs from nouns. These adverbs indicate direction toward a part of the body: **dextrad,** toward the right side (*dextra,* the right hand); **sinistrad,** toward the left side (*sinistra,* the left hand); **cephalad,** toward the head (Greek *kephalē,* head). (See the Etymological Notes in this lesson.)

DIMINUTIVE SUFFIXES

Some suffixes in Latin form diminutive nouns from other nouns. These diminutives are first or second declension nouns, ending in *-us, -a,* or *-um,* depending on the gender of the noun to which they are affixed, and they are all characterized by the presence of a single or double *l.* They usually appear in English in their original Latin form, but the final *-us* is sometimes changed to *-e, -culus* to *-cle,* and *-illa* to *-il.* A diminutive suffix expresses the idea of smallness, as in **fibril,** meaning a small fiber.

Examples of Diminutive Suffixes

-cle	ventricle	**-culus**	ventriculus
-ella	rubella	**-ellum**	cerebellum
-il	fibril	**-illa**	fibrilla
-ola	roseola	**-olus**	alveolus
-ule	globule	**-ulus**	calculus

DIMINUTIVE SUFFIXES

Diminutive suffixes are characterized by the presence of a single or double *l* and express the idea of smallness.

Words such as **rubella** (*ruber,* red) and **roseola** (*roseus,* rosy, reddish) are New Latin formations from Latin adjectives of the first and second declensions. These particular words are neuter plural in form. Rubella, or German measles, is named for the "little red things," the eruptions that accompany this disease. Roseola, a skin condition marked by maculae or red spots, is named for the "little reddish things" that characterize this condition. **Variola** (*varius,* spotted), smallpox, and **varicella** (an irregularly formed diminutive from *varius*), chickenpox, are similar formations. Often, a new genus of bacteria is named by adding the neuter plural suffix **-ella** to the surname of its discoverer: *Salmonella* (Daniel E. Salmon, 1850–1914), *Brucella* (Sir David Bruce, 1855–1931), *Shigella* (Kiyoshi Shiga, 1870–1957).

NOTE: A word may have more than one suffix: **adiposity, morbidity.** Greek prefixes and suffixes may be used with Latin words: **adipositis, periocular.** Greek and Latin words may be combined in a single term: **cardiopulmonary** (Greek *kardia*, heart, Latin *pulmō, pulmōnis*, lung). Such words are known as **hybrids** (Latin *hybrida*, mongrel). A child born of a Roman father and a foreign mother, or one born of a freeman and a slave, was known as a *hybrida*, a word probably borrowed from the Greek *hybris* (insolence).

Many Latin words and expressions are used in medical terminology in their original form: **medulla oblongata** (*medulla*, marrow; *oblongata* [New Latin], elongated), referring to the lowest part of the brainstem; **cerebellum** (*cerebellum*, little brain), the portion of the brain forming the largest part of the rhombencephalon; **auricle** (*auricle*, little ear), the portion of the external ear not contained within the head.

VOCABULARY

NOTE: Beginning with this lesson, combining forms of Latin words will be printed in **bold italics**.

Latin	Combining Form(s)	Meaning	Example
abdōmen, abdōminis	***ABDOMIN-***	belly, abdomen	**abdomin**-ocentesis
adeps, adipis	***ADIP-***	fat	**adip**-ose
auris	***AUR-***	ear	**aur**-icular
bacillus	***BACILL-***	[rod, staff] bacillus	**bacill**-emia
bursa (Medieval Latin)	***BURS-***	[leather sack] bursa	**burs**-itis
calx, calcis	***CALC-***	stone, calcium, lime (salts)	**calc**-iferous
calor	***CALOR-***	heat, energy	**calor**-ic
caput, capitis	***CAPIT-***	head	de-**capit**-ate
cerebrum	***CEREBR-***	brain	**cerebr**-al
costa	***COST-***	rib	**cost**-algia
dens, dentis (Fig. 8-1)	***DENT-***	tooth	**dent**-ist
dorsum	***DORS-***	back (of the body)	**dors**-al
externus, -a, -um	***EXTERN-***	outer	**extern**-al
fibra	***FIBR-***	fiber, filament	**fibr**-ous
fistula	***FISTUL-***	(tube, pipe) fistula, an abnormal tubelike passage in the body	**fistul**-ectomy
frīgus, frīgoris	***FRIG-, FRIGOR-***	cold	re-**frig**-erate
insula	***INSUL-***	island*	**insul**-in
internus, -a, -um	***INTERN-***	inner	**intern**-al
meātus	***MEAT-***	passage, opening, meatus (pronounced mee-ate'-us)	**meat**-oplasty
nāsus	***NAS-***	nose	**nas**-al
pus, puris	***PUR-***	pus	**pur**-ulent
rādix, rādīcis	***RADIC-, RAD-, RADIX***	root	**radic**-es
rēn, rēnis	***REN-***	kidney	**ren**-ovascular
sanguis, sanguinis	***SANGUI(N)-***	blood	**sanguin**-opurulent
sonus	***SON-***	sound	**son**-ogram
synovia (New Latin)	***SYNOV-***	synovial fluid, synovial membrane or sac	**synov**-ium
tuba	***TUB-***	[trumpet] tube	**tub**-outerine
tussis	***TUSS-***	cough	anti-**tuss**-ive
vacca	***VACC-***	cow†	**vacc**-ine
vīrus (Fig. 8-2)	***VIR-, VIRUS-***	[poison, venom] virus‡	**vir**-al
viscus, visceris (plural, *viscera*)	***VISCUS-, VISCER-***	internal organ(s)	**viscer**-al

*See Etymological Notes in this lesson.
†Words containing vaccin- have to do with vaccine.
‡Words like virulent are from the Latin adjective *virulentus*, strong, powerful (literally, full of poison).

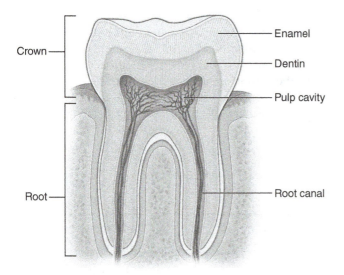

Figure 8-1. Tooth structure (longitudinal section). (From Henry, R. K., and Goldie, M. P., *Dental Hygiene: Applications to Clinical Practice*, F. A. Davis, 2016, with permission.)

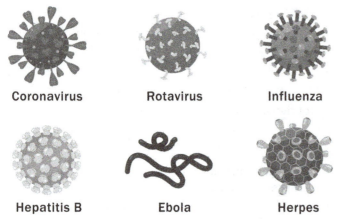

Figure 8-2. Viruses. (Courtesy of Elena Istomina, iStock/Getty Images Plus.)

LATIN PRONUNCIATION

In Latin, all consonants and vowels are pronounced, with no silent letters. The sound of the consonants is the same as in English, except that *c* and *g* are always "hard"; thus, *cancer* is pronounced "kanker," and the *g* of *genus* is pronounced like the *g* of gate. The letter *t* is always pronounced like the *t* in tin and never has the sound of the *t* in nation. It is customary to pronounce *i* like the *y* in yes and *v* like the *w* in win. Vowels may be long or short and are pronounced as follows:

Short Vowels	Long Vowels	Diphthongs
a as in adrift	*ā* as in father	*ae* as ie in tie
e as in bet	*ē* as in they	*au* as ou in house
i as in tin	*ī* as in machine	*ei* as ei in eight
o as in hot	*ō* as in tone	*oe* as oi in boil
u as oo in look	*ū* as in rude	

Latin words are accentuated on the penult, the next to last syllable, if that syllable is long. A long syllable is one that contains a long vowel or a diphthong, or one in which the vowel is followed by two consonants, whether long or short. If the second of two consonants is *l* or *r*, the syllable need not be considered long; *cerebrum* is accented on the antepenult. If the penult is short, the syllable before that, the antepenult, receives the accent.

NOMINATIVE SINGULAR

The nominative singular, the vocabulary form, of some words (e.g., *radix*, *tussis*, *abdomen*, *auris*, and *viscus*) is used in medical terminology.

ETYMOLOGICAL NOTES

As spoken Latin gradually became French, a number of sound changes took place. The sound of an initial Latin *c*, when followed by *a*, usually developed into *ch* in French: Latin *caballus* (horse), French *cheval*; Latin *caldus* (hot), French *chaud*; Latin *castus* (pure), French *chaste*. Latin *cancer* (crab, ulcer) became French *chancre*, which is used with the same spelling in English. A **chancre** is a venereal ulcer, an outward manifestation of syphilis. This disease takes its name from Syphilus, the hero of the medical poem entitled *Syphilis sive Morbus Gallicus* (Syphilis, or the French Disease) by the Italian physician and poet Girolamo Fracastoro (1484–1553). In this poem, Syphilus suffered from an infectious disease that Fracastoro named syphilis, perhaps from the Greek verb *philein* (love).

Insulin (*insula*, island) takes its name from the islets of Langerhans, cell clusters in the pancreas. The islets of Langerhans were named after the German pathologist Paul Langerhans (1847–1888), who first realized their existence and function. These cells are of three types: alpha, beta, and delta. The beta cells produce the protein hormone insulin, which regulates the metabolism of carbohydrates in the body. Deficient production or utilization of insulin causes **hyperglycemia** (Greek *glykys*, sweet), the characteristic of the disease **diabetes mellitus** (Latin *mel*, *mellis*, honey). Diabetes mellitus (DM) type 1 is caused by the destruction of pancreatic beta cells and is thought to result from autoimmune destruction of those cells. Development usually occurs in childhood or adolescence. Because insulin is required to manage type 1 DM, it is often called insulin-dependent diabetes. Type 2 DM, formerly called adult-onset diabetes, results from a combination of insulin resistance (cells do not respond to circulating insulin produced by the beta cells) and abnormal gluconeogenesis (glucose production) (Fig. 8-3). A third type of diabetes, type 1.5, also called latent autoimmune diabetes in adults, is a form of diabetes with characteristics of both type 1 and type 2 diabetes.

Comparison of Type 1 (Insulin-Dependent) Diabetes Mellitus and Type 2 (Non–Insulin-Dependent) Diabetes Mellitus

	Type 1	Type 2
Age at onset	Usually under 30	Usually over 40
Symptom onset	Abrupt	Gradual
Body weight	Normal	Obese–80%
HLA association	Positive	Negative
Family history	Common	Nearly universal
Insulin in blood	Little to none	Some usually present
Islet cell antibodies	Present at onset	Absent
Prevalence	0.2%–0.3%	8%
Symptoms	Polyuria, polydipsia, polyphagia, weight loss, ketoacidosis	Polyuria, polydipsia, peripheral neuropathy
Control	Insulin, diet, and exercise	Diet, exercise and often oral hypoglycemic drugs or insulin
Vascular and neural changes	Eventually develop	Will usually develop
Stability of condition	Fluctuates, may be difficult to control	May be difficult to control in poorly motivated patients

Figure 8-3. Diabetes table. (From Venes, D., *Taber's Cyclopedic Medical Dictionary*, 24th ed., F. A. Davis, 2021, pg. 668, with permission.)

The words **vaccine** and **vaccination** come from the Latin *vacca* (cow). In 1789, Edward Jenner, an English country physician, announced to the world his discovery that injection of the cowpox virus into humans (i.e., vaccination) provided immunity against smallpox. It was known then that people who were employed on dairy farms and who happened to contract the bovine disease cowpox became immune to smallpox. Jenner began his experimentation in 1796 by inoculating a healthy young boy with matter taken from an ulcerating sore on the hand of a milkmaid suffering from cowpox. Later, this boy was inoculated with the smallpox virus and resisted the disease. This was the first vaccination. In 1959, the World Health Organization (WHO) began a global immunization campaign to eradicate smallpox. In May 1980, WHO declared smallpox was eradicated worldwide.*

The incidence of many illnesses has been greatly reduced or eliminated by vaccines. A vaccine developed recently to protect against several types of the human papilloma virus (HPV) infection has the potential to eradicate cervical cancer caused by cell changes related to HPV infection of the cervix.

Vaccine refusal is the unwillingness to allow oneself or a family member to be immunized against a preventable contagious disease. It occurs most often in people who fear adverse reactions, who have religious or philosophical objections, or who have had allergic reactions to some component of a vaccine. Vaccine refusal has contributed to outbreaks of previously eradicated diseases.

The English words **viscous** and **viscid** bear no relationship to the internal organs—the viscera—but are derived from Latin *viscum* (mistletoe) (Fig. 8-4). The ancient Romans prepared a sticky substance from the berries of the mistletoe plant that they spread on branches of trees. Unfortunate birds that perched on those branches were

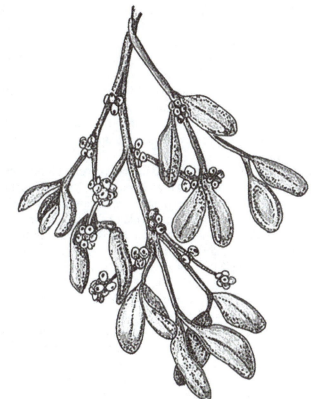

Figure 8-4. Mistletoe. (Drawing by Laine McCarthy, 2001.)

caught and held fast by this glutinous substance, which we call birdlime. The Roman poet Virgil writes of the olden days when men had to toil for their living and hunt for their food:

> It was then that men found a way to snare wild beasts in nets, to trap birds with birdlime *(viscum)* and to surround the huge groves of trees with hounds [*Georgics* 1.139–140].

---
*https://www.cdc.gov/smallpox/history/history.html

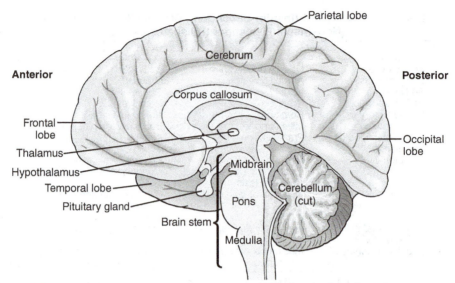

Figure 8-5. Midsagittal section of brain as seen from left. (From Lippert, L., *Clinical Kinesiology and Anatomy*, 6th ed., F. A. Davis, 2017, with permission.)

The adverb-forming suffix **-ad** indicates direction toward a part of the body, as in the words **dextrad,** toward the right; **sinistrad,** toward the left; or **cephalad,** toward the head. Early in the 19th century **-ad** entered the English language after a proposal by the British scholar James Barclay in his work *New Anatomical Nomenclature* (1803) that **-ad** be used as an equivalent of -ward in English: **homeward, forward,** and so forth. The suffix **-ad** did not exist in Latin and seems to have been an adaptation of the prefix *ad-* (toward).

Aureolus Theophrastus Bombastus von Hohenheim (1493–1541), better known as Paracelsus, has been called the "precursor of chemical pharmacology and therapeutics, and the most original medical thinker of the 16th century."* The name Paracelsus is thought to have been bestowed upon him as an indication of his superiority to the Roman physician Celsus. The son of a physician, he became professor of medicine at Basle in 1527. He was a pioneer in chemistry who wrote extensively (in Latin) on medicine during a stormy career that ended in a tavern brawl in Salzburg. The word **synovia** is first found in his writing and seems to have been coined by him, perhaps from the Latin *ōvum* (egg) because of the viscous quality of this colorless fluid. Paracelsus considered synovia the nutritive fluid of the body, but its use by later physicians was restricted to the lubricating fluid secreted within synovial membranes of joints, bursae, and tendon sheaths. Synovia has no etymology; it seems to have been the invention of Paracelsus.

The word **bursa** is first found in Medieval Latin and is derived from the Greek *byrsa* (skin, hide of an animal). This word meant a leather bag or sack. Later, the term *bursa mucosa* was applied to a sac or cavity found in connective tissue and containing synovial fluid. One of the original senses of the word, a bag to hold money, is retained in the English words purse (where the letter *p* is unexplained), burse (a scholarship for school or university), bursar, disbursement, and so forth. It is also found in the French *bourse*, meaning purse, and *Bourse*, the stock exchange of Paris. The Burse was the original Royal Exchange in London.

The Latin words *occipitium* and *occiput, occipitis* are compounds of the prefix *ob-* and *caput, capitis* (head), and meant the back part of the head, the **occiput** (Fig. 8-5). Latin *sinciput* was an abbreviated form of *semi-caput* and in Latin meant half of a head, in particular the smoked cheek or jowl of a hog. **Sinciput** now means the fore and upper part of the cranium, or the upper half of the skull. The words *occiput* and *sinciput* show a reduction of the *a* of *caput* to *i* in the nominative case and of the *u* to *i* in the genitive case. This is believed to be because of a strong stress accent on the first syllable of Latin words that occurred during an early period of the development of the language. Other examples of this vowel reduction can be seen in **biceps,** two-headed, and **triceps,** three-headed, which are also from *caput*. This change can be seen more clearly in Latin verbs and in their derivatives in English.

The word *fistula* (tube, pipe) was used by Ovid in the *Metamorphoses* in a simile to describe how the blood of the unhappy lover Pyramus spurted from his body when he took his own life with a sword. Pyramus and Thisbe were a young couple of Babylon who lived next door to one another. They fell in love, but their parents forbade them to meet. However, they spoke to one another through a chink in the common wall that separated their houses, and, at length, the lovers decided to meet under a mulberry tree that was laden with snow-white berries at the nearby tomb of Ninus, an ancient king of Babylon. The young girl, Thisbe, arrived first at the appointed place that night. As she waited, a lioness came along, fresh from the kill, to quench her thirst at a nearby pool. Thisbe fled in terror,

*Garrison FH. *An Introduction to the History of Medicine.* 3rd ed. Saunders; 1927.

dropping the thin cloak that she had brought along. When the lioness had drunk her fill, the beast found the cloak and mangled it with her bloodied jaws. Pyramus arrived shortly after and, seeing the bloodstained cloak and thinking that Thisbe had met a cruel death, drew his sword and fell upon it. As he lay there dying,

Cruor emicat alte,
non aliter quam cum vitiato fistula plumbo
scinditur et tenui stridente foramine longas
eiculatur aquas atque ictibus aera rumpit.

[*Metamorphoses* 4.121–124]

The blood gushed forth, just as water bursts through a broken pipe *(fistula)* and, with a strident sound, spurts through the air.

Ovid goes on to say that the fruit of the mulberry tree was stained with the crimson blood. Thisbe came out of her hiding place and found Pyramus with his life's blood ebbing. She fitted the point of the sword to her own breast and fell forward on the blade that was still warm from the blood of her lover. From that day on, the fruit of the mulberry tree reddens as it ripens, a remembrance of the lovers' blood that was shed there.

Exercise 1: Analyze and Define

Analyze and define each of the following words. In this and in succeeding exercises, analysis should consist of separating the words into prefixes (if any), combining forms, and suffixes or suffix forms (if any) and giving the meaning of each. Be certain to differentiate between nouns and adjectives in your definitions. Consult a medical dictionary for the current meanings of these words. Use a separate paper if you need more room for an answer.

1. abdominoplasty _____

2. adipokinesis _____

3. adrenalinemia _____

4. auricula _____

5. auriculotherapy _____

6. bacillary _____

7. biceps _____

8. bursae _____

9. calcipexy _____

10. calculogenesis _____

11. calorimeter _____

12. capitulum _____

13. cerebellum _____

14. costochondral _____

15. dentist _____

16. dorsal _____

17. externalize _____

18. fibromyalgia _____

19. fistula _____

20. frigostabile _____

21. insulinase _____

22. internal _____

23. leiomyofibroma _____

24. meatotomy _____

25. myelofibrosis _____

26. myofibril _____

27. nasoscope _____

28. neurotropic virus _____

29. nonose _____

30. occiput _____

31. pararenal _____

32. pertussis _____

33. polyradiculitis* _____

34. postnasal _____

35. purulent _____

36. quadriplegia _____

_____

*Words containing radic- and radicul- usually refer to roots of spinal nerves.

37. radiculalgia _____

38. radix _____

39. renogram _____

40. retrovirus _____

41. sanguineous _____

42. synoviocyte _____

43. tenosynovitis _____

44. tuboplasty _____

45. tussive _____

46. ultrasonogram _____

47. vaccine _____

48. virusemia _____

49. viscerotrophic _____

50. viscus _____

Exercise 2:   Word Derivation

Give the word derived from Greek and/or Latin elements that matches each of the following. Verify your answer in a medical dictionary. **Note that the wording of the dictionary definition may vary from the wording used here.**

1. Knife or shears for cutting through a rib (or cartilage) _____

2. Small toothlike projection _____

3. Toward the back _____

4. Surgical removal of (all or part of) a tube _____

5. Tumor composed of mucous and fibrous elements _____

6. Pertaining to the nose _____

7. Head shaped _____

8. Calculus formed in a bursa _____

9. Inflammation of the spinal nerve roots _____

10. Presence of viruses in the blood _____

11. Pertaining to the production of heat or energy _____

12. Science of the development, administration and use of vaccines _____

13. Tumor arising from a synovial membrane _____

14. Development of fibrous tissue _____

15. Presence of (rod-shaped) bacteria in the blood _____

16. Any disease of the brain _____

17. Fatty _____

18. (Relative or absolute) excess of insulin (in the blood) _____

19. (Through, into, or) across the abdomen or abdominal wall _____

20. Generalized enlargement of the internal [abdominal] organs _____

Exercise 3:   Drill and Review

Analyze and define each of the following words. Analysis should consist of separating the words into prefixes (if any), combining forms, and suffixes or suffix forms (if any), and give the meaning of each. Be certain to differentiate between nouns and adjectives in your definitions. Using the elements in the word determine its meaning. Consult a medical dictionary for the current meanings of these words. Use a separate paper if you need more room for an answer.

1. adipectomy _____

2. adipocyte _____

3. aural _____

4. aviremia _____

5. bacillar _____

6. binauricular _____

7. binotic _____

8. bursotomy _____

9. calculus _____

10. calorimetry _____

11. cerebral _____

12. chondrocostal _____

13. costalgia _____

14. costochondritis _____

15. decimeter _____

16. dentin _____

17. external _____

18. fibromyoma _____

19. fistuloenterostomy _____

20. frigid _____

21. hypercalcemia _____

22. hyperinsulinemia _____

23. infrarenal _____

24. insulinemia _____

25. intercostal _____

26. internalize _____

27. myeloradiculopathy _____

28. nasogastric _____

29. nontoxic _____

30. occipital _____

31. periradicular _____

32. postvaccinal _____

33. predentin _____

34. purulent synovitis _____

35. radiculomeningomyelitis _____

36. renal calculus _____

37. retronasal _____

38. sanguine _____

39. semisynthetic _____

40. sincipital _____

41. sonography _____

42. subcostal _____

43. supervirulent _____

44. supradiaphragmatic _____

45. suprarenal _____

46. synovectomy _____

47. tuboabdominal _____

48. tuborrhea _____

49. viscerosomatic _____

50. virustatic _____

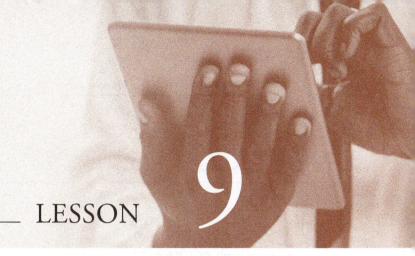

LATIN VERBS

*I would have given the name insectology to that part of natural history which has insects as its object: that of
entomology . . . would undoubtedly have been more suitable . . . but its barbarous sound terrify'd me.*

[Bennet's *Contemporary Natural History*, London 1776]

*Earache and disorders of the ear are cured by the urine of a wild boar that has been kept in a glass jar, or by the gall of
a wild boar or of a pig or an ox with equal portions of citrus and rose oil added. But the best cure of all is warm gall
of a bull with leek juice. If there are suppurations, honey should be added, and if there is a foul odor the gall should be
warmed with the rind of a pomegranate.*

[Pliny the Elder, *Natural History* 28.48.173]

Most Latin verbs have four principal parts, as illustrated by
secō, secāre, secuī, sectus (to cut).

Principal Part	Example	Meaning
1st: Present Active Indicative	*secō*	I cut
2nd: Present Active Infinitive	*secāre*	to cut
3rd: Perfect Active Indicative	*secuī*	I cut, have cut
4th: Perfect Passive Participle	*sectus*	having been cut

Latin verbs are divided into four classes, or groups, called
conjugations. This classification is based on the stem vowel
of the present infinitive, the second principal part of the verb.
The ending of the present infinitive in the first conjugation is
-āre; in the second, *-ēre;* the third, *-ere;* and in the fourth, *-īre.*

Latin verbs have three stems on which the various
tenses are formed: the present, the perfect active, and the
perfect passive. Only the first and third of these have been
productive in furnishing English derivatives, and these are
the only ones considered here. The first stem is that of
the infinitive, and the third is that of the perfect passive

participle, an adjective of the first and second declension
with the endings *-us*, *-a*, or *-um*, indicating masculine, feminine, or neuter gender, respectively. In this manual, the
perfect passive participle is given with the ending *-us*, the
form in which all such adjectives are cited here.

Thus, Latin verbs have two combining forms. The first
is formed by dropping the ending of the infinitive and the
second by dropping the *-us* of the perfect passive participle. The verb *dūcere, ductus* (lead, bring) has two combining
forms, DUC- and DUCT-, giving the stem of such English
derivatives as **induce, reduce, induction,** and **reduction.**
As with Greek verbs, Latin verbs are customarily cited in
Latin dictionaries and grammars in the form of the first
person singular (*ducō*, I lead; *cadō*, I fall). English dictionaries usually cite Latin verbs in the form of the present
infinitive, and that is how they are cited in this manual.

Some verbs appear only in the passive form but with active
meanings. These are known as **deponent** verbs. The infinitives
of the four conjugations of deponent verbs end in *-ārī, -ērī, -ī,*
and *-īrī.* The combining form is found by dropping these endings. The deponent verb *patior, patī, passus sum* (endure, suffer)
gives us such words as **patient, patience,** and **passion.**

Conjugation	Present Indicative	Present Infinitive	Perfect Indicative	Perfect Passive Participle
1st	*secō* (cut)	*secāre*	*secuī*	*sectus*
2nd	*habeō* (have)	*habēre*	*habuī*	*habitus*
3rd	*fundō* (pour)	*fundere*	*fūdī*	*fūsus*
4th	*sciō* (know)	*scīre*	*scīvī*	*scītus*

SUFFIXES

Many suffixes are added only to the stems of verbs. Latin suffixes often undergo some changes in English words. They are presented here in the form in which they appear in English.

-able: adjective-forming suffix: capable of (being), able to:

ten-**able**   dur-**able**

-ation: noun-forming suffix indicating an action or process: the act of (being), the result of (being), something that is:

gest-**ation**   form-**ation**

-ce: noun-forming suffix: the act of (being), the state of (being):

patien-**ce**   innocen-**ce**

-cy: noun-forming suffix: the act of (being), the state of (being):

constan-**cy**   hesitan-**cy**

-ible: adjective-forming suffix: capable of (being):

aud-**ible**   divis-**ible**

-id: adjective-forming suffix: in a state or condition of:

flu-**id**   tep-**id**

-ile: adjective-forming suffix: capable of (being), like:

fac-**ile**   infant-**ile**

-ion: noun-forming suffix: the act of:

tens-**ion**   correct-**ion**

-ive: adjective-forming suffix: pertaining to:

act-**ive**   nat-**ive**

-ment: noun-forming suffix: agent or instrument:

liga-**ment**   instru-**ment**

-or: noun-forming suffix: agent or instrument:

abduct-**or**   invent-**or**

-orium:* noun-forming suffix: place for something:

audit-**orium**   script-**orium**

-ory:* **(1)** adjective-forming suffix: pertaining to:

exposit-**ory**   compuls-**ory**

(2) noun-forming suffix: place for something:

dormit-**ory**   laborat-**ory**

-ure, -ura: noun-forming suffix: result of an action:

fiss-**ure**, fiss-**ura**   script-**ure**

ENGLISH SUFFIX -E

Note the use of the English suffix **-e** to form verbs from Latin infinitives: **reduce** (*dūcere*, lead), **excite** (*excitāre*, rouse), **inspire** (*spirāre*, breathe), and so forth.

PRESENT PARTICIPLES

The Latin present participle is a third declension adjective that is formed on the stem of the present infinitive. The forms of the nominative and genitive singular are *-āns*, *-antis* for the first conjugation; *ēns*, *-entis* for the second and third; and *-iēns*, *-ientis* for some of the third and for the fourth conjugation. The combining form of participles is found by dropping the *-is* ending of the genitive case. In some instances, this combining form becomes an English adjective translated with -ing added to the meaning of the verb, as in the following table:

sonant (*sonāre*, sound)	sounding
latent (*latēre*, lie hidden)	lying hidden
cadent (*cadere*, fall)	falling
incipient (*incipere*, begin)	beginning
sentient (*sentīre*, feel)	feeling

In other instances, this combining form becomes an English noun meaning a person or thing that does something, as in the following table:

inhabitant (*inhabitāre*, inhabits)	a person who inhabits
rubefacient (*ruber*, red and *facere*, make)	an agent that reddens the skin

Most English derivatives of Latin present participles are abstract nouns ending in -ce or -cy. These endings represent the *-t* of the present participle stem plus the abstract noun-forming suffix *-ia*; the resultant *-tia* becomes

---

*The suffixes -arium and -ary, with the same meaning as -orium and -ory, are usually found with nouns: sanitarium (*sānitās*, health), library (*liber*, book).

either -ce or -cy in English. These noun-forming suffixes mean the act of (being) or the state of (being), as in the following:

redundancy (*redundāre*, be superfluous)	the state of being redundant or superfluous
reverence (*reverērī*, revere)	the state of being revered
sequence (*sequī*, follow)	the act of following
science (*scīre*, know)	the state of knowing

Sometimes words have been formed in English as if from Latin present participles, although such verbs did not exist in Latin. Some of these words have been formed from Greek nouns and verbs: **intoxicant** (and **intoxicate**, as if from a Latin verb *intoxicāre, intoxicātus*). Note that intoxicant, as well as other similar formations, although structurally adjectives, are now used as nouns.

INCEPTIVE VERBS

The letters **-sc-** inserted between the stem and the ending of the Latin infinitive denote the beginning of an action. Example: *valēre*, be well, *valescere*, begin to get well. The present participles of inceptive verbs give us many English derivatives. English: **convalescent**, beginning to get well.

VOWEL WEAKENING

During the prehistoric period in the development of the Latin language, there seems to have been a strong stress accent on the first syllable of words; consequently, vowels in internal syllables became weakened, both quantitatively and qualitatively. The effects of this weakening can be seen in both nouns and verbs. The *-u-* of *caput* (head) becomes weakened to *-i-* in cases other than the nominative singular: *caput, capitis. Virgō* (maiden) loses the final *-n-* of the nominative singular, and the long *-o-* of the final syllable is reduced to short *-i-*: *virgō (n), virginis; pater* (father) and *mater* (mother) drop the *-e-* of the final syllable: *patris, matris.*

This phenomenon is most apparent with verbs, especially when prefixes are added: *caedere, caesus* (cut): *incīdere, incīsus, dēcīdere, dēcīsus; capere, captus* (seize): *incipere, inceptus, recipere, receptus; facere, factus* (make): *efficere, effectus, inficere, infectus.* Sometimes the perfect passive participle is not affected by this change: *cadere, cāsus*, fall: *incidere, incāsus.* In the vocabularies in this manual, the verbal stems that undergo these changes are indicated by a dash before the stem in question: *facere, factus,* make: FAC-, FIC-, -FECT, and so forth.

Latin verbs often take on new and different meanings when compounded with prefixes. The verb *capere, captus,* means to take; the compound verb *incipere, inceptus,* means to take in hand, to undertake, and thus, to begin. The word incipient is from the present participle of this verb.

The Latin compound verb *inficere, infectus,* meaning to stain, dye, spoil, corrupt, gives us the word **infection.**

VOCABULARY

Note: Latin combining forms appear in ***bold italics***.

Latin	Combining Form(s)	Meaning	Example
anterior	***ANTER-***	front, in front	**anter-**ior
brāchium (Fig. 9-1)	***BRACHI-***	(upper) arm	**brachi-**um
caedere, caesus	***-CID-, -CIS-***	cut, kill	in-**cis-**or
capere, captus	***-CIP-, -CEPT-***	take	in-**cept-**ion
crescere, crētus	***CRESC-, -CRET-***	(begin to) grow	ex-**cresc-**ence
digitus	***DIGIT-***	finger, toe	**digit-**al
dūcere, ductus	***DUC-, DUCT-***	lead, bring, conduct	ab-**duct**
facere, factus	***FAC-, -FIC-, -FECT***	make	tume-**fac-**tion
faciēs	***FACI-, -FICI-, FACIES***	face, appearance, surface	super-**fici-**al
febris	***FEBR-, FEBRIS***	fever	**febr-**ile
ferre, lātus	***FER-, LAT-***	carry, bear	odori-**fer-**ous
flectere, flexus	***FLECT-, FLEX-***	bend	re-**flex**
fungus	***FUNG-***	[mushroom] fungus	**fung-**al
fundere, fūsus	***FUS-****	pour	dif-**fus-**e
gignere, genitus	***GENIT-***	bring forth, give birth	**genit-**al
gerere, gestus	***GER-, GEST-***	carry, bear	di-**gest**
immūnis	***IMMUN(I)-***	[exempt] safe, protected	**immun-**ologist

*Both principal parts of Latin verbs do not always produce English derivatives.

Latin	Combining Form(s)	Meaning	Example
inferior	**INFERIOR-**	below	**inferior**-ity
lābī, lapsus	**LAB-, LAPS-**	slide, slip	re-**laps**-e
latus, lateris	**LATER-**	side	**later**-al
ōs, ōris	**OR-, OS**	mouth, opening	**or**-al
ossa	**OSS-**	bone	**oss**-ify
pediculus	**PEDICUL-**	louse	**pedicul**-osis
posterior	**POSTER-, -POSTERIOR**	behind, in back	**poster**-olateral
secāre, sectus	**SECT-**	cut	re-**sect**
somnus	**SOMN-**	sleep	**somn**-olence
stabilis	**STABIL-, STABL-**	stable, fixed	**stabil**-e
superior	**SUPERIOR-**	above	**superior**-ity
tūmēre	**TUM(E)-**	be swollen	**tum**-or

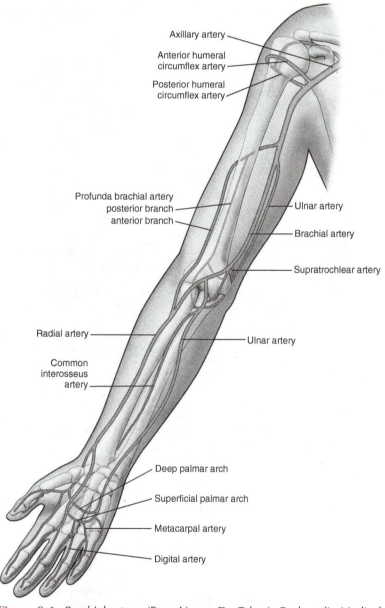

Figure 9-1. Brachial artery. (From Venes, D., *Taber's Cyclopedic Medical Dictionary*, 24th ed., F. A. Davis, with permission.)

PLANES OF THE BODY

A plane (Latin plānum) of the body is a flat surface formed by making an imaginary cut through the body. Planes are used as points of reference by which positions of parts of the body are indicated (Fig. 9-2). There are three principal planes of the body, all based on the assumption that the body is in an upright position:

sagittal plane (Latin sagitta, arrow), also called the **median** plane: a vertical plane dividing the body into two equal and symmetrical right and left halves

frontal plane (Latin frons, frontis, front), also called the **coronal** plane (Latin corōna, crown, borrowed from the Greek, korōnē): a vertical plane at right angles to the sagittal plane dividing the body into anterior and posterior portions

transverse plane (Latin trans-, across, versus, turned), also called the **horizontal or axial plane:** a horizontal plane across the center of the body and at right angles to the sagittal and frontal planes, dividing the body into a top and bottom portion

Abduction of a limb is movement away from the median plane of the body; **adduction** is movement toward the median plane (Fig. 9-3). An **abductor** is a muscle that draws a part away from the median plane when contracted; an **adductor** is a muscle that draws a part of the body toward the median plane.

ETYMOLOGICAL NOTES

Aristotle and Pliny the Elder discuss insects:

> There are creatures called insects, as their name (entoma) indicates. They have incisions either on their upper or lower parts, or on both. They have neither separate bony parts (ostōdes) nor fleshy parts (sarkōdes) but consist of

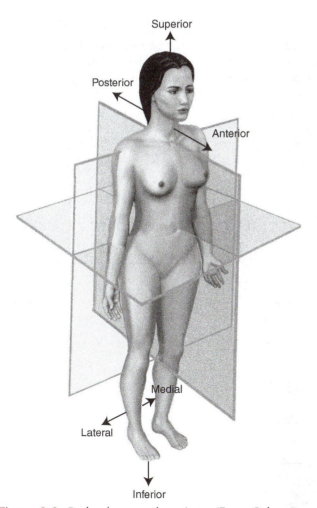

Figure 9-2. Body planes and sections. (From Gylys, B. and Masters, R., Medical Terminology Simplified, 7th ed., F. A. Davis, 2023, with permission.)

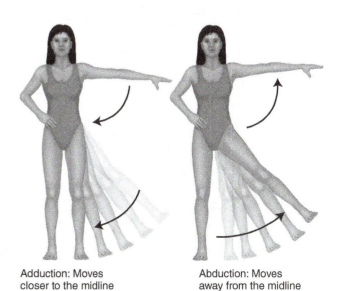

Adduction: Moves closer to the midline

Abduction: Moves away from the midline

Figure 9-3. Abduction and adduction of limbs. (From Gylys, B. and Masters, R., Medical Terminology Simplified, 7th ed., F. A. Davis, 2023, with permission.)

something intermediate, as their bodies, both inside and outside, are uniformly hard (*skleron*).

[Aristotle, *History of Animals* 4.523b 13–18]

There are living creatures *(animalia)* of immeasurable minuteness which some people maintain do not breathe and are actually bloodless. There are great numbers and many kinds of these, some living on land and some in the air, some winged—bees, for example—some lacking wings—centipedes, for example—and some having the characteristics of both—ants, for example—and some lacking both wings and feet. All of these are correctly named insects *(insecta)*, because of the incisions which encircle the necks of some, the chests or stomachs of others, and, in others, which separate their limbs from their bodies, these being connected by a slender tube *(fistula)*. With some of these the incision does not encircle the entire body, but lies like a wrinkle on the belly or higher up. They have vertebrae that are flexible like gutter-tiles, displaying nature's craftsmanship in a more remarkable fashion than anywhere else.

[Pliny the Elder, *Natural History* 11.1.1.1] (Fig. 9-4)

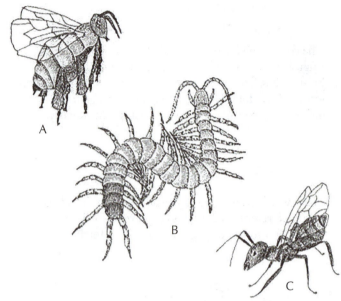

Figure 9-4. Insects. (*A*) Bee. (*B*) Centipede. (*C*) Ant. (Drawings by Laine McCarthy, 2001.)

Exercise 1:   Analyze and Define

Analyze and define each of the following words. In this and in succeeding exercises, analysis should consist of separating the words into prefixes (if any), combining forms, and suffixes or suffix forms (if any) and giving the meaning of each. Be certain to differentiate between nouns and adjectives in your definitions. Consult a medical dictionary for the current meanings of these words.

1. abduct _____

2. ablation _____

3. adduct _____

4. afferent _____

5. antebrachium _____

6. anteroposterior _____

7. biocide _____

8. brachial _____

9. calcification _____

10. contralateral _____

11. decalcify _____

12. dentofacial _____

13. detoxification _____

14. digestion _____

15. digiti _____

16. dissection _____

17. dorsiflection _____

18. dorsolateral _____

19. excise _____

20. excrescence _____

21. febrifacient _____

22. frigolabile _____

23. fungi (pronounced funj'eye) _____

24. fungicide _____

25. genitalia _____

26. gestosis _____

27. immunochromatography _____

28. inception _____

29. incipient _____

30. incisor _____

31. infusion _____

32. ingestant _____

33. insomnia _____

34. introflexion _____

35. intumesce _____

36. labile _____

37. nematocide _____

38. orad _____

39. orifice _____

40. ossification _____

41. pedicular _____

42. quadrisection _____

43. reflexogenic _____

44. relapse _____

45. somnology _____

46. stabile (pronounced stay'bile) _____

47. subfebrile _____

48. superficial _____

49. tumescence _____

50. virulent _____

Exercise 2:   Word Derivations

Give the word derived from Greek and/or Latin elements that matches each of the following. Verify your answers in a medical dictionary. **Note that the wording of the dictionary definition may vary from the wording used here.**

1. (In anatomy) located in front and to one side _____

2. Absence of reflexes _____

3. Division into two parts by cutting _____

4. Producing heat _____

5. (Intense) pain in the arm _____

6. Having or containing teeth _____

7. Agent that destroys a virus _____

8. To remove the toxic quality of a substance _____

9. Located behind and above a part _____

10. Transfer away from (a central organ or part) _____

11. Pertaining to fever; feverish _____

12. Containing calcium _____

13. Person affected by insomnia _____

14. Capable of inducing an immune response _____

15. To become bone (tissue) _____

16. Infestation with lice _____

17. Not changed or destroyed by heat _____

18. Falling down or dropping down of an organ or internal part _____

19. (Opposite to or) away from the mouth _____

20. On the same side _____

Exercise 3:   Drill and Review

Analyze and define each of the following words. Analysis should consist of separating the words into prefixes (if any), combining forms, and suffixes or suffix forms (if any), and give the meaning of each. Be certain to differentiate between nouns and adjectives in your definitions. Using the elements in the word determine its meaning. Consult a medical dictionary for the current meanings of these words. Use a separate paper if you need more room for an answer.

1. aborad _____

2. adoral _____

3. afebrile _____

4. brachiocephalic _____

5. calcemia _____

6. calcigerous _____

7. collapsotherapy _____

8. concrescence _____

9. cystigerous _____

10. cytocide _____

11. decalcification _____

12. deferent _____

13. deflection _____

14. digitate _____

15. digitation _____

16. dorsiflexion _____

17. ductogram _____

18. ductule _____

19. excision _____

20. exsanguination _____

21. facial _____

22. faciobrachial _____

23. flexor _____

24. fungistasis _____

25. fungoid (pronounced fung'oid) _____

26. hemifacial _____

27. hypogenitalism _____

28. immunology _____

29. incise _____

30. indigestible _____

31. ingestion _____

32. lateral _____

33. leukocidin _____

34. microbicide _____

35. oral _____

36. ossicle _____

37. ossific _____

38. pedicular _____

39. perfusion _____

40. receptor _____

41. reflex _____

42. reflexology _____

43. resectable _____

44. sanguinopurulent _____

45. section _____

46. somnipathy _____

47. somnogen _____

48. thermolabile _____

49. translation _____

50. tumefacient _____

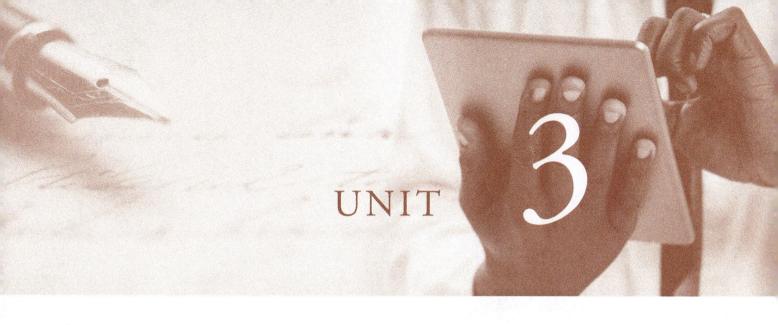

BODY SYSTEMS

UNIT 3

CARDIOVASCULAR SYSTEM

RESPIRATORY SYSTEM

DIGESTIVE SYSTEM

OPTIC SYSTEM

FEMALE REPRODUCTIVE SYSTEM

GENITOURINARY SYSTEM

CARDIOVASCULAR SYSTEM

If you kill a living animal by severing its great arteries, you will find that the veins become empty at the same time as the arteries. This could never happen unless there were anastomoses between them.

[Galen, *On the Natural Faculties* 3.15]

Advances were made in the field of medicine at the great institutions of learning in Alexandria: the Museum and the Library. Both were established in the early third century BC by Ptolemy I, a former Macedonian general of Alexander the Great and the founder of the Ptolemaic dynasty in Egypt. The medical school (as well as the other institutes) in Alexandria became the focal point for men of learning for many centuries. In the middle of the second century AD, the physician Galen went there after studying at the Asclepium, the famed medical school in his native city of Pergamum in Asia Minor. Galen's theory of the movement of the blood in the human body influenced and even ruled medical thinking until the 17th century, when William Harvey discovered that blood circulates. Harvey found that all blood that leaves the heart, after passing to the organs and parts of the body, returns to its point of departure, and then begins the process all over again. This discovery revolutionized medical thought and formed the basis for modern scientific medicine.

Galen believed that food was converted in the intestines into a fluid that he called chyle (Greek *chylos*, juice) [*On the Use of the Parts* 4.3]. This fluid was then carried to the liver, where it was transformed into blood and charged with a vapor or spirit. Unaware of the circulatory movement of the blood, Galen thought this supercharged blood was then carried from the liver through the veins to the various parts of the body in a forward and backward movement. One part of Galen's theory on the movement of the blood

is of special interest. He believed that some blood was carried by the veins to the right ventricle of the heart instead of flowing back through the veins to the liver. This blood then passed through a septum—a wall or partition dividing two body cavities—into the left ventricle through small passages between the right and left heart.

> The thinnest portion of the blood is drawn from the right cavity *(koilia)* of the heart into the left through passages in the septum *(diaphragma)* between these parts. These passages can be seen for the most part of their length; they are like pits with wide openings, but they keep getting narrower and it is not possible to see the end of them because of both their small size and the fact that the animal being dead, all of its parts are cold and shrunken.

[Galen, *On the Natural Faculties* 3.15]

Rigid adherence to the theory that blood passed directly through the septum from the right to the left ventricle prevented the realization of the true nature of the circulation of the blood for 15 centuries.

One man, the theologian Michael Servetus, dared to challenge the theories of Galen concerning the nature of the movement of the blood. Servetus was born in 1511 in Spain, studied theology at Toulouse in France, and then went to Paris to study medicine. This was early in the period of the Reformation, and Servetus held views that were considered almost heretical by both Catholics and

Protestants. Along with his religious tracts, he wrote a work on physiology, the content of which was clothed in the title *Christianismi restitutio* (Restitution of Christianity). In this work, which was published in 1553, Servetus challenged Galen's theory regarding the presence of a certain natural spirit that entered the blood in the liver. In addition, he maintained that the blood did not pass through the septum from the right to the left ventricle. Instead, he wrote, the blood passed from the right ventricle to the lungs, where it was purified by inspired air and then, lighter in color, was conveyed to the left ventricle. Servetus was arrested, tried for heresy, found guilty, and burned alive at Geneva on October 27, 1553. Although Servetus's book was burned with him, a few copies survived, and his theories undoubtedly influenced later scientists. Three-quarters of a century passed before the actual circulation of the blood in the human body was perceived and made known.

In 1628, William Harvey, a fellow of the Royal College of Physicians in London, published his great work *Exercitatio anatomica de motu cordis et sanguinis* (An Anatomical Treatise on the Motion of the Heart and Blood), written in Latin. Harvey's work was flawless as far as it went. It stopped short of completion because the microscope at that time was not capable of producing a clear image at high power. Marcello Malpighi's microscopic examination of the circulatory system of the frog revealed the action of the network of capillaries in joining the arterioles to the venules. His work, *De Pulmonibus* (On the Lungs), was published at Bologna in 1661.

CIRCULATION OF BLOOD

Blood begins its journey through the body as it is pumped from the upper end of the left ventricle into the great artery: the aorta (Figs. 10-1, 10-2). The aortic valve prevents the blood from flowing back into the ventricle (**aortic regurgitation**). Blood flows away from the heart through the arterial network. The **coronary arteries** supply blood to the muscle of the heart. **Myocardial infarction** (MI) is the injury of living heart muscle as a result of **coronary artery occlusion** and lack of oxygenation of cardiac muscle tissue. MI usually occurs when an atheromatous plaque in a coronary artery ruptures and the resulting clot obstructs the injured blood vessel. Perfusion of the muscular tissue that lies downstream from the blocked artery is lost. If blood flow is not restored within a few hours, the heart muscle is damaged and can no longer contract effectively or conduct electricity properly. MI can be diagnosed by classic clinical symptoms of chest pain, by specific enzymes released during cardiac muscle injury, and by specific changes on an electrocardiogram (ECG).

As the arteries branch, they become increasingly smaller and are called **arterioles** until they unite in a network of tiny vessels to form the **capillaries.** Here the oxygenated blood from the left side of the heart delivers needed oxygen to the tissues of the body. From these microscopically small vessels, blood passes into the **venules,** very small veins, and then into the venous system. The blood finally enters the right atrium through the two **venae cavae.** The superior vena cava returns blood from the organs and parts above the diaphragm (except the lungs). The inferior vena cava returns blood from organs and tissues below the diaphragm.

From the right atrium, the blood passes through the tricuspid valve into the right ventricle where the blood begins another journey, the pulmonary or lesser circulation. Deoxygenated blood from the venous system returns to the heart and flows through the pulmonary circulation, where it is oxygenated in the capillary networks of the lung. The deoxygenated blood passes into the pulmonary artery, the only artery that carries deoxygenated blood, which then branches out in the lungs, becoming smaller and smaller. The arterioles unite with capillaries, which in turn unite with the pulmonary venules that carry blood into the left atrium through the left superior and inferior pulmonary veins. From the left atrium, the blood enters the left ventricle through the mitral or bicuspid valve to start its journey again. Contractions of the cardiac muscle, which pumps about four quarts of blood per minute, are controlled by the vagus nerve, which slows the contraction rate, and the sympathetic nervous system, which accelerates it. Regulation is achieved by way of the sinoatrial node, the body's natural pacemaker. If this natural pacemaker is defective, an artificial or electrical pacemaker can be attached externally or inserted internally to control the heartbeat through rhythmic electrical discharges. For patients who have suffered a cardiac arrest, an **implantable cardioverter defibrillator** (ICD) can be implanted to respond to abnormal cardiac rhythms. Defects and malfunctions, either congenital or acquired, along this complicated network of vessels and valves can cause numerous potentially fatal disorders that we call heart disease.

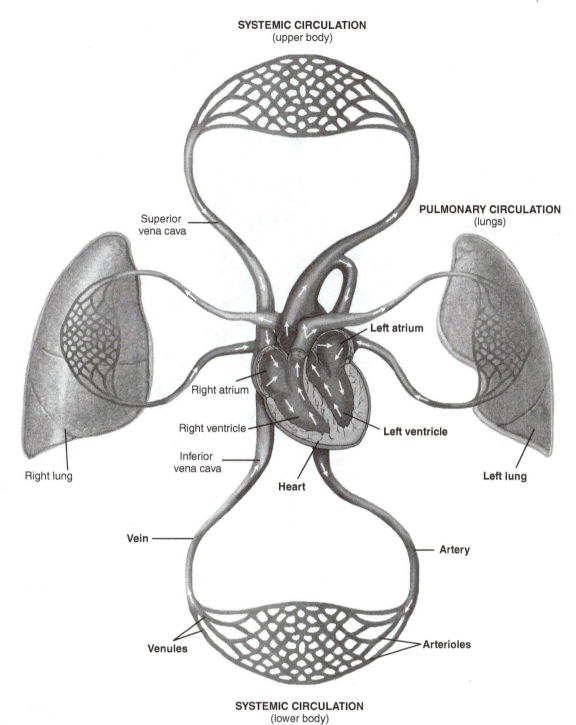

SYSTEMIC CIRCULATION
(upper body)

PULMONARY CIRCULATION
(lungs)

Superior
vena cava

Left atrium

Right atrium

Right ventricle

Left ventricle

Inferior
vena cava

Right lung

Heart

Left lung

Vein

Artery

Venules

Arterioles

SYSTEMIC CIRCULATION
(lower body)

Figure 10-1. Circulation of blood through heart and major vessels. (From Gylys, B. A., and Wedding, M. E., *Medical Terminology Systems: A Body Systems Approach*, 8th ed., F. A. Davis, 2017.)

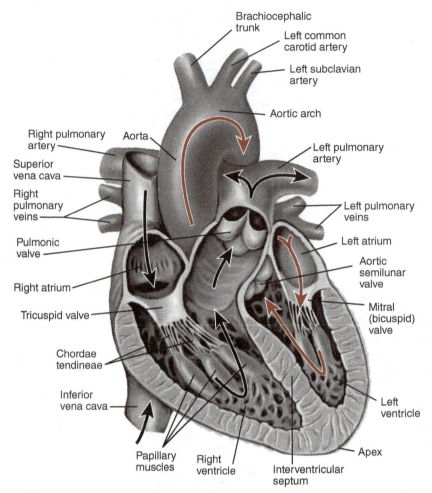

Figure 10-2. The heart. (A) Anterior view. (B) Frontal section. (From Gylys, B. A., and Wedding, M. E., *Medical Terminology Systems: A Body Systems Approach*, 8th ed., F. A. Davis, 2017.)

VOCABULARY

Life is short, the Art lasting, opportunity elusive, experiment perilous, judgment difficult. The physician must be ready not only to do what is necessary, but to see to it that his patient, the attendants, and all external arrangements are ready.

[Hippocrates, *Aphorisms* 1.1]

Note: Latin combining forms appear in ***bold italics***.

Greek or Latin	Combining Form(s)	Meaning	Example
amylon	**AMYL-**	starch	**amyl-**in
angina	***ANGIN-***	choking pain, angina pectoris	***angin-***a
aortē	**AORT-**	aorta	**aort-**ostenosis
arctāre, arctātus	***ARCT(AT)-***	compress	aort-**arct-**ia
athērē	**ATHER-**	[soup] fatty deposit	**ather-**oma
ātrium	***ATRI-***	[entrance hall] atrium	**atri-**oventricular
bolē	**BOL-**	a throwing	em-**bol-**us
capillus	***CAPILL-***	[hair] capillary	**capill-**ary
kirsos	**CIRS-**	dilated and twisted vein, varix	**cirs-**otomy
claudere, clausus	***-CLUD-, -CLUS-***	close	oc-**clus-**ion
cor, cordis	***COR, CORD-***	heart	**cord-**ate
corōna	***CORON-***	crown	**coron-**al

Greek or Latin	Combining Form(s)	Meaning	Example
cuspis, cuspidis	*CUSP, -CUSPID*	point	bi-**cuspid**
dexter	*DEXTR-*	right (side)	ambi-**dextr**-ous
forma	*-FORM*	shape	coli-**form**
gurgitāre, gurgitātus	*GURGIT-, GURGITAT-*	flood, flow	re-**gurgit**-ant
pectus, pectoris	*PECTOR-*	breast, chest	**pector**-al
phleps, phlebos	*PHLEB-*	vein	**phleb**-otomy
pulmō, pulmōnis	*PULM(ON)-*	lung, pulmonary artery	**pulmon**-ary
rhythmos	*RHYTHM-*	[steady motion] heartbeat	ar-**rhythm**-ic
saeptum	*SEPT-*	wall, partition	**sept**-um
sinus	*SIN-, SINUS-*	[curve, hollow] sinus	**sinus**-itis
sinister	*SINISTR-*	left (side)	**sinister**-ad
sphygmos	*SPHYGM-*	pulse	**sphygm**-ometer
stellein	*STAL-, STOL-*	send, contraction	sy-**stol**-ic
tendere, tensus	*TENS(I)-*	stretch	hyper-**tens**-ive
thrombos	*THROMB-*	blood clot	**thromb**-osis
topos	*TOP-*	place	**top**-ical
vagus	*VAG-*	[wandering] the vagus nerve	**vag**-olysis
varix, varicis	*VARIC-, VARIX*	dilated and twisted vein, varix	**varic**-es
vās	*VAS-*	(blood) vessel; vas deferens	**vas**-ectomy
vēna	*VEN-*	vein	**ven**-ostat
venter, ventris	*VENTR-*	belly, abdomen, abdominal cavity	**ventr**-al

ETYMOLOGICAL NOTES

The Hippocratic Oath, attributed to the Greek physician Hippocrates (c. 460–375), is "sworn by physicians and other health care professionals to practice medicine according to a code of ethics."* The Hippocratic Oath begins:

> I swear by Apollo the healer, by Asclepius, by Hygieia, by Panacea and by all the gods and goddesses as witnesses, that I will fulfill this oath and covenant.

Apollo had many attributes, among them the ability to heal the sick as well as to rain down destruction and death upon the wicked. He was often called Paean, the name of the Physician of the Gods in Homer's *Iliad*. Apollo's son Asclepius, born to the nymph Coronis, exceeded his father's healing skills. Asclepius received his medical education from the famed centaur Chiron. He became so skilled that he not only was able to heal the sick but also acquired the ability to bring the dead back to life. Like his father, Asclepius was also called Paean in tribute to his great healing powers.

Once, when Asclepius was pondering how to bring Glaucus, son of King Minos of Crete, back to life, a snake coiled itself around his staff. He struck the creature and killed it. Later, a second snake came carrying a leaf in its jaws. The snake placed the leaf on the head of the dead snake, and the serpent came to back to life. Asclepius used the same medicament to restore Glaucus. A snake curled around the staff of Asclepius became the symbol of this great healer and is a symbol of medicine and healing to this day (Fig. 10-3).

Asclepius's gift for restoring life to the dead, however, did not please Hades, the ruler of the Home of the Dead, who complained to his brother Zeus that Asclepius's healing skills were returning to life dead souls he felt were rightfully his. Zeus, worried that Asclepius's healing power was upsetting the normal balance of life and death, used his lightning bolt to strike Asclepius down. Zeus, however, recognized Asclepius's service to humanity and turned him into the constellation Serpens, in which Asclepius is forever holding a giant snake.

The words **systole** and **diastole** are from the Greek verb *stellein* (send). Systole refers to the period of contraction of the heart when the blood is sent through the aorta and the pulmonary artery. Diastole is the period of expansion when the heart dilates and the atria and ventricles fill with blood from the venae cavae and the pulmonary vein. Blood pressure is taken by means of an inflatable cloth cuff known as a **sphygmomanometer** (Greek *manos*, occurring at intervals), which is placed around the upper arm. Air is pumped into the sphygmomanometer (commonly referred to as a blood pressure cuff), compressing the patient's arm. This compression causes a column of mercury to rise, indicating the pressure within the cuff. Once the pressure is sufficient to stop the flow of blood through the brachial artery, which is detected by listening to the heartbeat through a stethoscope pressed against the patient's arm, the pressure is released. When the

---

*Venes, D., *Taber's Cyclopedic Dictionary*, 23rd ed. F. A. Davis, 2017, p. 1132, with permission.

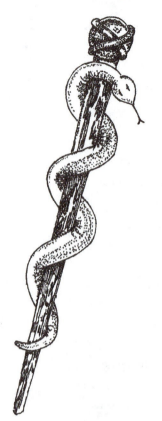

Figure 10-3. The Staff of Asclepius. (Drawing by Laine McCarthy, 2002.)

heartbeat is once again audible, the level of the column of mercury indicates the systolic pressure. As more air is let out of the cuff, the pulse fades. The level of the mercury at this point indicates the diastolic pressure.

The **mitral valve** of the heart lies between the left atrium and the left ventricle and allows passage of blood from the atrium into the ventricle. It is also called the bicuspid valve because it has two cusps. The mitral valve is meant to be a one-way valve. A mitral defect can cause the blood to flow backwards, a condition called **mitral regurgitation.** The Latin word *mitral* comes originally from the Greek word *mitra*, referring to a type of turban worn by certain people of Asia Minor. In Virgil's *Aeneid*, the Moorish king Iarbas was scorned by Dido, a Phoenician princess who had recently settled in North Africa. On hearing that Dido and Aeneas, a wanderer from Troy, were openly flaunting their love, Iarbas prayed to Jupiter for vengeance, referring contemptuously to Aeneas as another Paris:

> *et nunc ille Paris cum semiviro comitatu,*
> *Maeonia mentum mitra crinemque madentem*
> *subnixus, rapto potitur.*

> And now that Paris with his band of half-men,
> his chin and oiled hair bound with a
> Maeonian miter, possesses what he has stolen.

[*Aeneid* 4.215–217]

The modern medical term mitral comes directly from the word miter or mitre, a tall, cleft, pointed hat worn by bishops of the Western church. The word valve comes from the Latin *valvae*, a plural word meaning a particular kind of door that folds within itself.

There are many and various causes of what is referred to as a heart attack (myocardial infarction). The site of the initial attack is usually either a coronary artery, so called because these vessels form a crown (*corōna*) over and around the heart, or the cerebrovascular system (Fig. 10-4).

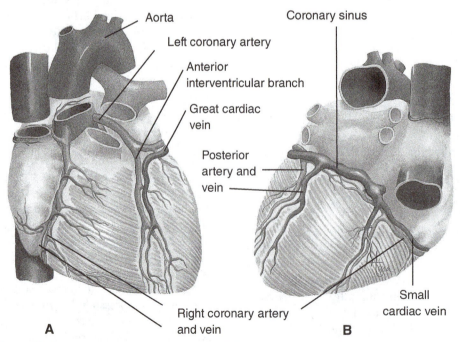

Figure 10-4. Coronary arteries. (*A*) Anterior. (*B*) Posterior. (From Scanlon, V. C., and Sanders, T., *Essentials of Anatomy and Physiology*, 8th ed., F. A. Davis, 2020., with permission.)

Coronary artery disease results from the narrowing or closing of the coronary arteries, usually as a result of either **atherosclerosis** or the presence of a **thrombus** or an **embolus.** An embolus may be formed from clotted blood and thus is a form of thrombus. An embolus can also be formed from a portion of a cardiac tumor, such as a myxoma, or from any foreign substance such as fibrous matter, fat, or gas. The artery is then unable to carry the blood that is pumped into it by the cardiac muscle. The resulting condition, called **coronary occlusion** or **coronary thrombosis,** can and often does lead to **myocardial ischemia,** a temporary deficiency of blood flow, which can cause **myocardial infarction,** cardiac arrest, and sudden death.

An **aneurysm** (Greek *ana-*, up, *eurys*, wide, *-m(a)*, noun-forming suffix) is the local distention of the wall of a blood vessel, usually an artery, and often the aorta (Fig. 10-5). The dilation is caused by a weakening of the vascular wall, often as a result of arteriosclerosis coupled with hypertension. Aortic aneurysms may occur anywhere along this great artery. They often occur in the abdominal region (**abdominal aortic aneurysm,** AAA) or in the area of the pulmonary arteries (**thoracic aortic aneurysm,** TAA). Rupture of an aneurysm with subsequent massive hemorrhage is a common cause of death.

Stroke is the sudden loss of neurologic function caused by loss of blood flow to an area of the brain. Cerebral infarction causes 80% of strokes, and cerebral hemorrhage causes most other strokes.

The Greek verb *ballein* (throw) has many derivatives. For instance, the science of projectiles is **ballistics.** But it is in the form BOL-, from the noun *bolē* (a throwing), that it is most relevant in medicine. An **embolism** is the blockage of a blood vessel by any mass of undissolved matter, a blood clot, or an air bubble. **Metabolism** is the sum of the processes of **anabolism.** Anabolism is the constructive phase of metabolism, the process by which cells take nutrients from the blood required for repair and growth of tissue. **Catabolism** is the process by which complex compounds are reduced to simpler ones, often accompanied by the release of energy.

The verb *diaballein,* meaning throw across, had the secondary meaning of slander, make a false accusation. From this verb, the noun *diabolē* (slander) was formed. The noun *diabolos* meant one who slanders, an evil person. This word

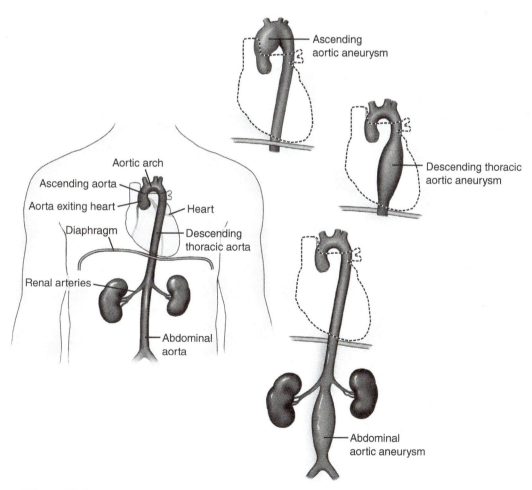

Figure 10-5. Aortic aneurysms. (From Hoffman, J., and Sullivan, N., *Medical-Surgical Nursing: Making Connections to Practice,* 2nd Edition, F.A. Davis, 2020.)

is found in the Septuagint (I Chronicles, 21:1) meaning the enemy, or Satan. Matthew (4:1) writes, "At that time, Jesus was led into the wilderness by the Spirit, and there he was tempted by the devil *(diabolos)*."* When the Scriptures were translated into Old English, the Latin *diabolus* of the Vulgate was translated as *deofol* (devil). *Diabolos* remains in English in the word **diabolic** (devilish).

Exercise 1: Analyze and Define

Analyze and define each of the following words. In this and in succeeding exercises, analysis should consist of separating the words into prefixes (if any), combining forms, and suffixes or suffix forms (if any) and giving the meaning of each. Be certain to differentiate between nouns and adjectives in your definitions. Consult a medical dictionary for the current meanings of these words.

1. ambidextrous _____

2. amyloid _____

3. amylolysis _____

4. anginous _____

5. aortarctia _____

6. aortocoronary _____

7. arteriovenous _____

8. atherogenesis _____

9. atheroma _____

10. atrioventricular _____

11. capillarectasia _____

12. capillariasis _____

13. cirsectomy _____

14. coliform _____

15. cordate _____

---

*The Bible, King James version.

16. corona dentis _____

17. coronary _____

18. cusp _____

19. dorsoventral _____

20. ectopia cordis _____

21. embolism _____

22. endaortitis _____

23. entopic _____

24. expectoration _____

25. extravasation _____

26. formation _____

27. hypertension _____

28. hypotensive _____

29. intrapulmonary _____

30. nasosinusitis _____

31. nonseptate _____

32. occlude _____

33. pansinusitis _____

34. phlebosclerosis _____

35. pulmonologist _____

36. regurgitant _____

37. sinistrad _____

38. sinogram _____

39. sinusoid _____

40. sphygmograph _____

41. systole _____

42. tachyarrhythmia _____

43. tensiometer _____

44. thrombasthenia _____

45. topical _____

46. topographical _____

47. tricuspid _____

48. vagotonia _____

49. varices _____

50. vasotomy _____

Exercise 2:   Word Derivations

Give the word derived from Greek and/or Latin elements that matches each of the following. Verify your answer in a medical dictionary. **Note that the wording of the dictionary definition may vary from the wording used here.**

1. Having two cusps (or projections) _____

2. Puncturing of a vein or the surgical opening of a vein (to withdraw blood) _____

3. Production of starch _____

4. Inflammation of a sinus _____

5. Irregularity or loss of rhythm, especially of the heart _____

6. Pertaining to or involving the lungs _____

7. Capillary disorder or disease _____

8. Resembling pus _____

9. (Surgical) destruction of the vagus nerve _____

10. Removal of all or a segment of the vas deferens _____

11. Having the heart on the right side of the body _____

12. Any disease that affects the (function or structure of) the aorta _____

13. Stone within a vein _____

14. Agent that promotes the clearance of mucus (from the respiratory tract) _____

15. Instrument for measuring the pulse _____

16. Act or process of stretching _____

17. Capable of producing a blood clot _____

18. Small varix _____

19. Contraction of a vein _____

20. Flowing backward _____

Exercise 3:   Drill and Review

Analyze and define each of the following words. Analysis should consist of separating the words into prefixes (if any), combining forms, and suffixes or suffix forms (if any), and give the meaning of each. Be certain to differentiate between nouns and adjectives in your definitions. Using the elements in the word determine its meaning. Consult a medical dictionary for the current meanings of these words. Use a separate paper if you need more room for an answer.

1. amyloidosis _____

2. anginoid _____

3. antithrombin _____

4. aortostenosis _____

5. asystolia _____

6. atheromatosis _____

7. atrial _____

8. bradyarrhythmia _____

9. capillary _____

10. cardiovascular _____

11. cirsoid _____

12. cirsotomy _____

13. coarctate _____

14. coronavirus _____

15. coronoidectomy _____

16. cuspid _____

17. dextral _____

18. diastole _____

19. dysrhythmia _____

20. ectopia _____

21. ectopotomy _____

22. exclusion _____

23. interatrial _____

24. interventricular _____

25. pectoral _____

26. pericoronitis _____

27. peristalsis _____

28. phlebography _____

29. preformation _____

30. pulmonic _____

31. septorhinoplasty _____

32. sinistrality _____

33. sinonasal _____

34. sphygmogram _____

35. systolic _____

36. tensor _____

37. thrombectomy _____

38. thrombocytopoiesis _____

39. topography _____

40. topology _____

41. vagolytic _____

42. vagovagal _____

43. varicomphalus _____

44. varicophlebitis _____

45. vascularization _____

46. vasculitis _____

47. vasohypertonic _____

48. vasorrhaphy _____

49. venectasia _____

50. ventricular _____

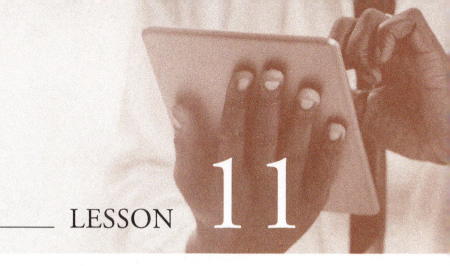

LESSON 11

RESPIRATORY SYSTEM

It is through the veins that we take in most of our breath, for they are the vents of the body, taking in the air and bringing it to the smaller vessels where it is cooled and then released.

[Hippocrates, *The Sacred Disease* 7]

All organs, tissues, and cells of the body require oxygen to function. The purpose of the respiratory system is to oxygenate the blood so the blood can carry oxygen to all parts of the body. In all cells of the body, oxygen is exchanged for carbon dioxide, which is carried in the bloodstream to the lungs and discharged into the atmosphere. The process of the inspiration (breathing in, or inhaling) of oxygen and expiration (breathing out, or exhaling) of carbon dioxide is called **respiration.** This is one of the vital processes of life (Fig. 11-1).

Air enters the body through the nose and mouth and travels downward through the pharynx and larynx, past the vocal cords, and into the trachea, or windpipe. The trachea branches into two tubes, the right and the left bronchi, which enter the lungs. After these bronchial tubes enter the lungs, they branch off into increasingly smaller tubes called bronchioles where the process ends. The inner surface of the lungs is lined with innumerable tiny sacs called alveoli, which become filled with air at each inspiration (Fig. 11-2). The pulmonary arteries from the heart branch off into arterioles in the lungs and then into capillaries. Blood in the capillaries receives the oxygen from the alveoli as the hemoglobin molecules in the blood become saturated with oxygen from the alveoli. Hemoglobin saturated with oxygen is called **oxyhemoglobin.** As the blood becomes oxygenated, it discharges carbon dioxide, which passes to the alveoli and is then exhaled. The oxygenated blood passes from the capillaries into the pulmonary veins and is carried back to the heart and pumped to all parts of the body to exchange oxygen for carbon dioxide. The process then

starts over again. This exchange, the crucial part of the process of respiration, normally takes place about 18 times per minute in the human body, from the moment of birth to the instant of death. Of anatomic note, the pulmonary vein is the only vein in the body that carries oxygenated blood, whereas the pulmonary artery is the only artery that carries deoxygenated blood.

Each lung is enclosed within a sac called the pleura, which has two layers: the inner, or visceral, and the outer, or parietal (pronounced par-eye'-et-al, Latin *pariēs, pariētis*) wall. Normally, there is no space within these two layers except a thin film of lubricating fluid. In certain lung diseases, however, a space is created between these layers by the accumulation of fluid, called **hydrothorax,** a type of plural effusion; the accumulation of blood, called **hemothorax,** caused by the rupture of small blood vessels in pulmonary disorders; or the accumulation of air, called **pneumothorax,** caused by perforation of the pleura that allows air to enter and fill this pleural space.

The lungs, with their pleural sacs, are separated from one another by a cavity called the **mediastinum.** The word mediastinum is a New Latin formation meaning in the middle, from Medieval Latin *mediastanus* (intermedial), from Latin *medius* (middle). Beneath the lungs lies a muscular membrane—the diaphragm—which flattens and contracts during inspiration, allowing air to be drawn into the lungs and expelling air from the lungs. The entire area between the diaphragm and the base of the neck is called the thorax. The thoracic cavity contains the heart, the lungs, and the origins of the great blood vessels.

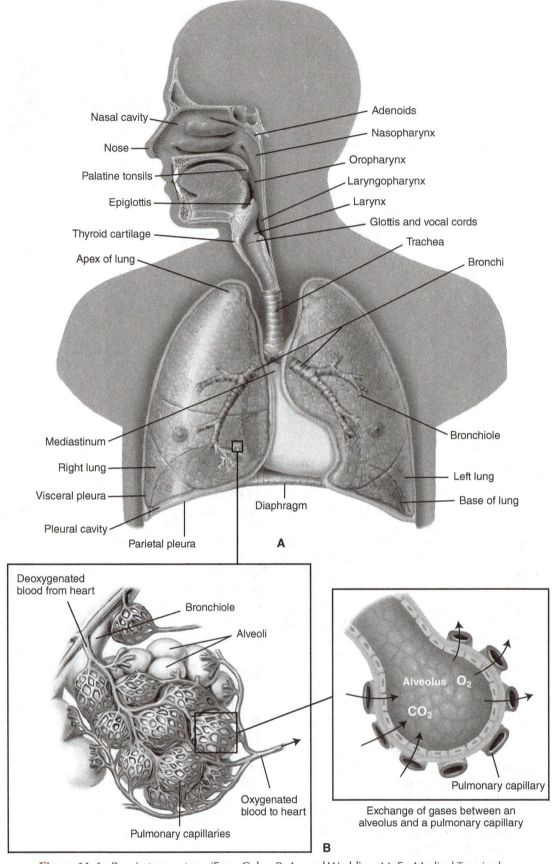

Figure 11-1. Respiratory system. (From Gylys, B. A., and Wedding, M. E., *Medical Terminology Systems: A Body Systems Approach*, 8th ed., F. A. Davis, 2017, with permission.)

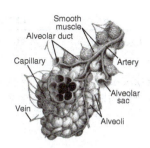

Smooth
muscle
Alveolar duct
Capillary
Artery
Alveolar
sac
Vein
Alveoli

Figure 11-2. Lungs. (From Eagle, S., and Brassington, C., *The Professional Medical Assistant, An Integrative Teamwork-Based Approach*, F. A. Davis, 2009.)

Any interference with the flow of air into and out of the lungs is a potential cause of pulmonary disease; any interference with the exchange of oxygen and carbon dioxide is a potential cause of respiratory failure. Interference with the process of respiration can result from disorders of the central nervous system; chemical changes in the blood; bacterial, fungal or viral infection; sedation; and physical changes in the respiratory organs caused by inhaling irritating material, such as asbestos or smoke.

VOCABULARY

I especially approve of a physician who in the acute diseases, those which are fatal to the majority of the people, shows a certain amount of superiority over the others.

These acute diseases are those which the ancients have named pleurisy, pneumonia, phrenitis, intense fever, and other diseases in which fever is generally unremitting.

[Hippocrates, *Regimen in Acute Diseases* 5]

Note: Latin combining forms are shown in ***bold italics***.

Greek or Latin	Combining Form(s)	Meaning	Example
alveus	**ALVE-***	hollow, cavity	**alve**-us
amygdalē	**AMYGDAL-**	[almond] tonsil	**amygdal**-ine
anthrax, anthrakos	**ANTHRAX, ANTHRAC-**	coal; anthrax	**anthrac**-osis
auxein	**AUX-, AUXE-,† -AUXIS**	grow, increase	**aux**-in
baktērion‡	**BACTER(I)-**	[small staff] bacterium	**bacteri**-a
bronchos	**BRONCH(I)-§**	[windpipe] bronchus	**bronchi**-al
kapnos	**CAPN-**	[smoke] carbon dioxide	hypo-**capn**-ia
kokkos	**COCC-, -COCCUS**	[berry] coccus (a type of spherical bacterium)	strepto-**coccus**
konis	**CONI-, KONI-**	dust	**coni**-ofibrosis
labium	***LABI-***	lip	**labi**-odental
larynx, laryngos	**LARYNX, LARYNG-**	larynx	**laryng**-itis
paresis¶	**PARESIS**	slackening of strength, paralysis	para-**paresis**
pharynx, pharyngos	**PHARYNX, PHARYNG-**	[throat] pharynx	**pharyng**-eal
physa	**PHYS-**	air, gas	em-**phys**-ema
pleura	**PLEUR-**	[side] pleura	**pleur**-itis
pnein	**PNE-**	breathe	a-**pne**-a
pneuma, pneumatos	**PNEUM(AT)-**	[breath] air, gas	**pneumat**-ocele
pneumōn	**PNEUM(ON)-**	lung	**pneumon**-ia
sidēros	**SIDER-**	iron	**sider**-openia
spīrāre, spīrātus	***SPIR(AT)-***	breathe	a-**spirat**-or
staphyle	**STAPHYL-**	[bunch of grapes] uvula, palate; staphylococci (microorganisms that cluster together like a bunch of grapes)	**staphyl**-ococcus

*Words containing the diminutive form alveol- refer to alveoli of the lungs or to dental alveoli.
†These forms of aux-, auxe-, and -auxin indicate nouns meaning increase in size, abnormal growth of a part.
‡*Bacterium* (plural, *bacteria*) is the Latinized form of this word.
§Words beginning with, ending with, or containing bronchi- are from *bronchia*, the bronchial tubes.
¶The Greek noun *paresis* is formed from the preposition *para* and the verb *hienai* (send, throw). The compound verb *parienai* meant to let fall, and thus the noun *paresis* meant falling or slackening (of strength).

Greek or Latin	Combining Form(s)	Meaning	Example
sternon	**STERN-**	chest, breast, breastbone	**stern**-ocostal
stēthos	**STETH-**	chest, breast	**steth**-oscope
streptos	**STREPT-**	[twisted] streptococci (microorganisms that form twisted chains)	**strept**-ococcal
sūdor	*SUD(OR)-*	sweat, fluid	tran-**sud**-ate
thōrax, thōrakos	**THORAX, THORAC-**	chest cavity, pleural cavity, thorax	pneumo-**thorax**
trachys	**TRACH(E)-, TRACHY-**	[rough] trachea	**trache**-ostomy

ETYMOLOGICAL NOTES

In the winter occur pleurisy, pneumonia, colds, sore throat, coughs, pains in the side, chest, and hip, headache, dizziness, and apoplexy.

[Hippocrates, *Aphorisms* 23]

Those with hemorrhoids do not get pleurisy or pneumonia.

[Hippocrates, *Humors* 20]

Diphtheria (Greek *diphthera*, leather) takes its name from a leatherlike false membrane composed of pus and dead cells that forms on the mucous surfaces of the air passages. The disease is caused by the diphtheria bacterium *Corynebacterium diphtheriae*, from the Greek *korynē*, club, because of the clublike shape of these bacteria. These bacteria lodge in the throat and trachea, producing exotoxins that are lethal to the cells of the adjacent tissues. As the disease progresses, this leatherlike false membrane causes difficulty swallowing. If the air passages become sufficiently swollen, **tracheostomy** and **intubation** may be necessary to provide a temporary passage for mechanical respiration. The word **trachea** is from Greek *tracheia*, the feminine form of this adjective, originally modifying the feminine noun *artēria* (artery). The ancient Greek anatomists thought that the arteries carried air (*aēr*, air, *tērein*, guard). The windpipe, or trachea, was called the "rough artery" because of the rings of cartilage that surround it. Before vaccines were developed, diphtheria was a leading cause of death in children worldwide.

Emphysema, a condition that results most often from cigarette smoking or exposure to other pollutants, takes its name from the Greek *emphysēma*, meaning a swelling or inflation, from the verb *emphysan* (inflate). Emphysema is a form of chronic obstructive pulmonary disease (COPD), which affects millions of smokers. The significance of the name is that the disease is characterized by an increase in the size of the terminal air spaces, which causes an excess of air in the lungs (hyperinflation) and destruction of the alveolar walls. The lung loses its normal elasticity, and inspiration and expiration require muscular effort. **Hypoventilation** then results in impaired gas exchange, leading to **hypoxia** and **hypercapnia.**

Influenza, commonly called flu, is a contagious respiratory viral infection; symptoms of flu are coryza (inflammation of the nasal mucous membrane with profuse discharge from the nostrils), cough, sore throat, myalgia, and general weakness. It takes its name from the Italian *influenza*, influence (literally, a flowing upon). In the 16th century and later, the name was applied to various epidemic diseases afflicting the people of Italy, which were thought to descend from the heavens. In 1743, it was applied specifically to the disease that we know as influenza, then called *la grippe*, which was ravaging Western Europe.

Pneumonia is an inflammation of the lungs usually resulting from infections caused by bacteria, viruses, or other pathogenic organisms. The most common of the bacterial agents are **streptococci, staphylococci,** and certain atypical bacteria. Pneumococcal or lobar pneumonia (usually caused by **pneumococci**) usually invades one or more lobes of the lungs. Signs of pneumococcal pneumonia include chills, cough, chest pain, expectoration of rust-colored sputum, and, as the disease progresses, tachypnea, tachycardia, and cyanosis. Prompt treatment with appropriate antibiotics generally ensures early recovery. Although pneumococci used to be uniformly sensitive to treatment with penicillins, drug-resistant strains are exceptionally common, making the choice of antibiotic therapy increasingly difficult. Pneumonias in immunocompromised individuals are sometimes caused by *Pneumocystis carinii* (*P. carinii*) or by fungal species such as *Aspergillus* or *Candida*. *P. carinii*, also known as PCP. PCP has historically been a common cause of death in patients with AIDS. The development of active antiretroviral drug regimens has restored immune function to AIDS patients and reduced the incidence of PCP. Pneumonia caused by influenza and SARS-CoV-s virus are major causes of mortality in the young, the elderly, and those with multiple comorbid medical conditions.

Sir Alexander Fleming (1881–1955), a British bacteriologist, applied the term **penicillin** to a culture of certain molds he observed inhibiting the growth of bacteria. These molds were two of the genus *Penicillium*, named from the Latin *pēnicillum* (brush), because of the brushlike or broomlike appearance of the mold under microscopy. The Latin *pēnicillum* is a diminutive of *pēnis*, the original meaning of which was tail.

Anthrax is a highly infectious disease caused by the spore-forming bacteria *Bacillus anthracis.* Anthrax commonly attacks hoofed animals, particularly goats, horses, sheep, and cattle. Humans can acquire anthrax from exposure to infected animals or their hair and wool, hide, or waste matter. One manifestation of the disease in humans is cutaneous anthrax (Latin *cutis,* skin). This is characterized by the eruption of reddish carbuncles (Latin *carbunculus,* diminutive of *carbō, carbōnis,* coal) called anthrax boils, accompanied by localized erythema of the skin. The disease gets its name from the color of the inflammation, which looks like burning coal or charcoal. Another form of this disease is inhalation anthrax, which attacks the mediastinum, causing hemorrhage and pulmonary edema, and may also involve the gastrointestinal tract. Inhalation anthrax is also called **rag-sorter's disease.** Although anthrax is a potential agent for use in **biological warfare** or bioterrorism, most experts have concluded that it is technologically difficult to use effectively as a weapon on a large scale because anthrax cannot be spread from person to person.

A number of respiratory diseases are caused by exposure to occupational pulmonary irritants. These usually lead to a fibrotic interstitial lung disease such as **anthracosis,** also known as black lung, a disease often suffered by coal miners. Anthracosis is characterized by carbon deposits within the lungs due to inhalation of smoke or coal dust. **Byssinosis** affects those who work in cotton mills. **Silicosis** affects those who work in granite and sandstone industries. Bronchial carcinoma can result from **asbestosis** in those who are exposed for any length of time to the fibers of asbestos. **Siderosis** affects iron and steel workers and welders. **Silo filler's disease,** which affects those who work in grain silos, is caused by exposure to nitrogen dioxide and is characterized by irritation of the eyes and pharynx and damage to the lungs.

Tuberculosis (TB) is a disease caused by *Mycobacterium tuberculosis.* It usually affects the respiratory system but may attack other body systems. In pulmonary TB, the most common form of the disease, early signs are the development of lesions of the lung tissues. These lesions, collections of giant cells, are called **tubercles** (little swellings), from which the disease gets its name. Pulmonary TB is also known as **consumption.** It has been called "the great imitator" because of its various clinical presentations and the multiplicity of organs affected. Pulmonary TB was known to the ancient Greek physicians as *phthisis* (a wasting illness).

In the case of those who are afflicted with phthisis, if the sputum that is coughed up has an offensive smell when poured upon hot coals, and if the hair falls from the head, the disease will be fatal.

[Hippocrates, *Aphorisms* 5.11]

The incidence of TB declined steadily from the 1950s until about 1990, when the AIDS epidemic, an increase in the homeless population, an increase in immigrants from endemic areas, and a decrease in public surveillance caused a resurgence of the disease. Populations at greatest risk for TB include individuals infected with HIV, Asian and other immigrants, the urban homeless, people who abuse alcohol and other substances, people incarcerated in prisons or psychiatric facilities, nursing home residents, patients taking immunosuppressive drugs (as is the case with organ transplant recipients), and people with chronic respiratory disorders, diabetes mellitus, renal failure, or malnutrition. People from these risk groups should be assessed for TB if they develop pneumonia. All health-care workers should be tested annually.

Pertussis, commonly known as whooping cough, is caused by the bacillus *Bordetella pertussis,* first isolated and identified by Jules Bordet (1870–1961), a Belgian physician and bacteriologist, and Octave Gengou (1875–1957), a French bacteriologist, and named after Bordet. Routine immunization beginning at 2 months of age prevents this disease. Adults also require booster immunizations in later life.

The Greek word *sphygmos* (pulse) had the alternate form *sphyxis,* most commonly found in the word **asphyxia,** lack of a pulse. This word has now come to mean a condition caused by insufficient intake of oxygen. Its adjectival form, **asphyxial,** means affected with asphyxia. Modern derivatives of Greek *asphyxia* include **asphyxiate, asphyxiator,** and **asphyxiation,** all having to do with suffocation, the lack of oxygen.

Exercise 1:   Analyze and Define

Analyze and define each of the following words. In this and in succeeding exercises, analysis should consist of separating the words into prefixes (if any), combining forms, and suffixes or suffix forms (if any) and giving the meaning of each. Be certain to differentiate between nouns and adjectives in your definitions. Consult a medical dictionary for the current meanings of these words.

1. alveobronchitis _____

2. amygdaloid _____

3. anthracosis _____

4. antibacterial _____

5. apnea _____

6. apneumatosis _____

7. aspiration _____

8. auxotrophic _____

9. bacteriolysin _____

10. bacteriophage _____

11. bronchiolectasis _____

12. capnometry _____

13. coccobacilli _____

14. coniofibrosis _____

15. costopneumopexy _____

16. diplococcus _____

17. dyspnea _____

18. emphysema _____

19. epipharynx _____

20. expiratory _____

21. hemilaryngectomy _____

22. hydropneumothorax _____

23. hypercapnia _____

24. labioplasty _____

25. laryngismus _____

26. meningococcemia _____

27. mycobacterium _____

28. orotracheal _____

29. otolaryngologist _____

30. parasternal _____

31. paresis _____

32. pharyngoplasty _____

33. pleurodynia _____

34. pleuropneumonia _____

35. pneumatosis _____

36. pneumocephalus _____

37. pneumolysin _____

38. pseudobacteremia _____

39. respiration _____

40. siderophore _____

41. spirogram _____

42. staphylococcus _____

43. staphylolysin _____

44. sternad _____

45. stethoscope _____

46. streptococcal _____

47. sudorific _____

48. thoracic _____

49. tracheocele _____

50. transudate _____

Exercise 2:   Word Derivation

Give the word derived from Greek and/or Latin elements that matches each of the following. Verify your answer in a medical dictionary. **Note that the wording of the dictionary definition may vary from the wording used here.**

1. Pertaining to a tonsil _____

2. Substance that promotes growth (in plant cells and tissues) _____

3. Pertaining to the lips and teeth _____

4. Any fungal infection of the bronchi or bronchial tubes _____

5. Swelling containing gas or air _____

6. Study of dust (and its effects) _____

7. Iron deficiency in the blood _____

8. Surgical opening of the trachea _____

9. Inflammation of the alveoli _____

10. (Congenital) absence of the lungs _____

11. Oozing of a fluid (through pores or interstices) _____

12. Decreased amount of carbon dioxide (in the blood) _____

13. Resembling a bacterium _____

14. Presence of staphylococci in the blood _____

15. Science of the ear, nose and larynx _____

16. Plastic surgery to alter the (size and shape of the) chest wall _____

17. Suture of a lung _____

18. Excision of (part of) the pleura _____

19. Instrument used to open the trachea _____

20. Across the thorax _____

 ## Exercise 3:   Drill and Review

Analyze and define each of the following words. Analysis should consist of separating the words into prefixes (if any), combining forms, and suffixes or suffix forms (if any) and giving the meaning of each. Be certain to differentiate between nouns and adjectives in your definitions. Using the elements in the word determine its meaning. Consult a medical dictionary for the current meanings of these words. Use a separate paper if you need more room for an answer.

1. abrachia _____

2. alveolar _____

3. alveolate _____

4. amygdalin _____

5. anthrax _____

6. antistreptolysin _____

7. aspirator _____

8. asternia _____

9. auxology _____

10. bacteriotherapy _____

11. bacteriotoxin _____

12. bradypnea _____

13. bronchiolitis _____

14. capnography _____

15. cephalothoracic _____

16. coccobacteria _____

17. coniosis _____

18. emphysematous _____

19. episternum _____

20. hemiparesis _____

21. hemithorax _____

22. hemosiderin _____

23. hemisiderosis _____

24. inspiration _____

25. labial _____

26. laryngomalacia _____

27. laryngopharyngeal _____

28. laryngoscopist _____

29. monoparesis _____

30. oropharynx _____

31. peribronchiolar _____

32. peripharyngeal _____

33. pleurodesis _____

34. pleuropulmonary _____

35. pneumatics _____

36. pneumocyte _____

37. pneumonectomy _____

38. rhinopharyngocele _____

39. spirograph _____

40. spirometry _____

41. staphylococci _____

42. staphyloma _____

43. stereogram _____

44. streptococcus _____

45. streptolysin _____

46. thoracoscope _____

47. thoracostomy _____

48. tracheopathy _____

49. trachychromatic _____

50. transudation _____

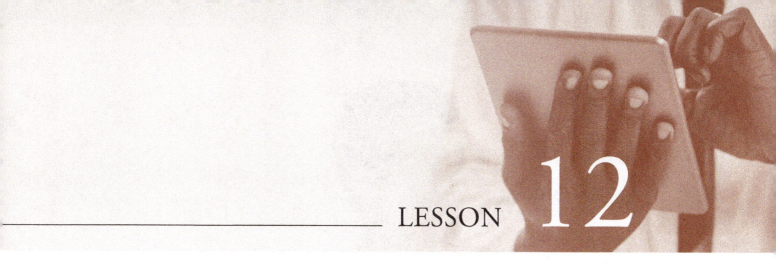

DIGESTIVE SYSTEM

There is but one entrance, the mouth, for the various kinds of food. But what is nourished is not one single part, but many, and they are widely separated. And so, do not be surprised at the great number of organs which Nature has created for the purpose of nutrition.

[Galen, *On the Natural Faculties* 1.10.23]

Every part of the body needs nutrition to function and to repair and replace damaged cellular tissue. Cells receive their nutrition from the circulating blood, which carries the usable material from digested food in the intestine to all parts of the body. When the cells receive this digested food, it is changed into other compounds for use by the body. This is called **metabolism** and involves two processes: **anabolism** and **catabolism. Anabolism,** the constructive phase of metabolism, is the process by which simple substances are converted into complex substances and then into protoplasm—that is, the conversion of non-living material into living cellular material. **Catabolism,** the destructive phase of metabolism, is the process by which complex substances are converted into simpler substances; it is usually accompanied by the release of energy. The sum of anabolism and catabolism maintains, builds up, and repairs the cellular structure of the body and provides energy for the body to function properly. All of this depends on nutrition.

Nutrition is achieved in the body through the various processes of ingestion, digestion, absorption, and metabolism (Fig. 12-1). The first three of these processes take place in the alimentary tract. This passage begins at the mouth and ends at the anus, where undigested, unabsorbed, and unused wastes are eliminated from the body. Ingested food is softened by mastication and by the addition of saliva. Three pairs of glands secrete and supply saliva: the parotid, the submandibular, and the sublingual. The masticated,

moistened, and softened food, called a bolus, is swallowed (a process called **deglutition**) and passes through the pharynx into the esophagus. A thin structure of membranous cartilage called the epiglottis folds over the larynx during deglutition to prevent food from entering the larynx and moving into the respiratory passage.

The esophagus is a tube about 10 inches long; its only function is to convey food to the stomach. At the juncture of the esophagus and the stomach is a muscle called the cardiac sphincter (also known as the lower esophageal sphincter). It lies at the entrance to the upper orifice of the stomach, called the cardia (Greek, *kardia*, heart) because of its proximity to the heart. This sphincter muscle prevents the reflux of food and acid from the stomach into the esophagus. If the cardiac sphincter malfunctions and food and acid, used to break down food in the stomach, regurgitate into the esophagus, the gastric acid irritates the esophageal mucosa. This condition is called gastroesophageal reflux disease (GERD), which causes heartburn or **pyrosis.** Damage to the esophageal mucosa caused by long-term reflux of gastric acid is called Barrett's esophagus, named for British surgeon Norman Barrett (1903–1979). Barrett's esophagus is considered a premalignant condition and is associated with the development of esophageal adenocarcinoma.

Most of the organs of the alimentary tract lie in the area known as the abdominopelvic cavity, which is lined with a serous membrane called the **peritoneum.** The outer surface of this membrane is called the **parietal** (Latin

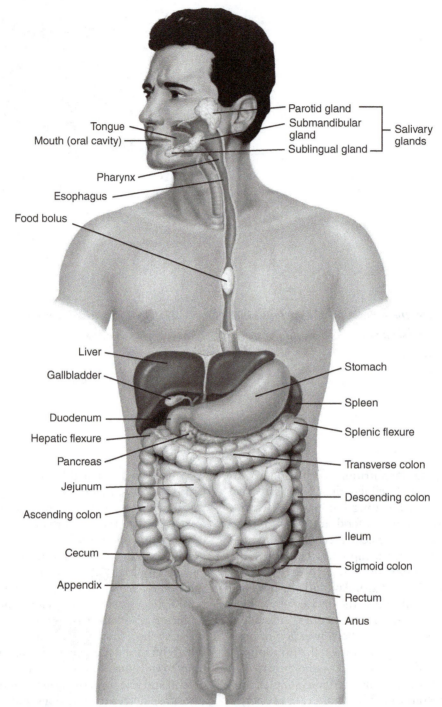

Figure 12-1. The digestive system. (From Gylys, B. A., and Wedding, M. E., *Medical Terminology Systems: A Body Systems Approach*, 8th ed., F. A. Davis, 2017, with permission.)

paries, parīetis, wall) peritoneum; the inner surface covering the visceral organs is called the **visceral** peritoneum. Inflammation of this membrane is the condition known as **peritonitis,** which can originate from inflammation or infection of any of the peritoneal organs. Peritonitis causes abdominal pain and the collection of fluid within the peritoneal cavity. Sampling of this fluid by paracentesis provides information about the cause of peritonitis (infection vs. inflammation). Each portion of the alimentary canal lying within the enclosure of the peritoneum

is attached to the posterior wall of the body by a double fold of peritoneal membrane known as the **mesentery.** Individual mesenteries are named for the specific organ to which each is attached, for example, the **mesogastrium,** the **mesoduodenum,** and so forth. Two other double folds of the peritoneum, called the **omenta** (plural of omentum), lie between the stomach and two other abdominal viscera: the greater or gastrocolic omentum, which is attached to the colon, and the lesser or gastrohepatic omentum, which is attached to the liver. Organs of the abdominal cavity that

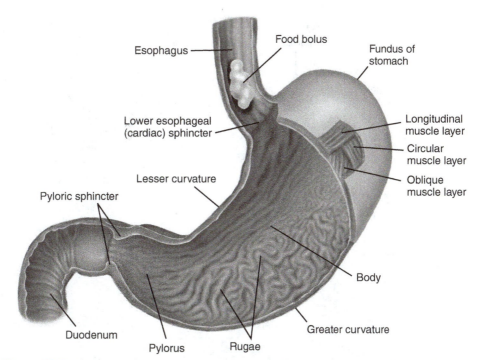

Figure 12-2. The stomach, anterior view, sectioned. (From Gylys, B. A., and Wedding, M. E., *Medical Terminology Systems: A Body Systems Approach*, 8th ed., F. A. Davis, 2017, with permission.)

are not held in position by mesenteries, but lie behind the peritoneum, are called retroperitoneal organs. The kidneys are retroperitoneal organs.

Undigested food enters the stomach through the cardiac sphincter (Fig. 12-2). Here proteins are digested by pepsin—the chief enzyme of gastric juice—and hydrochloric acid. The mass of digesting food, called chyme, is propelled forward to the lower end of the stomach, the pylorus. The force that propels food through the digestive tract from the esophagus to the anus is **peristalsis.** Peristalsis is the involuntary wavelike series of contracting and relaxing motions of the walls of the organs through which the digesting and digested food pass. At the juncture of the stomach and the duodenum is the pyloric sphincter, which is normally closed but relaxes and opens to allow partially digested food to pass into the duodenum.

The small intestine has three divisions: the **duodenum,** the **jejunum,** and the **ileum.** The process of digestion is completed here. When fats enter the duodenum, the gallbladder sends bile through the bile duct to emulsify the fat. Bile is manufactured in the liver and sent through the hepatic duct to the gallbladder to be stored until fatty substances enter the duodenum, stimulating its release. Bile and other juices, including pancreatic juice and juice from the intestine itself, *succus entericus*, complete the process of digestion. The nutrients of digested food pass into the bloodstream in the small intestine. The mucous lining of the small intestine contains thousands of minutely small projections called villi (plural of villus). The villi contain a network of capillaries that carry the nutrients from the digested food to the arterial capillaries, which then unite with the venous capillaries to join the venules and venous system.

The residue of digested food passes through the ileocecal sphincter into the large intestine, which consists of the **cecum, colon,** and **rectum.** The rectum ends at the anal opening (Fig. 12-3). The colon itself consists of four segments: the ascending colon, the transverse colon, the descending colon, and the sigmoid colon. In addition to these organs is the appendix, a dead-end tube that extends from the cecum. It has no apparent function and makes itself known only when it becomes inflamed, a condition called appendicitis. The large intestine forms fecal matter from the waste food after digestion, lubricates it with mucus, absorbs water from it, and carries the waste to the colon and the anal area for defecation. There are two anal sphincters: the first, or internal, is involuntary, and the second, or external, is voluntary.

The **liver,** one of the vital organs of the body, produces **bile,** which is carried through the hepatic ducts to the gallbladder for storage (Fig. 12-4). Other important functions of the liver include elimination of toxins, production of proteins, storage of glucose, and production of blood-clotting factors. Bile is stored in the gallbladder and becomes concentrated by absorption of water. If the bile becomes too concentrated, minerals or cholesterol in the bile may precipitate and form gallstones. If one or more of these stones is carried into the common bile duct and obstructs that passageway, the condition known as **choledocholithiasis** occurs and can result in **jaundice** (see Etymological Notes, Lesson 3, for the etymology of this word). Cellular degeneration in the liver due to fatty deposits is called **steatohepatitis. Nonalcoholic fatty liver disease (NAFLD)** is a common syndrome affecting approximately 20% of the adult population and is sometimes asymptomatic. Patients

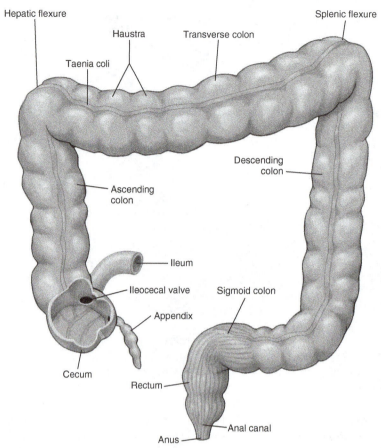

Figure 12-3. The colon and rectum. (From Venes, D., ed., *Taber's Cyclopedic Medical Dictionary*, 24th ed., F. A. Davis, 2021, p. 524, with permission.)

may have mild elevation of liver enzymes, which leads to the diagnosis.

Bile is carried from the liver by the left and the right hepatic ducts, which unite to form the common hepatic duct. This duct branches off into the cystic duct, which carries bile to the gallbladder to be concentrated and stored until needed for digestion. Inflammation of the left or right hepatic ducts or the cystic duct is known as **cholangitis.** Radiographic examination of any of these ducts, a procedure known as **cholangiography,** has been replaced by **ultrasonography.** Surgery to remove stones in the gallbladder or common bile duct **(cholangiotomy)** can sometimes be performed laparoscopically.

Bile leaving the gallbladder enters the hepatic duct, which descends into the duodenum and becomes the common bile duct. The Greek word *dochos* (receptacle) is used in naming it. Thus, inflammation of the common bile duct is called **choledochitis.** As this duct is about to enter the duodenum, it is joined by the pancreatic duct carrying pancreatic digestive enzymes. Control over the entry of bile and the pancreatic juices is exercised by a muscle called the sphincter of Oddi, named for Ruggero Oddi, a 19th-century Italian physician. If concretions (gallstones) form in the gallbladder, the condition is known as **cholelithiasis.** If cholelithiasis becomes symptomatic

with abdominal pain after eating fatty foods, a **cholecystectomy** may be performed.

The entire alimentary, or gastrointestinal (GI), tract is lined with a mucus-secreting membrane called the mucosa. Inflammation or erosion of the gastric mucosa causes the condition known as **gastritis.** Gastric ulcers are defined as mucosal destruction that extends through the muscularis mucosae, the muscular layer of the GI tract.

The term peptic ulcer disease (PUD) refers to ulcerations of the stomach, duodenum, or both, but ulcerations can occur in any portion of the GI tract. Zollinger-Ellison syndrome (named for American surgeons Robert M. Zollinger [1903–1992] and Edwin H. Ellison [1918–1970]) is caused by neuroendocrine tumors, usually in the pancreas, which stimulate the stomach to secrete excessive amounts of hydrochloric acid and pepsin. This condition, called a hypersecretory state, can cause peptic ulcer disease. Treatment of PUD has evolved from dietary management and use of antacids to gastric acid suppression with H_2 blockers (H_2-receptor antagonists) and proton (Greek *protos*, first) pump inhibitors, and now to eradication of *Helicobacter pylori (H. pylori)*. *H. pylori* is a gram-negative bacterium that is etiologically related to most peptic ulcers and to gastritis. The eradication of *H. pylori* requires antibiotics as well as therapy to suppress gastric acid secretion.

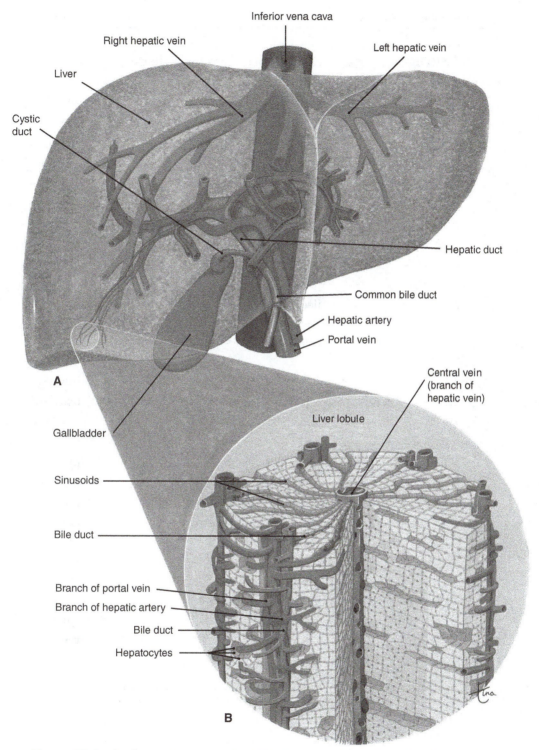

Figure 12-4. The liver. (*A*) Liver and gallbladder. (*B*) Lobule. (From Scanlon, V. C., and Sanders, T., *Essentials of Anatomy and Physiology*, 8th ed. F. A. Davis, 2020, with permission.)

VOCABULARY

When the more lax intestine, which is named the colon, tends to be painful, and when the pain is nothing more than flatulence, one should endeavor to promote digestion by reading aloud and other exercises. Hot baths and hot food and drinks are helpful, but all cold foods, all manner of cold, all sweets, all kinds of beans and whatever else contributes to flatulence should be avoided.

[Celsus, *De Medicina* 1.6.7]

Note: Latin combining forms are shown in ***bold italics.***

Greek or Latin	Combining Form(s)	Meaning	Example
bīlis	**BILI-**	bile	**bili**-rubin
kardia*	**CARDI-**	cardia (upper orifice of the stomach)	**cardi**-oesophageal
caecus	**CEC-**	[blind] cecum	**cec**-um
klyzein	**CLY(S)-**	rinse out, inject fluid	**cly**-sis
kopros	**COPR-**	excrement, fecal matter	**copr**-olith
kreas, kreatos	**CREAT-**	flesh	pan-**creat**-ic
dochos	**-DOCH-**	duct	chole-**doch**-al
duodēnī	**DUODEN-**	[12] duodenum	**duoden**-um
oisophagos	**ESOPHAG-**	esophagus	**esophag**-ismus
faex, faecis	**FEC-**	[sediment] excrement, fecal matter	**fec**-es
geuein	**GEUS(T)-**	taste	a-**geust**-ia
gingīva	**GINGIV-**	gum (of the mouth)	**gingiv**-itis
glōssa	**GLOSS-**	tongue	**gloss**-ectomy
īleum	**ILE-**	ileum	**ile**-um
jējūnus	**JEJUN-**	[empty] jejunum	**jejun**-um
liēn (pronounced in two syllables: lie'-en)	**LIEN-**	spleen	**lien**-omyelomalacia
lingua	**LINGU-**	tongue	**lingu**-al
osmē	**OSM-**	sense of smell; odor	**osm**-esthesia
peptein	**PEPS-, PEPT-**	digest	dys-**peps**-ia
proktos	**PROCT-**	anus	**proct**-oscopy
pylē	**PYLE-**	[gate] portal vein	**pyle**-thrombosis
pylōros	**PYLOR-**	[gatekeeper] pylorus	**pylor**-ic
rectus	**RECT-**	[straight] rectum	**rect**-al
skōr, skatos	**SCAT-**	excrement, fecal matter	**scat**-ology
sialon	**SIAL-**	saliva, salivary duct	**sial**-olith
sigma	**SIGM-**	[sigma, the Greek letter s] sigmoid colon	**sigm**-oid
sphinctēr	**SPHINCTER-**	sphincter muscle	**sphincter** ani
splanchnon	**SPLANCHN-**	internal organ, viscus	**splanchn**-a
typhlos	**TYPHL-**	[blind] cecum	**typhl**-enteritis
zymē	**ZYM-**	[leaven] ferment, enzyme, fermentation	en-**zym**-e

*kardia is the Greek word for heart; it is also used to designate the upper orifice of the stomach connecting with the esophagus. It is so named because of its proximity to the heart.

ETYMOLOGICAL NOTES

Celsus, a first-century AD Roman physician, was aware of the shape, size, and position of the internal organs, knowledge that he acquired, seemingly, by dissection. In his discussion of these organs, after a description of the liver, he turns his attention to the digestive tract:

These are the locations of the visceral organs. The gullet (*stomachus*), which is the beginning of the intestines, is sinewy and begins at the seventh vertebra of the spine. It joins the stomach (*ventriculum*) in the region of the precordia. The stomach, which is the receptacle of food, is comprised of two coats, and it is located between the spleen and the liver, with both of these organs overlapping it a little. There are also thin membranes by which the stomach, the spleen, and the liver are connected, and they are joined to that membrane which I have described above as the transverse septum.

The lowest part of the stomach turns a little to the right and narrows as it enters the top of the intestine. This entry is called by the Greeks *pylorus* because, like a gateway, it allows through to the lower parts whatever is to be excreted.

From this point begins the *jejunum intestinum,* which is not folded upon itself as much. It is called the empty intestine because it does not retain what it has received, but immediately passes it along to the lower parts.

After that comes the thinner intestine, folded into many loops, which are connected to the more internal parts with membranes. These loops are turned toward the right, ending in the region of the hip, occupying, however, mostly the upper parts.

Then this intestine joins crosswise with another, which, beginning on the right side, is long, and on the left it is pervious but on the right it is not and so it is called *caecum intestinum.*

But that one which is pervious . . . bending backward and to the right, descends straight downwards to the place of excretion, and for this reason is called the *rectum intestinum.*

The omentum, which lies over all these organs, is smooth and compact at its lower part, but at the top is softer. It produces fat, which, like the brain and bone marrow, is without feeling.

[*De Medicina* 4.1.6–10]

The duodenum is so named because it is about the length of 12 finger widths. Actually, it varies in length from 8 to 11 inches, the average being 10 inches.

Salmonella is a form of gastroenteritis that is produced by ingesting food containing one or more of the *Salmonella* organisms. The disease was named after the American pathologist Daniel E. Salmon (1850–1914), who first isolated the genus of these organisms. **Typhoid fever,** a severe intestinal disease found in developing countries with poor sanitation, is caused by the organism *Salmonella typhi.*

Diverticula (Latin *di-,* apart, aside, *vertere,* turn, and *-cula,* the plural of *-culum,* the diminutive suffix) are small pouches or sacs formed by herniation of the wall of a canal or organ, occurring most frequently in the colon (Fig. 12-5). This condition, called **diverticulosis,** is most commonly found in patients over the age of 40 and may be asymptomatic. If

these pouches fill with digested wastes, inflammation often accompanied by abdominal pain (usually in the left lower quadrant of the abdomen) and fever, a condition called diverticulitis, can develop. Treatment is usually antibiotics. However, if antibiotics do not alleviate the condition, and especially if the inflammation spreads, surgery may be necessary to remove the affected area of the intestine. Sometimes, a **colostomy**—an incision into the intestine to create an opening to the surface of the abdomen through which fecal matter can be eliminated—may be necessary.

The pancreas gland was so named because it is entirely constituted of flesh without muscular tissues. John Banister (1540–1610), in *The History of Man* (London, John Daye, 1578), wrote of the pancreas: "This body is called Panchreas, that is, all carnous or fleshy, for that it is made and contexted of Glandulous flesh." Both Aristotle and Galen used the word *pankreas* to refer to this organ.

The word hiatus means an opening. A hernia is the protrusion of an organ or part of the organ through the wall of the canal or cavity in which it is normally contained. A **hiatal hernia** is the protrusion of any organ, usually the stomach, upward through the esophageal hiatus of the diaphragm, that is, the opening of the diaphragm through which the esophagus passes. More common types of hernia are umbilical and inguinal.

The Greek noun *zymē* means leaven (Latin *levāre,* raise), any substance that causes fermentation in bread dough, fruit juice, and so forth. Words containing *zym-* refer to fermentation or to the presence of enzymes. **Enzymes,** complex proteins, are catalysts (Greek *kata-,* down, *lyein,* break), agents that induce chemical changes in other substances without being altered themselves. Enzymes are found in digestive juices and act on the mass of ingested food as it passes along the alimentary tract, breaking it down into simpler compounds. Each enzyme has a more or less specific function: **ptyalin,** secreted in the salivary glands, hydrolyzes starch; **pepsin** and **rennin,** in the gastric

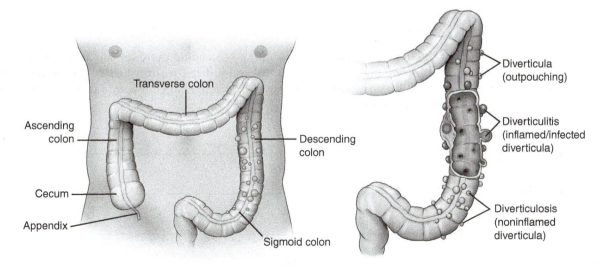

Figure 12-5. Multiple diverticula of the colon. (From Hoffman, J., and Sullivan, N., *Medical-Surgical Nursing: Making Connections to Practice,* 2nd Edition, F.A. Davis, 2020, with permission.)

juice, act on protein; and **steapsin,** an enzyme present in pancreatic juice, hydrolyzes fat. Thus, ptyalin is an amylase, or amylolytic enzyme, and steapsin is a lipase, or lipolytic enzyme. A list of the principal enzymes can be found in your medical dictionary.

Zymogen is a substance that develops into an enzyme, or ferment, an obsolete term for enzyme. **Zymology** is the science of fermentation. **Zymolysis** refers to the changes produced by an enzyme. Biblical scriptures refer to the festival of Passover and Unleavened Bread. In the Septuagint (the Greek translation of the Old Testament), reference is made in Exodus 29.2 to loaves of unleavened bread, *artous* (accusative plural of *artos*, bread) *azymous*, and unleavened cakes, *lagana* (plural of *laganon*, a thin broad cake) *azyma*.

The Greek noun *sphinctēr*, from which the sphincter muscles take their name, is related to the verb *sphingein* (bind tight). Also related to this verb is the noun *sphinx* (strangler, destroyer). In Greek mythology, a dreadful calamity befell the kingdom of Thebes. A monster, the Sphinx, was sent by Hera, queen of the gods, to ravage the land. Apollodorus, the mythographer and author of *The Library*, described the Sphinx: She had the face of a woman; the breast, feet, and tail of a lion; and the wings of a bird. She posed a riddle to the Thebans (which she had learned from the Muses): What has one voice and becomes four-footed, two-footed, and three-footed? While the Thebans were pondering the riddle, she snatched them one by one and devoured them. Finally, Oedipus came along and found the answer, declaring that man as an infant is four-footed, as an adult is two-footed, and as an old man gains a third foot in a staff. The Sphinx killed herself, and Oedipus was asked to wed the late king's widow, Jocasta, and become the ruler of the land. Although it was unknown to both at the time, Jocasta was his mother. And so begins the tragic tale of Oedipus the King.

The portal vein, which carries blood to the liver, is formed by the union of several veins of the visceral area. It enters the liver at the porta hepatis, a fissure on the undersurface of the liver where the hepatic artery also enters this organ and where the right and left hepatic ducts leave it. In medical terminology, the portal vein is referred to by the Greek word *pylē* (gate or entrance). **Pylemphraxis,** a term not frequently used in medical literature, means an occlusion of the portal vein. **Pylethrombosis,** commonly known as portal vein thrombosis, is a condition that can lead to massive gastrointestinal bleeding. The word *pylē* is generally found in the plural form *pylai* in Greek. In this form, it meant the gates of a city or the entrance to an area. Perhaps the most famous of these gates in Greek history was a narrow mountain pass in the northern part of Greece, Thermopylae, the "hot gate" (*thermos*, hot), so called because of the hot sulphur springs there. Thermopylae was thought to be the northern entry into Greece, and it was here that a famous battle was fought in 480 BC. The Greek forces, after holding the pass for 2 days against the huge Persian army that was invading Greece from the north, were forced to abandon their position when a Greek traitor showed Xerxes, the Persian king, a way around the pass. Leonidas, the Spartan king, and 300 of his men, together with 700 Thespians, are said to have perished here while making a symbolic stand against the barbarian army.

Botulism, a form of food poisoning caused by eating foods contaminated with *Clostridium botulinum*, especially prevalent in preserved meats, takes its name from the Latin word for preserved meat, *botulus* (stuffed intestine or sausage). The poison responsible for botulism damages the nervous system by blocking the release of acetylcholine at the neuromuscular junction. This is the cause of the paralysis associated with botulism.

Exercise 1: Analyze and Define

Analyze and define each of the following words. In this and in succeeding exercises, analysis should consist of separating the words into prefixes (if any), combining forms, and suffixes or suffix forms (if any) and giving the meaning of each. Be certain to differentiate between nouns and adjectives in your definitions. Consult a medical dictionary for the current meanings of these words.

  1. ageustia _____

  2. anosmia _____

  3. aortoiliac _____

  4. biliary _____

5. cardioesophageal _____

6. cardiospasm _____

7. cecopexy _____

8. cecostomy _____

9. cholangiotomy _____

10. choledochoenterostomy _____

11. coprolith _____

12. coproscopy _____

13. creatorrhea _____

14. defecation _____

15. diglossia _____

16. dolichosigmoid _____

17. duodenojejunostomy _____

18. dyspepsia _____

19. esophagismus _____

20. fecaloid _____

21. feculent _____

22. gingivitis _____

23. glossectomy _____

24. ileocecal sphincter _____

25. ileocolic _____

26. ileocolostomy _____

27. jejunostomy _____

28. labiogingival _____

29. lienal _____

30. lingula _____

31. pancreatic _____

32. pepsin _____

33. postlingual _____

34. proctologist _____

35. proctosigmoiditis _____

36. pylethrombosis _____

37. pylorospasm _____

38. rectoclysis _____

39. rectostenosis _____

40. retrolingual _____

41. scatology _____

42. sigmoiditis _____

43. sigmoidoscope _____

44. sphincteroplasty _____

45. sphincterotome _____

46. splanchnic _____

47. splanchnicectomy _____

48. typhlectasis _____

49. zymogen _____

50. zymolysis _____

Exercise 2:   Word Derivation

Give the word derived from Latin and/or Greek elements that matches each of the following. Verify your answer in a medical dictionary. **Note that the wording of the dictionary definition may vary from the wording used here.**

1. Situated under the tongue _____

2. Vomiting of fecal material _____

3. Formation of a passage between the duodenum and the intestine _____

4. Pain in the esophagus _____

5. Injection (of a nutrient or medicinal liquid) into the bowel _____

6. Formation of a passage between two parts of the jejunum _____

7. Suture repair of the common bile duct _____

8. Softening of the spleen and bone marrow _____

9. Incision into the ileum _____

10. Inflammation of the colon and rectum _____

11. Presence of stones in the salivary duct _____

12. Operation to repair (or alter) the pylorus _____

13. Incision of the bladder through the rectum _____

14. Excision of a sphincter muscle _____

15. Pertaining to digestion _____

16. Cyst or tumor of a salivary gland _____

17. Study of the viscera _____

18. Power of perceiving and distinguishing odors _____

19. Impairment or perversion of the sense of taste _____

20. Pain in or around the anus _____

Exercise 3:   Drill and Review

Analyze and define each of the following words. Analysis should consist of separating the words into prefixes (if any), combining forms, and suffixes or suffix forms (if any) and giving the meaning of each. Be certain to differentiate between nouns and adjectives in your definitions. Using the elements in the word determine its meaning. Consult a medical dictionary for the current meanings of these words. Use a separate paper if you need more room for an answer.

1. ageusia _____

2. anosmic _____

3. bilious _____

4. biloma _____

5. calorifacient _____

6. capnophilic _____

7. cardialgia _____

8. cardiopyloric _____

9. cecoptosis _____

10. choledochal _____

11. coprolalia _____

12. coprophilic _____

13. duodenorrhapy _____

14. dyspeptic _____

15. esophagocele _____

16. gingivostomatitis _____

17. glossoptosis _____

18. heterotaxia _____

19. ileoproctostomy _____

20. immunotherapy _____

21. intraduodenal _____

22. lingulae _____

23. mesenteritis _____

24. mesojejunum _____

25. osteophlebitis _____

26. oxychloride _____

27. pachyonychia _____

28. pancreatitis _____

29. pancreatoduodenectomy _____

30. pylethrombophlebitis _____

31. pyloromyotomy _____

32. rectocolitis _____

33. rectopexy _____

34. retroesophageal _____

35. sialadenosis _____

36. sialorrhea _____

37. sigmoidoscopy _____

38. somnolent _____

39. sphincterotomy _____

40. splanchna _____

41. splanchnocranium _____

42. stereognosis _____

43. stomatogastric _____

44. typhlenteritis _____

45. typhlitis _____

46. vascularize _____

47. venoclysis _____

48. viscerosomatic _____

49. zymase _____

50. zymolytic _____

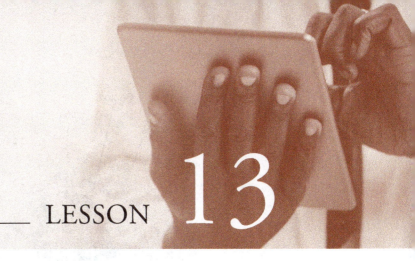

Optic System

There is a certain weakness of the eyes in which people see well in the daytime but not at all at night. This condition does not exist in women whose menstruation is regular. Those who suffer with this disability should anoint their eyeballs with the drippings from a liver while it is roasting—preferably that of a he-goat; if that is not possible, one from a she-goat; and the liver itself should be eaten.

[Celsus, *De Medicina* 6.6.38]

The globe of the eye is surrounded by three layers of tissue (Fig. 13-1). The outermost layer—the **sclera**—is a tough, fibrous coat that forms a protective covering for the delicate nerves and membranes beneath. The **cornea** is the anterior, visible, and transparent portion of the sclera. The sclera and the cornea form one continuous coat. The anterior portion of the sclera is covered with a transparent mucous membrane called the **conjunctiva,** an extension of the lining of the eyelids. The portion of the conjunctiva that lines the eyelids is called the **palpebral conjunctiva** (Latin *palpebra,* eyelid); the membrane covering the sclera is the **bulbar conjunctiva;** the loose fold connecting the two is the **fornix conjunctivae** (Latin *fornix,* arch).

The episclera is a thin layer of tissue covering the exterior surface of the sclera that contains blood vessels that nourish the sclera. **Episcleritis** is a common disease of the sclera. Although the cause may not be clear in most cases, episcleritis generally afflicts people with inflammatory diseases such as rheumatoid arthritis and Crohn's disease. Treated with topical corticosteroids, lubricant eye drops, cold compresses, and NSAIDs such as ibuprofen, episcleritis usually clears in 7 to 10 days.*

The cornea is subject to bacterial, viral, and fungal infection as well as to injury by foreign bodies. Ulceration and abrasion of the cornea are common. Minor abrasions will generally resolve within 24 to 72 hours; pain relief with topical or oral analgesics can reduce discomfort. Eye patching was commonly recommended. However, a meta-analysis published in 1998 found no difference in healing time with or without eye patching, and that patching increased discomfort.† *Streptococcus pneumoniae* is another common cause of bacterial corneal ulcers called **keratitis.**

Herpes simplex virus (HSV) is the most common viral cause of corneal ulcers, called HSV keratitis or **herpetic keratitis.** The global incidence of HSV keratitis is roughly 1.5 million per year, 40,000 of which are new cases of severe monocular visual impairment or blindness.‡ Contact lens wearers are at increased risk for HVP keratitis. The Centers for Disease Control and Prevention (CDC) recommends proper cleaning and regular replacement of both lenses and lens cases to reduce the incidence of HPV keratitis.§ Infectious mononucleosis is another cause of keratitis.

Hypopyon keratitis, a serpent-like ulcer with pus in the anterior chamber of the eye, can be a complication of both bacterial and viral ulceration. Other causes of keratitis

---

*Episcleritis. Healthline. https://www.healthline.com/health/episcleritis. Accessed February 6, 2021.

†Flynn CA, D'Amico F, Smith G. Should we patch corneal abrasions? A meta-analysis? *J Fam Pract.* 1998, 47:264-270.

‡Zagaria MAE. HSV Keratitis: An Important Infectious Cause of Blindness. *US Pharm.* 2015;40(4):16-18.

§Healthy contact lens wear and care. Centers for Disease Control and Prevention. https://www.cdc.gov/contactlenses/fast-facts.html. Accessed February 6, 2021.

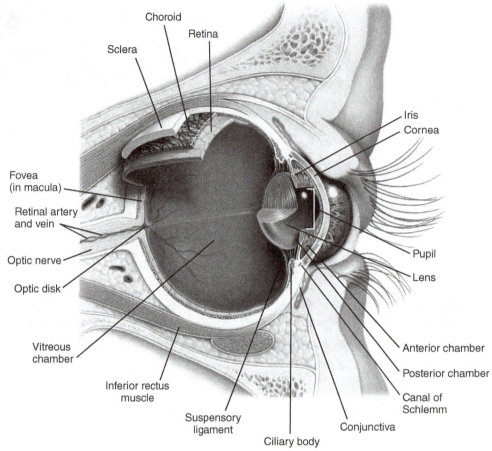

Figure 13-1. Anatomy of the eye. (From Gylys, B. A., and Wedding, M. E., *Medical Terminology Systems: A Body Systems Approach*, 8th ed., F. A. Davis, 2017.)

include Bell's palsy, which can result in dry-eye syndrome, and side effects from certain drugs.

Fungal keratitis, also called fungal corneal ulcers, is an infection that can cause rapid loss of vision and pain. As with HSV keratitis, contact lens wearers are more susceptible to fungal corneal ulcers, as are people with long-term contact with soil and plant materials, such as farm workers. Other risk factors include eye surgery, topical steroid use, and immunosuppression. Individuals with fungal keratitis may be treated with antifungal eye drops, antifungal medication in pill form, or for more serious infections, with antifungals administered intravenously or injected into the eye. Use of topical steroids are not effective for fungal infections and may increase susceptibility to other infections.*

Corneal ulceration may be caused by avitaminosis A, the lack of vitamin A, as a result of either dietary deficiency or impaired absorption and utilization from the gastrointestinal tract. Avitaminosis A can cause a hardening and drying of the epithelium throughout the body, a condition known as **xerosis.** Xerosis of the conjunctiva and cornea is called **xerophthalmia.** Corneal ulceration caused by avitaminosis A is characterized by a softening of the cornea

called **keratomalacia,** and often by necrosis, leading to perforation. Sources of vitamin A, such as dairy products, liver, fish, fortified cereals, carrots, broccoli, cantaloupe, and squash, are available in most markets. The National Institutes of Health (NIH) sets vitamin dosages by age groups. For more information about vitamin A, visit the NIH website.†

The middle layer of the eye, or vascular layer, is a dark brown tissue called the **uvea** because of its resemblance to a grape (Latin *ūva*). The uveal tract is composed of the iris, the ciliary body, and the choroid. The uveal tract contributes blood supply to the retina and is protected by the outer layer, the cornea, and the sclera. The choroid is the posterior portion extending to the point opposite the lens; the ciliary body is a thickened triangular structure; the iris is the anterior extension of the ciliary body.

The ciliary body secretes a fluid called the aqueous humor into the posterior chamber of the eye, the area behind the iris and in front of the vitreous body. The aqueous humor flows from the posterior chamber into the anterior chamber through the pupil, and leaves the eye through the trabecular (diminutive of Latin *trabs, trabis,* a beam of

---

*Treatment for fungal eye infections. Centers for Disease Control and Prevention. https://www.cdc.gov/fungal/diseases/fungal-eye-infections/treatment.html. Accessed February 6, 2021.

†Vitamin A and carotenoids. National Institutes of Health. http://ods.od.nih.gov/factsheets/VitaminA-HealthProfessional/#h2. Accessed February 6, 2021.

wood) meshwork named Schlemm's canal for the German anatomist Friedrich Schlemm (1795–1858). Schlemm's canal opens at the inner corner of the anterior chamber between the cornea and the iris. Approximately 30 collector channels leading from Schlemm's canal carry the aqueous humor into the venous system. Intraocular pressure (IOP) is controlled by the rate at which the aqueous humor leaves the eye through Schlemm's canal.

If aqueous humor fails to drain normally, IOP increases and gradually damages nerve fibers at the optic disc. Unchecked, this can lead to **glaucoma,** the third leading cause of impaired vision and blindness in the United States. Infection or inflammation can block Schlemm's canal. More often, normal drainage is impaired without infection or inflammation. Glaucoma is categorized by whether or not the angle between the posterior cornea and anterior iris is open or not. Two common forms of glaucoma are primary open-angle glaucoma (POAG) and closed-angle glaucoma. Glaucoma can be detected with a **tonometer,** an instrument that measures IOP. Extremely high IOP can cause blindness in a short time by damaging the optic nerve or by compressing the blood vessels of the retina to the point where the supply of blood is cut off. Early detection and treatment of glaucoma is decreasing the incidence of this disease. Treatment depends on the severity of the damage. Nonoperative treatment for glaucoma includes topical medications such as beta blockers. More serious disease may require surgery. Marijuana has been shown to alleviate symptoms of severe glaucoma by lowering IOP.* African Americans are at increased risk of developing glaucoma. Physicians recommend that all African Americans age 40 and over should have their eyes examined annually; earlier for individuals with a family history of glaucoma.†

The **retina,** an outgrowth of the optic nerve, is the innermost layer of the eye globe. It is a thin, semi-transparent sheet of neural tissue that lines the inner aspect of the posterior two-thirds of the globe. The retina receives visual images through the lens and transmits these images through the optic nerve to the proper receptors in the brain. The retina is composed of 10 layers of cells. The first of these—the inner coating—is made up of pigmented epithelial cells. The rods and cones, nerve receptors that respond to light, form the second layer. The rods, which control night vision **(scotopia),** depend on an adequate supply of vitamin A. Vitamin A deficiency can cause night vision deficiency **(nyctalopia).**

The cones of the retina are sensitive to color, and any interference with their normal transmission of visual images can result in one or more forms of color vision deficiency, also called color blindness or color deficiency. There are three types of cones, each sensitive to a different color of the light spectrum. Light has three primary colors: red, green, and blue. If the cones lack sensitivity to red, the person is said to have protanopia (Greek, *prōtos,* first) because red is the first of the primary colors. Green color

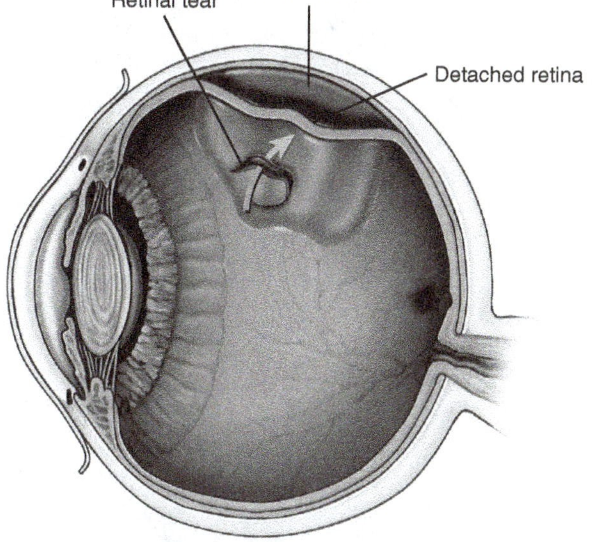

Figure 13-2. Retinal detachment. (From Hoffman, J., and Sullivan, N., *Medical-Surgical Nursing: Making Connections to Practice,* 2nd Edition, F.A. Davis, 2020.)

vision deficiency is called **deuteranopia** (Greek, *deuteros,* second). Color vision deficiency in which blue and yellow appear gray is called **tritanopia** (Greek, *tritos,* third).

The opposite of these conditions—an oversensitivity in the cones—causes defects in which the person sees everything either through a red haze **(erythropia),** a green haze **(chloropia),** or a blue haze **(cyanopia).** Color vision defects are usually hereditary.

Age-related macular (Latin, *macula,* spot) degeneration (ARMD; also AMD) is the most frequent cause of central visual field blindness in the United States affecting 1.8 million Americans over age 40. Factors contributing to ARMD include environment and genetics. Smoking is positively correlated to onset and progression of ARMD.‡

The condition known as detached retina occurs when the rod and cone layer of the retina (the sensory layer) become partially separated from the pigmented epithelial layer of the retina (Fig. 13-2). The upper exterior portion of the retina is the area most commonly affected, but any part may become detached. Retinal detachment usually occurs when a hole develops in the inner sensory layer of the eye that allows the vitreous humor—the jellylike, semifluid that fills the eyeball—to leak under the retina, pushing it up. This may be the result of head or eye trauma or cataract surgery; it may also appear in people who are very myopic. Other causes include choroiditis, retinitis, and malignant melanoma of the choroid. People with diabetes or sickle cell disease are at higher risk for retinal detachment. Some cases of retinal detachment are idiopathic, without apparent cause. This condition can usually be corrected by microscopic vitreous surgery, a procedure that

---

*Venes D, ed. *Taber's Cyclopedic Medical Dictionary*, 23rd ed., F.A. Davis, 2017, p. 1021.
†Venes D, ed. *Taber's Cyclopedic Medical Dictionary*, 23rd ed., F.A. Davis, 2017, p. 1022.

‡Age-related macular degeneration. Centers for Disease Control and Prevention. https://www.cdc.gov/visionhealth/basics/ced/index.html#a3. Accessed February 6, 2021.

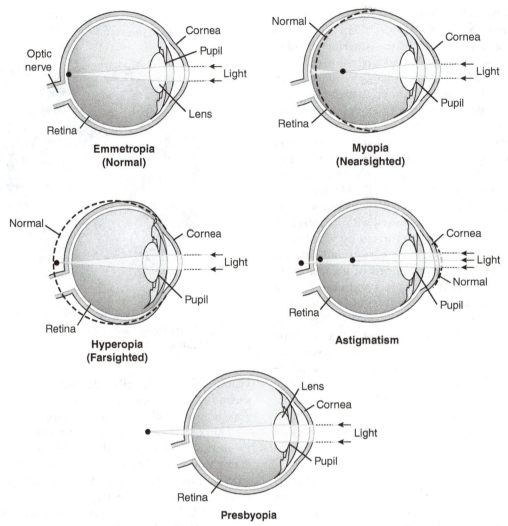

Figure 13-3. Emmetropia, myopia, and hyperopia. (From Hoffman, J., and Sullivan, N., *Medical-Surgical Nursing: Making Connections to Practice*, 2nd Edition, F.A. Davis, 2020.)

may include severing and removing tissue, diathermy, and laser photocoagulation.

The lens of the eye is held in place by bands of ligament (zonula ciliaris) connecting it to the ciliary body on either side. It lies between the aqueous humor in front and the vitreous humor behind. The purpose of the lens is to focus the light rays on the retina at the fovea centralis retinae, commonly called the **fovea**, by refracting them to the proper degree. When focusing is normal, the condition is called **emmetropia**, and no refractive errors are present. There are three fairly common abnormalities that interfere with normal focusing: **hyperopia** (hypermetropia), **myopia**, and **astigmatism** (Fig. 13-3).

Myopia, or nearsightedness, is caused by a larger-than-normal eye that lets light rays focus in front of the retina. Myopia is corrected by negative, or convex, eyeglasses or contact lenses. Increasing the amount of time children spend outside may reduce the incidence of myopia.*

Hyperopia, or farsightedness, results from the failure of light rays to focus directly on the retina. Hyperopic eyes tend to be small, with a shallow anterior chamber. Parallel rays of light entering the eye are focused behind the retina instead of on the retina. As in myopia, hyperopia can be corrected by the use of eyeglasses or convex contact lenses.

Astigmatism results when the lens or the cornea is egg-shaped rather than spherical, causing some of the light rays to focus behind the retina and some to focus in front of it. The condition is so named because those who suffer from it have difficulty in focusing their sight on a point (Greek *stigma*).

Surgery using lasers to correct these three common focusing conditions is called LASIK. The acronym stands for laser in situ keratomileusis (*in sitū*, Latin, in the place; *keratos*, Greek, cornea; *mileusis*, Greek, shaping). As the name suggests, the procedure involves using a laser to reshape the cornea into the proper configuration.†

Taber's Cyclopedic Medical Dictionary, ed 23. Philadelphia: F. A. Davis, 2017, p. 710.

†The LASIK Institute (http://www.lasikinstitute.org) (accessed February 6, 2021).

VOCABULARY

It is a bad sign if hiccough and redness of the eyes follows vomiting.

[Hippocrates, *Aphorisms* 7.2]

Note: Latin combining forms are shown in ***bold italics***.

Greek or Latin	Combining Form(s)	Meaning	Example
blepharon	**BLEPHAR-**	eyelid	**blephar-**ostat
chorioeidēs	**CHOROID-**	[skin-like] choroid	**choroid-**itis
korē	**COR(E)-**	[girl] pupil (of the eye)	**core-**oplasty
kyklos	**CYCL-**	circle; the ciliary body	**cycl-**oplegia
dakryon	**DACRY-**	tear; lacrimal sac or duct	**dacry-**ocystitis
herpēs, herpētos	**HERPES, HERPET-**	[shingles] herpes, a creeping skin disease	**herpet-**iform
iris, iridos	**IR(ID)-**	[rainbow] iris	**irid-**emia
jungere, junctus	***JUNCT-***	join	con-**junct-**ivitis
keras, keratos	**KERAT-**	[horn] cornea	**kerat-**itis
lacrima	***LACRIM-, LACHRYM-***	tear	**lacrim-**al
myein	**MY-**	close, shut	**my-**opia
oculus	***OCUL-***	eye	**ocul-**ar
ōps	**OP(S)-**	vision	dys-**ops-**ia
ophthalmos	**OPHTHALM-**	eye	**ophthalm-**ia
optos	**OPT-**	[seen] vision; eye	**opt-**ical
phakos	**PHAC-, PHAK-**	[lentil] lens	a-**phak-**ia
rēte, rētis	***RET-, RETIN-***	[net] retina; network, plexus	**retin-**a
stigma, stigmatos	**STIGM-, STIGMAT-**	point, mark, spot	a-**stigmat-**ism
xēros	**XER-**	dry	**xer-**osis

ETYMOLOGICAL NOTES

If the winter is dry and the winds are from the north, and if the spring is rainy and the winds are from the south, the summer will be laden with fever and will cause ophthalmia and dysenteries.

[Hippocrates, *Airs, Waters, and Places* 10]

The word *glaukōma* (Greek *glaukos*, gleaming, gray) was used by Aristotle, Galen, and others to indicate opacity of the lens of the eye called a cataract. The earliest examples of the word glaucoma in English mean cataract. It was not until 1705 that the difference between a true glaucoma and an ordinary cataract was recognized in dissection by the French physician Pierre Brisseau. The term **glaucoma**, as now used, refers to the condition of increased IOP. As IOP increases, the optic disc (the area of the retina where the optic nerve enters) atrophies and changes color from its natural pink to a light gray color. It is this progressive atrophy of the optic disc that causes blindness in absolute glaucoma, the final stage of this disease.

The ultimate etymology of the medical term **cataract** is uncertain. The Greek *kataraktēs*, found in Latin as *cataracta*, meant a waterfall, particularly a cataract of the Nile or Euphrates River. Later it came to mean a floodgate, as in the description of the flood in Genesis 7.11:

> In the six hundredth year of Noah's life, in the second month, the seventeenth day of the month, the same day were all the fountains of the great deep broken up, and the windows [or floodgates] of heaven were opened.

[*Bible*, King James version]

The Hebrew word for the "windows of heaven" is *Ārubot*, which was translated in the Septuagint (the Greek Old Testament) by *kataraktai* and in the Vulgate (Biblia Vulgāta, a late-fourth-century Latin translation of the Bible) by *cataractae*. *Ārubot* are also the "windows from on high" in Isaiah 24.18:

> And it shall come to pass, that he who fleeth from the noise of the fear shall fall into the pit; and he that cometh up out of the midst of the pit shall be taken in the snare: for the windows from on high are open, and the foundations of the earth do shake.

[*Bible*, King James version]

It is uncertain whether the Greek *kataraktēs* is from *katarassein* (dash down) or from *katarrhēgnynai* (break in pieces). The French surgeon Ambroïse Paré (1510–1590) was likely the first to use the word in its medical sense in a treatise in which he refers to a *cataracte* of the eye. Perhaps Paré, who developed artificial eye globes, had the idea that a cataract was a sort of gate that shut out the light. If so, more recent research has shown Paré to be correct: glare or light sensitivity is considered a symptom of cataracts. The modern surgical method for treatment of cataract by removal of the lens was introduced by the French surgeon Jacques Daviel (1696–1762).* Treatment of cataracts today builds upon the works of both of these surgeons: the cloudy lens of the eye is surgically removed and replaced with a clear, artificial lens.

The **herpes virus** takes its name from the Greek *herpēs* (shingles), an acute inflammatory eruption of the skin or mucous membrane, a term that was used with this meaning by Hippocrates. The noun *herpēs* is derived from the verb *herpein* (move slowly, creep), probably from the slow advance of the inflammation on the body. Pliny the Elder, in writing of ulcers and their treatment, says,

> "There is an animal which the Greeks call *herpes* by means of which all creeping ulcers are healed."

[*Natural History* 30.39.116]

It is not known what Pliny was referring to here because the Greek word meant only the inflammatory disease. He may have meant some sort of snake because the Latin noun *serpēns, serpentis* (Latin, *serpere*, creep) meant a serpent or snake. The etymological identity between the Latin and Greek verbs *serpere* and *herpein*, both meaning creep, would not have been lost on Pliny.

Cognate† words in Latin and Greek, if they show an initial *s-* in Latin, will show an initial "h" sound (the so-called rough breathing)‡ in Greek. Compare Latin *sēmi-* and Greek *hēmi-* (half); Latin *sex* and Greek *hex* (six); Latin *sūdor* (sweat) and Greek *hydor* (water), and so forth. The name for the acute infectious skin disease **herpes zoster** comes from the Greek noun *herpēs* plus the Greek *zōstēr* (belt). Herpes zoster is more commonly called shingles, from the Latin verb *cingere* (gird) with a noun *cingulum* (belt) formed from the verb. The word entered English through Old French *chengle*, with the alternate forms *cengle* and *sangle*. This skin infection was named by the ancient Greek physician Hippocrates because of the serpent-like scaly eruption and inflammation that generally encircles the trunk of the body. The varicella zoster virus causes shingles; it is the same virus that causes chickenpox. Shingles can affect people of any age, although it generally makes its unwelcome appearance in adulthood. There is no cure for shingles, but prompt intervention with prescription antiviral drugs, such as acyclovir, can speed healing and reduce complications.

Although there might seem to be no relationship between the trachea, a cartilaginous tube that connects the larynx to the bronchi of the lungs, and **trachoma,** an eye disease that has blinded millions of people, particularly in Asia and Africa, both terms are from the Greek adjective *trachys* (rough). The trachea is so named because of the rings of cartilage that surround it, giving that organ its characteristic rough surface. Trachoma is caused by the microorganism *Chlamydia trachomatis* (Greek *chlamys*, cloak) and is a form of conjunctivitis. It manifests itself by the presence of follicles (diminutive of Latin *follis*, bag), small secretory sacs that become hypertrophic and cause scarring of the palpebral conjunctiva. Ulceration of the cornea often ensues from secondary bacterial infections, which ultimately causes blindness.

Myopia, nearsightedness, does not take its name from Greek *mys*, muscle (with the combining form MY-) but from the verb *myein* meaning close or shut, for the characteristic squinting of those affected with myopia in an attempt to see more clearly.

The pupil of the eye was so called by the ancient Romans because the reflection seen by one looking at the pupil of another's eye appeared like a little dot (Latin *pūpilla*). The Greek word *korē* (girl, doll) was used by both Hippocrates and Galen to name the pupil of the eye. The combining form CORE-, coreometry, coreoplasty, is from *korē*.

Galen used the word iris to refer to the iris of the eye; Pliny used it to refer to a precious stone. But to the ancient Greeks and Romans, Iris was the many-hued goddess of the rainbow, who acted as a special messenger for both the king and the queen of the gods (Fig. 13-4). We meet her in

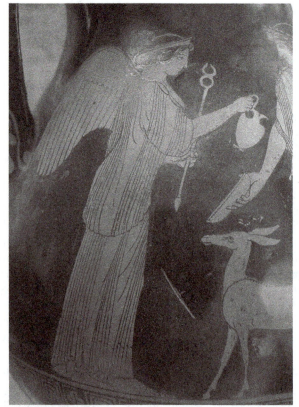

Figure 13-4. Iris, goddess of the rainbow. (Courtesy of Bibliothèque nationale de France.)

---

*Daviel's method was explained in an article in the Annals of the Royal Academy of Surgery (Paris), *Sur une nouvelle méthode de guérir la cataracte par l'extraction du cristallin*, in 1753.

†Just as the vocabularies of modern French, Spanish, Italian, and the other Romance languages are derived from Latin, so the vocabularies of Latin, ancient Greek, Sanskrit, and related ancient languages were derived from an earlier parent language, which we call Indo-European. Words in two (or more) Indo-European languages, each derived from the same presumed Indo-European word, are called cognates.

‡See Lesson 1 for a discussion of rough breathing.

Virgil's *Aeneid* at the end of the fourth book. The Phoenician queen Dido, exiled from her homeland, founded the city of Carthage in North Africa. In despair because her lover, Aeneas, deserted her after a year of intimacy, Dido attempted to take her own life by falling upon her sword. But her spirit would not leave her because Proserpina, the queen of the Underworld, had not taken a lock of hair from her head in order to permit her to enter the realms of the dead. Juno, the queen of the immortals, took pity on her and sent Iris to release her struggling soul from her body.

Ergo Iris croceis per caelum roscida pinnis,
mille trahens varios adverso sole colores,
devolat et supra caput adstitit. "Hunc ego Diti

sacrum iussa fero teque isto corpore solvo":
sic ait et dextra crinem secat; omnis et una
dilapsus calor atque in ventos vita recessit.

And Iris, all covered with dew, flew down
from heaven on saffron wings, trailing
a thousand colors reflected in the
rays of the sun, and stood above her head.
"As I have been ordered, I take this offering sacred to Dis*
and free you from your body."
So Iris spoke, and
with her hand cut the lock of hair.
All of a sudden the warmth left her,
and life faded into the winds.

(Aeneid 4.700–705)

Exercise 1: Analyze and Define

Analyze and define each of the following words. In this and in succeeding exercises, analysis should consist of separating the words into prefixes (if any), combining forms, and suffixes or suffix forms (if any) and giving the meaning of each. Be certain to differentiate between nouns and adjectives in your definitions. Consult a medical dictionary for the current meanings of these words.

1. achromatopsia _____

2. amblyopia _____

3. aphacia _____

4. astigmatism _____

5. binocular _____

6. blepharoptosis _____

7. blepharostat _____

8. chloropia _____

9. choroid _____

10. choroidoiritis _____

11. chromatoptometry _____

12. conjunctivoma _____

---

*Dis is another name for Hades or Pluto, king of the underworld.

13. corelysis _____

14. coreoplasty _____

15. cyclokeratitis _____

16. dacryocystorhinostomy _____

17. enophthalmos _____

18. erythropia _____

19. herpes facialis _____

20. herpetic _____

21. heterochromia iridis _____

22. hypermetropia _____

23. iridalgia _____

24. iridectropium _____

25. iridocystectomy _____

26. isocoria _____

27. keratomalacia _____

28. keratoprosthesis _____

29. lacrimation _____

30. macropsia _____

31. microphakia _____

32. micropsia _____

33. myopia _____

34. nasolacrimal _____

35. nyctamblyopia _____

36. ocularist _____

37. ophthalmologist _____

38. ophthalmoplegia _____

39. optometrist _____

40. orthoptic _____

41. presbyopia _____

42. purulent conjunctivitis _____

43. retinodialysis _____

44. rhinodacryolith _____

45. stigmatic _____

46. symblepharon _____

47. synoptoscope _____

48. varicoblepharon _____

49. xeropthalmia _____

50. xerostomia _____

Exercise 2: Word Derivation

Give the word derived from Greek or Latin elements that matches each of the following. Verify your answer in a medical dictionary. **Note that the wording of a dictionary definition may vary from the wording used here.**

1. Corneal rupture _____

2. Double vision _____

3. (Congenital) absence of all or part of the iris _____

4. Imperfect color vision _____

5. Absence of the (crystalline) lens of the eye _____

6. Inability to see well (in a faint light or at night) _____

7. Vision in which all objects appear to be blue _____

8. Discharge from the eye _____

9. Pertaining to tears _____

10. Narrowing of the pupil _____

11. Herpes of the eye _____

12. Excision of a portion of the cornea _____

13. Concerning the eyes and the face _____

14. Plastic surgery upon the eyelid _____

15. Concerning or affecting one eye _____

16. Resembling herpes _____

17. Paralysis of the ciliary muscle _____

18. (Roughness and) dryness of the skin _____

19. Pertaining to the retina and choroid _____

20. Protrusion of (a portion of) the iris _____

Exercise 3:   Drill and Review

Analyze and define each of the following words. Analysis should consist of separating the words into prefixes (if any), combining forms, and suffixes or suffix forms (if any) and giving the meaning of each. Be certain to differentiate between nouns and adjectives in your definitions. Using the elements in the word determine its meaning. Consult a medical dictionary for the current meanings of these words. Use a separate paper if you need more room for an answer.

1. abdominocentesis _____

2. alloantigen _____

3. antihydrotic _____

4. astigmia _____

5. astigmometer _____

6. blepharodiastasis _____

7. blepharotomy _____

8. brachiocephalic _____

9. capnography _____

10. chondroplasty _____

11. choroiditis _____

12. choroidocyclitis _____

13. conjunctiva _____

14. conjunctivoplasty _____

15. corectopia _____

16. coremorphosis _____

17. cyclectomy _____

18. cyclochoroiditis _____

19. dacryocystitis _____

20. dentolabial _____

21. dysopsia _____

22. ergonomics _____

23. erythropsia _____

24. flexile _____

25. herpes labialis _____

26. herpesvirus _____

27. hyperopia _____

28. immunotoxin _____

29. infusion _____

30. intubation _____

31. intumescent _____

32. iridemia _____

33. iridopathy _____

34. keratocele _____

35. keratomycosis _____

36. lachrymal _____

37. lachrymation _____

38. myope _____

39. oculonasal _____

40. oculoplastics _____

41. ophthalmodynamometry _____

42. ophthalmoscope _____

43. optogram _____

44. optometry _____

45. osmesthesia _____

46. posterolateral _____

47. sonic _____

48. synopsis _____

49. synoptophore _____

50. xerography _____

FEMALE REPRODUCTIVE SYSTEM

It is not easy for large creatures, whether animal or anything else, to reach full development in a short time. For this reason, horses and similar animals, although their life span is shorter than that of humans, have a longer period of gestation. The birth of horses occurs after a year; but in humans it is about ten months. For the same reason, birth takes a long time in elephants, whose gestation period is two years because of their great size.

[Aristotle, *Generation of Animals* 777b]

GYNECOLOGY

The principal organs of the female reproductive system are the **ovaries, fallopian tubes, uterus,** and **vagina.** The ovaries are two almond-shaped glands lying on either side of the cavity of the pelvis. The ovaries produce ova (Latin, plural of *ōvum*, egg) and hormones. These hormones, which include estrogen and progesterone, are responsible for the development and maintenance of female secondary sexual characteristics and the regulation of the menstrual cycle.

Within each ovary are hundreds of thousands of structures called **follicles** (*Latin folliculus*, diminutive of *follis*, bag), each consisting of epithelial cells surrounding a primitive ovum, the oogonium, which develops into an oocyte, and then into an ovum (Fig. 14-1). Approximately every 28 days during a woman's childbearing years, a single ovum matures and is released from the ovaries. This process, called **ovulation,** occurs about 14 days before each menstrual period. The mature ovum enters the fallopian tube and is transported toward the uterus. If sperm are present, the ovum may become fertilized; if not, the ovum degenerates and passes out of the body with the next menstruation.

Shortly after the follicle expels its ovum, the mass of cells of the follicle changes into a yellowish body called the **corpus luteum** (Latin *corpus*, body, and *lūteus*, yellow). If fertilization occurs, the corpus luteum forms a mass of cells in the ovary and produces the hormone progesterone. Progesterone's role is to improve blood and oxygen flow and support the growth of the uterus during the first 7 to 9 weeks of pregnancy. At about 10 weeks postfertilization, the corpus luteum begins to decrease in size and is gradually replaced by connective tissue.* If the ovum is not fertilized, the corpus luteum degenerates.

The two fallopian tubes, also called **oviducts** (often with the combining form OOPHOR- or SALPING-, from Greek *salpinx*, tube), extend from the uterus to each ovary. Their purpose is to transport the mature ovum from the ovary to the uterus, and spermatozoa from the uterus toward the ovary each month. The union of the ovum and sperm—fertilization—normally occurs in the fallopian tube. The fertilized ovum, or **zygote** (Greek *zygōtos*, yoked, from *zygon*, yoke), implants in the uterus and develops into the embryo. Occasionally, the zygote remains in the fallopian tube resulting in a tubal, or ectopic, pregnancy.

---

*Corpus luteum and the menstrual cycle. *MedicalNewsToday*. https://www.medical newstoday.com/articles/320433#corpus-luteum-and-the-menstrual-cycle. Accessed May 5, 2021.

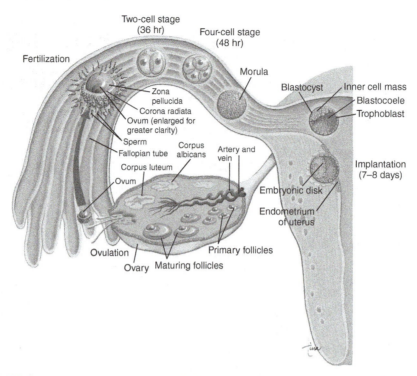

Figure 14-1. Human ovum. (From Ward, S. L., and Hisley, S. M. *Maternal-Child Nursing Care*, F.A. Davis, 2009, with permission.)

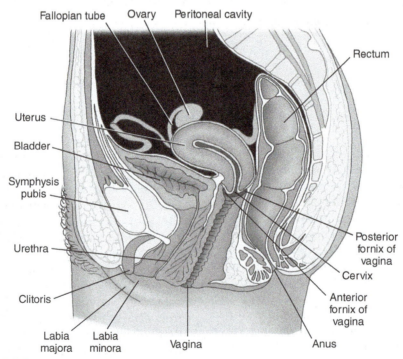

Figure 14-2. Female genital organs. Midsagittal section. (From Scanlon, V. C., and Sanders, T., *Essentials of Anatomy and Physiology*, 7th ed. F. A. Davis, 2015, p. 508, with permission.)

The uterus, or womb, is a hollow, muscular, pear-shaped and pear-sized organ that lies in the true pelvis between the bladder and rectum (Fig. 14-2). It consists of three parts: the **fundus** (Latin *fundus*, base, foundation) or uppermost portion; the **corpus** (Latin *corpus*, body), or central area; and the **endocervix,** the lowermost portion of the uterus, which opens into the vagina. The mucous membrane lining the inner surface of the uterus is called the endometrium

(Greek *mētra*, uterus); the muscular wall of the endometrium forming its main mass is called the myometrium. During a woman's childbearing years, from the beginning of menstruation (menarche) to the end (menopause), the uterine endometrium passes through the cyclic changes of menstruation each month.

The menstrual cycle consists of four phases: the menses; the proliferative phase, or follicular phase; the ovulatory phase; and the secretory phase, or luteal phase. During the proliferative phase, the endometrial lining proliferates, or thickens, in response to the main hormone of this phase, estrogen. In the ovulatory phase, the proliferative endometrium is transformed into the secretory endometrium at the time of ovulation. During the secretory phase, the endometrium is stabilized and prepared to receive the fertilized embryo. If the ovum is not fertilized and does not implant in the uterus, the lining of the endometrial cavity sloughs off through the endocervix and vagina (i.e., menstruation).

At birth, the inner lining of the endometrium, the decidua (Latin *dēciduus*, falling down, from *cadere*, fall), is shed. During pregnancy, the decidua basilis (New Latin, from Greek *basis*, base), the portion of the endometrium lying between the chorionic membrane enclosing the fetus and the myometrium, develops into the maternal portion of the placenta. Contractions of the uterine myometrium assist in expelling the fetus, placenta, and membranes.

The vagina (Greek *kolpos*, *koleon*, or *elytron*) is a muscular, membranous sheath extending from the cervix uteri to the vulva, the external genitalia. It serves as a passage for the entrance of the penis in coitus, for receiving semen, and for the discharge of the menstrual flow. It is the passageway, or birth canal, through which the fetus passes during labor and delivery.

The uterine cervix is the most inferior portion of the uterus and opens into the vagina. The **ectocervix** is the portion of the cervix visible through the vagina during gynecologic examination. **Dysplasia** of the cells of the ectocervix, if left untreated, can progress to cervical cancer. Human papillomavirus (HPV) infection is a known cause of cervical dysplasia. The **Papanicolaou test** (named for the Greek-born American scientist Nicholas Papanicolaou (1883–1962), commonly called a Pap test or Pap smear, is used to screen for the presence of cervical dysplasia. **Colposcopy** is a procedure used to evaluate abnormalities of the ectocervix.

VOCABULARY

If a woman is going to have a male child her complexion will be good; if a female child, her complexion will be bad.

[Hippocrates, *Aphorisms* 42]

The embryo of a male child is usually on the right and that of a female usually on the left.

[Hippocrates, *Aphorisms* 48]

Note: Latin combining forms are in **bold italics**.

Greek or Latin	Combining Form(s)	Meaning	Example
agōgos	**AGOG-**	leading, drawing forth	sial-**agog**-ue
archē	**ARCH-, -ARCHE**	beginning, origin	men-**arche**
cervix, cervīcis	***CERVIC-, CERVIX***	neck (of the uterus), cervix uteri	**cervic**-al
kolpos	**COLP-**	vagina	**colp**-oscopy
kyein	**CYE-**	be pregnant	**cye**-sis
eurynein	**EURY(N)-**	widen, dilate	an-**eury**-sm
gala, galaktos	**GAL-, GALACT-**	milk	**galact**-orrhea
(g)nascī, nātus	**-GN-, *NAT-***	be born	pre-**nat**-al
gonad*	**GONAD-**	sex glands, sex organs	**gonad**-otropin
gravidus†	***GRAVID-***	pregnant	primi-**gravid**-a
hymēn	**HYMEN-**	membrane; hymen	**hymen**-al
hystera	**HYSTER-**	uterus	**hyster**-ectomy
lac, lactis	***LACT-***	milk	**lact**-ation
mamma	***MAMM-***	breast	**mamm**-ography
mastos	**MAST-, MAZ-‡**	breast	**mast**-ectomy
mēn	**MEN-**	[month] menstruation	**men**-opause
mētra	**METR-, -METRA**	uterus	**metr**-itis
oophoron§	**OOPHOR-**	ovary	**oophor**-ectomy
ōvārium¶	***OVARI-***	ovary	**ovari**-an
ōvum	***OV-***	egg	**ov**-iduct
parere, partus	***PART-, -PARA***	give birth**	primi-**para**

*The word *gonad* did not exist in Greek or Latin; it is a modern formation as if from a Greek *gonas, gonados*, probably derived from the noun *gonē* (birth).
†The adjective *gravidus*, in the feminine singular form, gravida, was used as a noun to mean a pregnant woman.
‡In Greek *mazos* was an alternate form of the word *mastos:* micromazia.
§The compound word *oophoron* did not exist in Greek. It is a modern formation from Greek (*ōon*, egg, and *phor-*, from *pherein*, bear, carry)
¶ The word *ōvārium* did not exist in Latin, although there is a rare word, *ōvārius*, found only in an inscription, meaning an egg-keeper, that is, one who takes charge of newly laid eggs (Latin *ōvum*). The Latin suffix *-arium* meant "a place (for something)"; thus, *ōvārium*, "a place for the ovum," is a valid formation. Such formations are called New Latin.
**Words ending in -para indicate a woman who has given birth: primipara (Latin *prīmus*, first); nullipara (Latin *nullus*, none).

Greek or Latin	Combining Form(s)	Meaning	Example
pelvis	*PELV-*	[basin] pelvis	**pelv**-ic
pūbēs	*PUB-*	[signs of manhood] pubic hair, pubic bone, pubic region, pubis	**pub**-ic
pūbertās	*PUBER(T)-*	[manhood] puberty	**puber**-al
salpinx, salpingos	**-SALPING, -SALPINX**	[war trumpet] fallopian tube	**salping**-ography
syrinx, syringos	**SYRING-, -SYRINX**	[pipe] fistula, cavity, oviduct, sweat glands, syringe	**syring**-e
thēlē	**THEL(E)-**	nipple	**thel**-ium
tokos	**TOC-**	childbirth, labor	**toc**-olytic
uterus	*UTER-*	womb, belly, uterus	**uter**-ine
vāgīna	*VAGIN-*	[sheath] vagina	**vagin**-itis

ETYMOLOGICAL NOTES

The Amazons, legendary warrior women of Asia Minor, were said to have one breast removed so as not to interfere with the use of the bow; thus, their name: *a-mazon*. The Amazon River was discovered in 1500 by the Spanish explorer Vincente Pinzón, who named it *Rio Santa Maria de la Mar Dulce*. The first descent of the river from the Andes Mountains to the sea was made in 1541 by Francisco de Orellana, who renamed it the *Amazonas* from a battle that he and his followers had with a fierce tribe whose women fought alongside the men. de Orellana may have thought that these were indeed the Amazons described by the Greek writers.

The word *hymen* meant any of a variety of membranes; various writers used it to designate the pericardium, the peritoneum, the membrane that enclosed the brain, the nictitating (Late Latin* *nictitāre, nictitātus,* blink, wink) membrane (a third eyelid present in birds and some reptiles), parchment, and so forth. The ancients seem not to have used the word hymen in its modern anatomical meaning.

In Greek mythology, Hymen was the god of marriage and weddings, often invoked in a wedding song, *Hymenaeus,* the Hymeneal. In his great poem, the *Metamorphoses,* Ovid recites the story of a wedding that was attended by the god Hymen, but one to which he failed to bring his customary auspices. The bridegroom and bride were Orpheus and Eurydice (Fig. 14-3). Ovid tells us that the wedding torches of Hymen sputtered and smoked. However much they were swung about, they failed to blaze. In further witness of this ill-starred wedding, as Eurydice was crossing the lawn, she was bitten on the ankle by a poisonous serpent and perished on the spot. In the hope of being reunited with Eurydice, Orpheus went to the underworld and sang so persuasively to Hades and Proserpina, the rulers there, that he was permitted to lead his bride back to the upper

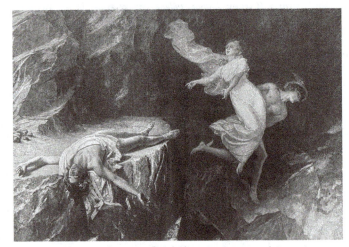

Figure 14-3. Orpheus and Eurydice. (Courtesy of Getty Images, clu, DigitalVision Vectors)

world. But, at the last moment, he failed to follow his instructions and looked back to make certain that Eurydice was following him. She was, indeed, but no sooner had he looked back than she turned and retraced her steps to the world of the dead.

Bracchiaque intendens prendique et prendere certans
nil nisi cedentes infelix arripit auras.
Iamque iterum moriens non est de coniuge quicquam
questa suo (quid enim nisi se quereretur amatam?).
Supremumque "vale," quod iam vix auribus ille
acciperet, dixit revolutaque rursus eodem est.

Stretching out his arms to embrace her and to feel her embrace he, unhappy one, grasped nothing but the empty air. And now, again dying, she had no complaint against her husband (for what could she complain of except that she had been loved?). Uttering a last *vale,* which he could scarcely hear she slipped back to that place she had just left.

[Ovid, *Metamorphoses* 10.58–63]

---

*Latin of the third and fourth centuries AD is usually called Late Latin.

The ancient Greeks believed that women were especially susceptible to emotional disorders and that these disorders arose from the womb. Galen used the word *hysterikos* (hysterical), and seems to have used it to refer to suffering in the womb and the emotional upheaval caused by this distress. Hippocrates says,

> When a woman suffers from hysterics or difficult labor, it is a good thing to sneeze.

[*Aphorisms* 5.35]

Two oviducts—the fallopian tubes—convey the ovum from the ovary to the uterus. The fallopian tubes were named for Gabriele Falloppio (1523–1562), an Italian anatomist who discovered the existence and the purpose of the ovaries and the tubes that bear his name. Like his teacher, Andreas Vesalius (1514–1564), the most important figure in European medicine after Galen and before Harvey, Falloppio was accused of vivisection of humans in his enthusiasm for research.

Another name for the fallopian tubes is the salpingian tubes, a term that is also used for the eustachian tubes of the ear (named for the 16th-century Italian anatomist Bartolommeo Eustachio). These two sets of tubes are named salpingian from the Greek word *salpinx, salpingos* (war trumpet) because of their shape. The common medical terminology for a complete hysterectomy, or removal of the uterus, fallopian tubes, and ovaries, is total abdominal hysterectomy bilateral salpingo-oophorectomy (TAH BSO).

The combining forms *syring-* and *-syrinx* have varied meanings in medicine but usually refer to a cavity or hollow area, a fistula, or some other tubelike passage. **Syringomyelia** is a disease of the spinal cord characterized by the development of cavities in the surrounding tissues. Syringectomy is the removal of the walls of a fistula. A syringocele is the central canal of the myelon or spinal cord. A **syringe** is an instrument for injecting fluids into body cavities, tissue, and vessels.

In Greek, the *syrinx* was the shepherd's pipe, or pipes of Pan. Ovid, in the *Metamorphoses*, tells how the pipes of Pan came into existence (Fig. 14-4).

> Once upon a time, there lived on the mountain slopes of Arcadia in Greece a young, beautiful woodland nymph named Syrinx. One day, Pan, that rustic divinity, saw Syrinx and pursued her. Pan almost caught the unwilling nymph when she prayed to her sisters for help. Pan caught her, but when he clutched her in his arms, he found that he held only a bunch of reeds. While Pan sighed over his disappointment, his breath blowing through the reeds made a pleasing sound. He bound a number of the reeds of unequal length together and called them the syrinx, the pipes of Pan.

> *"Hoc mihi concilium tecum" dixisse "manebit,"*
> *atque ita disparibus calamis conpagine cerae*
> *inter se iunctis nomen tenuisse puellae.*

> "This union with you, at least, will remain,"
> he said. And so pipes made of unequal
> lengths of reeds joined together with wax
> still keep the name of the nymph, *Syrinx*.

[Ovid, *Metamorphoses* 1.710–712]

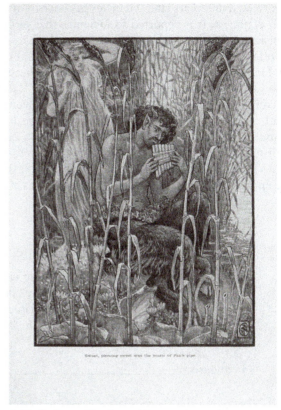

Sweet, piercing sweet was the music of Pan's pipe.

Figure 14-4. Pan with pipes of Pan.

Forms ending in **-agogue** entered English in the 14th century in words borrowed from Old French. Some of these words, like pedagogue and synagogue, had existed in Latin (*paedagōgous* and *synagōga*) and were borrowed from Greek (*paidagōgós*, a slave who took children to school or who taught them at home, and *synagōgē*, a place for gathering). The Greek words *agōgos* and *agōgē* are ultimately derived from the verb *agein* (lead, drive), which is cognate with the Latin verb *agere, actus*, with the same meanings. Words ending in -agogue usually refer to agents used to promote the flow or secretion of fluids within the body. A **sialagogue** is an agent that increases the flow of saliva.

The word **dyspareunia,** painful intercourse, has an interesting etymology. It is derived from the adjective *dyspareunos* (dys-, unpleasant, painful, and *pareunos*, a lying with or beside, from *para-*, alongside, and *eunazesthai*, go to bed) that meant "ill- or badly mated." This adjective is found in Greek literature in a passage describing a bed.

In Sophocles' tragedy *Trachiniae* (*Women of Trachis*, lines 794ff), Hyllus, the son of the great Heracles, has come to the city of Trachis to report to Deianira, wife of Heracles, that her husband is dying just outside of the city. Heracles' flesh had been burned away by a magic cloak that Deianira sent to him in ignorance of its dread powers. This cloak had been given to Deianira many years before by the centaur Nessus, whom Heracles had killed after he attempted violence on Deianira, then Heracles' bride. The centaur, dying, gave his cloak to the young bride and told her to give it to Heracles if she ever felt that his affections were fading. Now, many years later, Heracles has been away on a foreign conquest. It is reported to Deianira that he is on the outskirts of the city and has requested a cloak to wear when offering sacrifices to the gods for a successful campaign. He brought back with him as his prize the beautiful Iole, an Oechalian princess.

Deianira sent him the cloak that Nessus had given her, mindful of his advice. The cloak burned into the hero's flesh and, as he lay dying in the greatest agony, he cursed his "ill-mated" wedding bed *(dyspareunon lektron)* and Deianira herself. Zeus, at length, rescued him from his suffering and brought him up to Mount Olympus as a god,

with Hebe, the daughter of Zeus and Hera, as his companion for eternity.

Epithelium (Greek *epi-*, over, *thēlē*, nipple) is the layer of cells that forms the epidermis of the skin and the surface of mucous and serous membranes. It was first discovered by the German histologist Jacob Henle (1809–1885). It is not clear why this type of tissue was named "membrane over the nipple" except for the fact that epithelial tissue does cover the nipple of the breast. **Endothelium,** the layer of cells that lines the vessels and organs of the cardiovascular system, was named by the Swiss physician Wilhelm His (1831–1904).

Exercise 1:   Analyze and Define

Analyze and define each of the following words. In this and in succeeding exercises, analysis should consist of separating the words into prefixes (if any), combining forms, and suffixes or suffix forms (if any) and giving the meaning of each. Be certain to differentiate between nouns and adjectives in your definitions. Consult a medical dictionary for the current meanings of these words.

1. aneurism _____

2. antenatal _____

3. antepartum _____

4. celiohysterectomy _____

5. cervicovaginitis _____

6. cholagogue _____

7. colpocystocele _____

8. cyesis _____

9. endometrium _____

10. extrauterine _____

11. galactorrhea _____

12. gonadal dysgenesis _____

13. gynecoid pelvis _____

14. gynecomastia _____

15. hematosalpinx _____

16. hydrocolpos _____

17. hymenal _____

18. hymen septate _____

19. hyperemesis gravidarum _____

20. hysterosalpingography _____

21. hysterotrachelorrhaphy _____

22. inframammary _____

23. intrauterine _____

24. lactation _____

25. lactobacillus _____

26. mammogram _____

27. mastalgia _____

28. menarche _____

29. multigravida _____

30. neonatology _____

31. oligomenorrhea _____

32. oophoritis _____

33. opthalmia neonatorum _____

34. ovariotomy _____

35. oviduct _____

36. ovogenesis _____

37. pedagogy _____

38. pelvimetry _____

39. postpartum _____

40. pregnant _____

41. prepubescent _____

42. pubarche _____

43. puberty _____

44. pyosalpinx _____

45. syringoencephalomyelia _____

46. thelarche _____

47. tocodynamometer _____

48. uteropexy _____

49. uterotubal _____

50. vaginolabial _____

Exercise 2:   Word Derivation

Give the word derived from Greek and/or Latin elements that means each of the following. Verify your answer in a medical dictionary. **Note that the wording of a dictionary definition may vary from the wording used here.**

1. Inflammation of the cervix uteri _____

2. Pain in the vagina _____

3. Before birth _____

4. Surgical removal of one or both ovaries _____

5. Having the shape of an egg _____

6. Excision of the entire uterus _____

7. Pertaining to the pelvis _____

8. (Painful) spasms of the vagina _____

9. Instrument for examining the uterine cavity _____

10. Pertaining to a quick or sudden birth _____

11. Newborn infant (up to one month of age) _____

12. Inflammation (or infection) of the breast _____

13. (Occurring) after childbirth _____

14. Tumor of the sweat glands _____

15. Pertaining to the uterus and the cervix _____

16. Surgical removal of the breast _____

17. Substance that stimulates milk production _____

18. Period after puberty _____

19. Absence of menstruation _____

20. Pertaining to (the flow of) milk _____

Exercise 3:   Drill and Review

Analyze and define each of the following words. Analysis should consist of separating the words into prefixes (if any), combining forms, and suffixes or suffix forms (if any) and giving the meaning of each. Be certain to differentiate between nouns and adjectives in your definitions. Using the elements in the word determine its meaning. Consult a medical dictionary for the current meanings of these words. Use a separate paper if you need more room for an answer.

1. archenteron _____

2. astigmometer _____

3. cheirognostic _____

4. colpocystotomy _____

5. colpomicroscope _____

6. dysmenorrhea _____

7. endomastoiditis _____

8. endometriosis _____

9. expiration _____

10. galactopoiesis _____

11. gonadarche _____

12. gravida _____

13. hydrometra _____

14. hysterectomy _____

15. hysteromyoma _____

16. ileocystoplasty _____

17. ischidrosis _____

18. lactiferous _____

19. mammography _____

20. mastodynia _____

21. melanin _____

22. metritis _____

23. monocytopenia _____

24. natal _____

25. osmesthesia _____

26. ovariotubal _____

27. ovocyte _____

28. ovoid _____

29. oxytocin _____

30. partogram _____

31. pelves _____

32. poliovirus _____

33. polycythemia _____

34. prepuberal _____

35. prolactin _____

36. pseudoaneurysm _____

37. pseudophakia _____

38. psychopharmacology _____

39. quintipara _____

40. rectocele _____

41. retrocervical _____

42. retropubic _____

43. salpingo-oophoritis _____

44. salpingoscopy _____

45. sialagogue _____

46. sternomastoid _____

47. syringocarcinoma _____

48. thelium _____

49. tocolytic _____

50. vaginomycosis _____

GENITOURINARY SYSTEM

If a carbuncle forms on the penis, it should first be bathed with water through a syringe. Then it should be burned with a salve made of copper ore mixed with boiled honey, or with fried sheep's dung mixed with honey. When the carbuncle falls off, use the same salve for ulcers in the mouth.

[Celsus, *De Medicina* 6.18.5]

MALE REPRODUCTIVE SYSTEM

The principal organs of the male reproductive system are the **testes** (plural of testis) or **testicles,** the **epididymides** (plural of epididymis),* the **duct system,** the **penis,** and **accessory glands** (Fig. 15-1). The function of the male reproductive system is to manufacture sperm cells, or spermatozoa, and to convey these to the reproductive organs of the female through copulation. The two testes, the male gonads, are ovoid glands located in the scrotum that produce spermatozoa and the male hormone testosterone. Each testis is divided into numerous lobules, each containing one to three seminiferous tubules within which **spermatogenesis** takes place (Fig. 15-2).

The epididymis is a small structure located on the posterior surface of each testicle. It consists of a coiled mass of ducts enclosed within the tunica vaginalis. Spermatozoa are stored in the epididymides until they are released during ejaculation. From the epididymis, the sperm pass into the ductus deferens, or vas deferens. The two seminal vesicles located on either side of the prostate secrete a mucoid substance that empties into the ductus deferens at ejaculation. The prostate gland secretes a thin, opalescent, alkaline fluid that is added to the spermatozoa at ejaculation. The thick, sticky fluid containing the spermatozoa and the mixed product of the accessory glands, the prostate, and the seminal vesicles, is called **semen.** During ejaculation, semen passes into the ejaculatory duct, a short, narrow tube formed by the union of the ductus deferens and the excretory duct of the seminal vesicles. From there it travels into the **urethra,** a canal that extends from the bladder to the tip of the penis and serves as the passage for both urine and semen.

There are anywhere from 120 million to more than 500 million sperm in a normal amount of ejaculate (2 to 5 mL). The ejaculate must contain this large number of sperm for a single sperm to find and fertilize the ovum. When male sperm count falls substantially, infertility usually results.

During the development of the male fetus, the testes are lodged within the body. Before birth, in the late stages of fetal development, the testes descend into the scrotum. Spermatogenesis cannot occur in a testicle that remains within the body. Occasionally, this descent does not take place, or it occurs incompletely, so that one or both testes remain within the abdomen or somewhere along the line of descent. This is called **cryptorchidism,** or **undescended testes.** In 30% of premature and 3% of full-term male infants, one or both of the testicles will not have descended at birth. Most will descend spontaneously during the first 3 to 6 months of life; fewer than 1% of babies will have cryptorchidism by age 6 months.†

---

*From Greek *epi-*, upon, and *didymos*, testis.

†Undescended testicle (cryptorchidism). Harvard Health Publishing. https://www.health.harvard.edu/a_to_z/undescended-testicle-a-to-z. Published July 1, 2019. Accessed June 11, 2021.

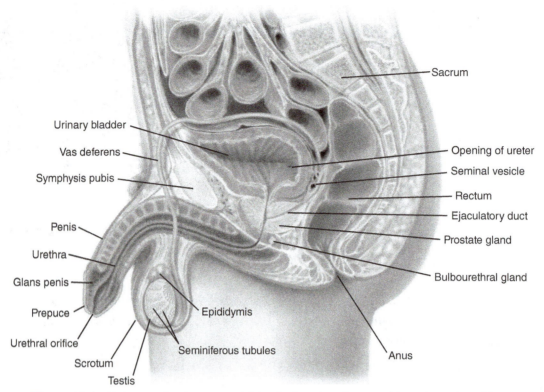

Figure 15-1. Male reproductive system. Midsagittal section. (From Gylys, B. A., and Wedding, M. E., *Medical Terminology Systems: A Body Systems Approach*, 8th ed. F. A. Davis, 2017, with permission.)

For infants who still have one or both testicles that remain in the abdomen, surgery is performed to relocate the undescended testicle or testicles into the scrotum. The surgeon sutures the undescended testicle to the tissue of the scrotum, a procedure called **orchidopexy** (formerly **orchiorrhaphy**).*

Damage or disease can destroy the epithelium of the seminiferous tubules of the testes.† Inflammation of one or both of the testes, called **orchitis** or **bilateral orchitis,** most commonly caused by mumps, may produce sufficient damage to result in sterility. Spermatogenesis is irreversibly damaged in 30% of cases of mumps orchitis. With the introduction of the mumps vaccine in 1967, the incidence of mumps orchitis in children has been reduced dramatically.‡ In postpuberty males, mumps is the most common cause of orchitis, affecting 20% to 30% of that population. Of those affected, 30% to 50% have some degree of testicular atrophy. Sexually transmitted diseases are also a cause of orchitis in this population.§

---

*Undescended testicle. Mayo Clinic. https://www.mayoclinic.org/diseases-conditions /undescended-testicle/diagnosis-treatment/drc-20352000. Accessed June 11, 2021.
†Seminiferous tubule. Science Direct. https://www.sciencedirect.com/topics/neuro science/seminiferous-tubule. Accessed June 6, 2021.
‡In 1971, the mumps vaccine was combined with measles and rubella as measles, mumps and rubella MMR.
§Orchitis. Mayo Clinic. https://www.mayoclinic.org/diseases-conditions/orchitis /symptoms-causes/syc-20375860. Published November 6, 2020. Accessed June 6, 2021.

URINARY SYSTEM

The kidneys are a pair of organs lying on the left and right side of the upper abdominal cavity behind the peritoneum. They are referred to as retroperitoneal organs (Fig. 15-3). By separating toxins from wastes, the kidneys filter wastes from the blood to maintain the proper acid-alkaline balance. End products of this process include the following: (1) those from proteins, mostly nitrogenous substances, such as urea and uric acid; (2) detoxified material from the liver, such as drugs, antibiotics, alcohol, and other toxins; (3) all substances in the circulating blood that are present in amounts greater than needed by the body, including sugars, alkalines, and acids; and (4) excess water.

On the medial side of each kidney is an indentation called the hilus. Three important structures enter each kidney at the hilus: the renal artery, the renal vein, and the ureter. After entering the hilus, the renal artery branches into smaller arteries that branch into arterioles. These arterioles enter the nephrons, the functional unit of the kidney. Each kidney contains about one million nephrons. Within each nephron is a cluster of capillaries called the **glomerulus.** The walls of these glomeruli comprise what is collectively called the glomerular membrane. Blood plasma passes through this membrane, with blood cells and most of the protein excluded. The fluid that passes through the glomerular membrane is called the glomerular filtrate.

The glomerular filtrate contains the metabolic wastes and other substances in amounts greater than are needed by the body for proper functioning. The glomerular filtrate also

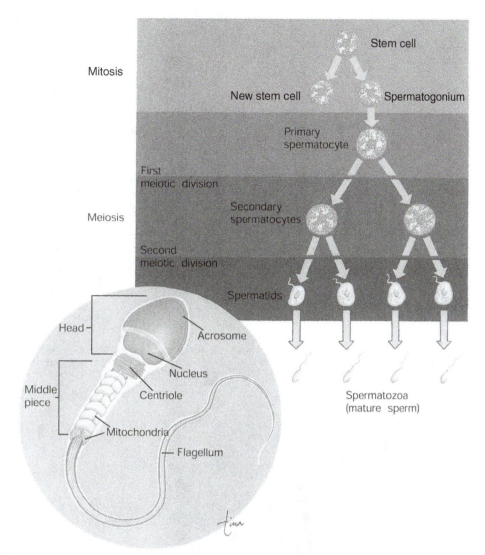

Figure 15-2. Spermatogenesis. (From Scanlon, V. C., and Sanders, T., *Essentials of Anatomy and Physiology*, 8th ed. F. A. Davis, 2017, with permission.)

contains substances the body needs, such as the small amount of protein that is not filtered out by the glomerular membrane, as well as glucose and certain salts and acids. These substances must be returned to the circulating blood. Within the nephron, the glomerular filtrate travels through a series of passages called tubules. All but a small portion of the glomerular filtrate is reabsorbed into the blood, first through the capillaries of the nephron, then into the venous system and the renal vein. The portion of glomerular filtrate that does not re-enter the circulating blood is made up of waste material. These wastes enter the large end of a funnel-shaped cavity in the hilus of the kidney called the renal pelvis. This fluid is now urine, which passes out of the renal pelvis into the ureter to be carried to the bladder. Kidney function is estimated by calculating the estimated Glomerular Filtration Rate (eGFR) using results from a patient's serum blood sample.

> Two veins, white in color, lead from the kidneys into the vesica; they are called by the Greeks ureters because they think that it is through them that the urine descends and flows into the vesica.
>
> [Celsus, *De Medicina* 4.1.10]

One ureter exits from each kidney. As urine enters the ureters, it is forced along by peristaltic contractions that occur at varying intervals from a few seconds to a few minutes. The urine enters the bladder through the ureteric orifices, which open to allow passage of the urine and then close to prevent a reflux. Renal calculi may occur in any location along the urinary tract. **Nephrolithiasis** (kidney stones) is a common renal disorder. The most common type of renal calculus, or stone, contains calcium oxalate. Factors that precipitate stone formation include **hypercalciuria, hyperoxaluria,** low urine volumes, dehydration and infections. Treatment for nephrolithiasis depends on the size of the kidney stone. For small stones, treatment may include drinking lots of water to dilute the urine, pain relievers to reduce discomfort, and alpha blockers to relax the muscles of the ureter and promote passing of the stone. More extensive treatments for large stones include sound waves to break up the stones and, if necessary, surgery, which involves using a "basket" to retrieve the large stone.*

---

*Kidney stones. Mayo Clinic. https://www.mayoclinic.org/diseases-conditions/kidney-stones/diagnosis-treatment/drc-20355759. Accessed June 17, 2021.

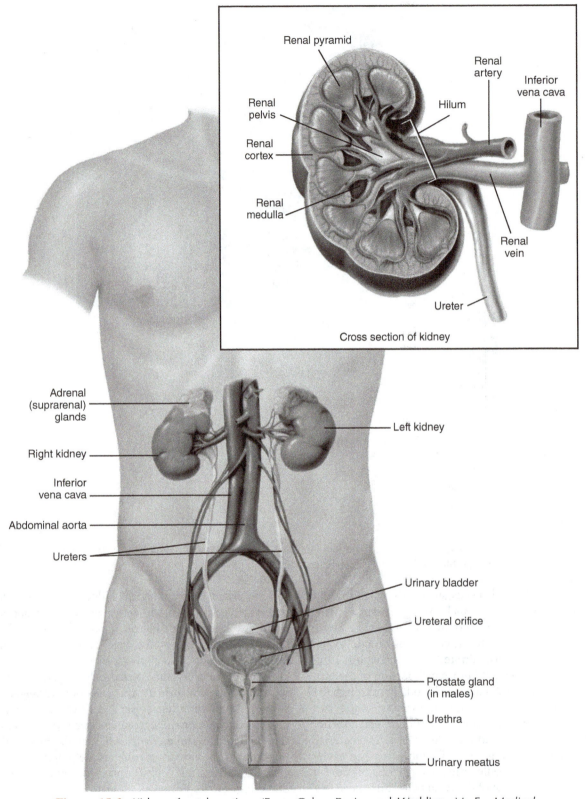

Figure 15-3. Kidney, frontal section. (From Gylys, B. A., and Wedding, M. E., *Medical Terminology Systems: A Body Systems Approach*, 8th ed. F. A. Davis, 2017, with permission.)

Urine is stored in the bladder until the volume reaches a certain amount. Then the internal and external urethral sphincters open to allow it to pass through the urethra. Emptying the bladder by passing urine through the urethra is called **micturition** (Latin *micturīre, micturītus,* urinate).

KIDNEY FUNCTION DISORDERS

Any damage to the kidneys that impairs their ability to filter metabolic wastes and toxins out of the blood results in abnormal kidney function, or renal insufficiency. Table 15-1 summarizes several causes of acute renal failure (ARF).

Table 15-1. **Causes of Acute Renal Failure**

Where	What's Responsible	Examples
Prerenal	Inadequate blood flow to the kidney	Severe dehydration; prolonged hypotension; renal ischemia or emboli; septic or cardiogenic shock
Renal	Injury to kidney glomeruli or tubules	Glomerulonephritis; toxic injury to the kidneys (e.g., by drugs or poisons)
Intrinsic Renal	Medical condition that obstructs urinary outflow	Kidney infections; blood clots in the kidney; medications such as rifampin, phenytoin, proton pump inhibitors; NSAIDs, such as ibuprofen.*

Source: From Venes, D., ed. *Taber's Cyclopedic Medical Dictionary*, 23rd ed. F. A. Davis, 2017, p. 888, with permission.
*What to know about acute renal failure. *MedicalNewsToday*. https://www.medicalnewstoday.com/articles/324627#causes. Reviewed March 5, 2019. Accessed June 15, 2021.

Some disorders are congenital. For example, in newborns, both kidneys may fail to form during gestation, a condition called **bilateral renal agenesis.** Without treatment, death will occur within a few days after birth. Unilateral agenesis in which one kidney forms is not necessarily fatal, as one kidney is sufficient to sustain life.

Acute loss of kidney function (ARF) often results immediately after kidney damage occurs and usually requires immediate admission to the intensive care unit. Serious kidney damage can result from (1) parenchymal damage to the kidney caused by toxins, such as contrast dye, or from infections, such as glomerulonephritis; (2) drugs, such as cyclosporine, angiotensin-converting enzyme (ACE) inhibitors for treating hypertension, or NSAIDs, all of which cause functional impairment; (3) decreased blood flow to the kidneys resulting in renal ischemia secondary to shock or dehydration; and (4) obstruction of the urinary outflow tract. Table 15-1 summarizes several causes of acute renal failure.

The immediate result of ARF is the rapid buildup of urea, uric acid, potassium, and other undesirable substances in the blood. The inability of the body to excrete nitrogenous wastes in urea and uric acid causes **uremia,** the rapid accumulation of metabolic by-products that normal kidneys excrete. **Azotemia** refers to increasing amounts of waste products, particularly urea, in the blood. **Hyperkalemia** results from abnormally high concentrations of potassium in the blood. Mild hyperkalemia can be treated with diuretics, diet, or dietary supplements. Severe hyperkalemia can cause severe cardiac dysfunction and requires immediate hospitalization and complete elimination of all potassium from the body.

Oliguria, urinary output less than 400 mL/day or 20 mL/hour, is present when daily urine volume is insufficient to remove the renal solute loads, which are the end products of metabolism. Oliguria results in ARF if not caught early and reversed.

Streptococcal infection, particularly in the respiratory tract, can result in acute glomerular nephritis, or **glomerulonephritis.** The infection itself does not damage the kidneys. The glomeruli react to antibodies the body makes to combat the infection and become inflamed. This causes malfunction of the nephrons, sometimes resulting in ARF. Usual symptoms of glomerulonephritis include **hematuria, proteinuria, albuminuria, oliguria,** red blood cell casts, pruritus, nausea, constipation, hypertension, and **edema.**

Rhabdomyolysis is a potentially fatal disease in which the by-products of skeletal muscle destruction accumulate in renal tubules, causing ARF. Rhabdomyolysis may result from crush injuries, toxic effects on skeletal muscles produced by drugs or chemicals, extremes of exertion, shock, sepsis, and severe hyponatremia (Greek, *hypo-*, deficient, New Latin, *natrium*, sodium, Greek, *haima*, blood). Rhabdomyolysis can also result from decreased concentration of sodium in the blood. Life-threatening hyperkalemia and metabolic acidosis may result from untreated rhabdomyolysis.

Inflammation of the renal pelvis is called **pyelitis,** but the disease invariably extends into the kidney itself, the renal parenchyma. The proper term for the disease when it affects both the pelvis and the body of the kidney is **pyelonephritis.** Almost any pyogenic bacterium can cause this disease, although in most cases, *Escherichia coli* is the responsible microbe. Prompt therapy with antibiotics is effective in most cases.† A health-care provider may request an x-ray to view the movement of blood through the renal veins. This procedure, called an **intravenous pyelogram** (IVP), involves injecting a radiopaque substance through the renal vein and taking a series of x-ray films to observe its progress. An IVP may reveal calculi, lesions, or deformities in the pelvic area.

Anemia is a disease associated with chronic renal insufficiency. **Erythropoietin** is a cytokine made by the kidneys that stimulates the proliferation of red blood cells. Insufficient kidney function results in insufficient erythropoietin production, with a consequent diminution in the number of erythrocytes. Synthetic erythropoietin is used to treat patients with anemia and renal failure.

RENAL DIALYSIS—THE ARTIFICIAL KIDNEY

In cases of kidney damage so severe that the kidneys cannot function efficiently enough to prevent fatal toxicity of the blood, renal dialysis may be initiated. Dialysis acts as an

†Herness J, Buttolph A, Hammer NC. Acute pyelonephritis in adults: rapid evidence review. *Am Fam Physician.* 2020;102(3):173-180. https://www.aafp.org/afp/2020/0801/p173.html. Accessed July 5, 2021.

artificial kidney with the filtering process occurring outside the body. The functional unit of the dialysis machine is a semipermeable membrane that allows all of the blood to flow through except erythrocytes and proteins. The circulating blood is withdrawn from the body via an artery, and is pumped through the dialysis machine, where it passes through the semipermeable membrane, leaving behind red cells and proteins. Once through the membrane, the plasma passes into a liquid called the dialyzing fluid, which contains most of the constituents of normal plasma except the waste products of metabolism, principally urea. The toxic wastes in the plasma diffuse into the dialyzing fluid and remain there when the plasma, now rid of most of the waste matter, is returned through the membrane into the body. To prevent coagulation of the blood in the artificial kidney, the anticoagulant heparin is infused into the blood before it enters the dialysis machine. Major advances in the science of renal dialysis now allow other forms of dialysis, such as continuous ambulatory peritoneal dialysis (CAPD), with improved outcomes and ease of administration.

DIABETES MELLITUS

Diabetes mellitus (DM) is a chronic disease characterized by the body's inability to metabolize carbohydrates. This is caused by inadequate production and secretion of insulin by the beta cells of the islets of Langerhans in the pancreas (named after Paul Langerhans, a German pathologist, 1847–1888). Another cause is resistance to the metabolic effects of insulin in the cells of the body. Manifestations of the disease are elevated blood sugar **(hyperglycemia)** and sugar in the urine **(glycosuria).** Symptoms include excessive thirst **(polydipsia),** excessive urination **(polyuria),** weight loss despite eating excessive amounts of food **(polyphagia),** and fatigue. When the course of diabetes is allowed to advance without proper treatment, diabetic ketoacidosis (DKA) and coma can result. DKA is characterized by severe nausea, vomiting, dyspnea, and delirium.

There are two types of diabetes mellitus (see Table 15-2). Type 1 diabetes mellitus, also called insulin-dependent diabetes mellitus (IDDM), is caused by insufficient insulin production. Type 1 diabetes mellitus was formerly known as juvenile diabetes because it begins early in life. Type 2 diabetes mellitus, called non–insulin-dependent diabetes mellitus (NIDDM), usually begins later in life and is characterized by resistance to the effects of insulin at the cellular level. Type 2 diabetes is by far the most common. Both types of diabetes lead to increased blood sugar levels.

For some patients with type 2 diabetes, the only treatment required is a well-balanced diet that is low in calories (1600 to 1800 calories per day) and carbohydrates. Tests for blood sugar (glucose) should be taken frequently. The development of Continuous Glucose Monitors (CGMs) greatly improves patient ability to monitor blood sugars. These devices are affixed to the skin and monitor blood glucose continuously, giving the patient readings every 10 minutes without the need for a fingerstick. If glucose concentration

Table 15-2. Comparison of Type 1 Insulin-Dependent Diabetes Mellitus and Type 2 Non–Insulin-Dependent Diabetes Mellitus

	Type 1	Type 2
Age at onset	Usually <30	Usually >40
Symptom onset	Abrupt	Gradual
Body weight	Normal	Obese (80%)
HLA association	Positive	Negative
Family history	Common	Nearly universal
Insulin in blood	Little to none	Some usually present
Islet cell antibodies	Present at onset	Absent
Prevalence	0.2% to 0.3%	6%
Symptoms	Polyuria, polydipsia, polyphagia, weight loss, ketoacidosis	Polyuria, polydipsia, peripheral neuropathy
Control	Insulin, diet, and exercise	Diet, exercise, and often oral hypoglycemic drugs or insulin
Vascular and neural changes	Eventually develop	Usually develop
Stability of condition	Fluctuates, may be difficult to control	May be difficult to control in poorly motivated

Source: From Venes, D., ed. *Taber's Cyclopedic Medical Dictionary*, 24th ed. F. A. Davis, 2021, p. 681, with permission.

remains high in the blood and urine, it may be necessary to prescribe medications, such as the sulfonylureas (or possibly newer medications), which stimulate the pancreas to release insulin. If blood glucose levels remain high after dietary modifications, it may be necessary to start medications to lower blood glucose levels. Older medications, such as the sulfonylureas (e.g., Glucotrol), increase the production of insulin in the pancreas but are used less frequently with the advent of newer oral agents. These newer agents have different mechanisms of actions to decrease blood glucose levels. Biguanides (e.g., Glucophage) inhibit the liver's release of glucose. Sodium-glucose co-transporter 2 (SGLT-2) inhibitors (e.g., Invokana) increase the kidney's removal of glucose through urination. Dipeptidyl peptidase-4 (DPP-4) inhibitors (e.g., Januvia) increase insulin production from the pancreas to decrease glucose levels. If oral agents do not control glucose levels, it may be necessary to start insulin therapy.

Insulin was discovered in 1921 by Canadian Drs. Frederick G. Banting, Charles H. Best, and James R. Macleod. For this discovery, Banting and Macleod were awarded the 1923 Nobel Prize in Medicine. This landmark discovery has made it possible for people with diabetes to lead normal lives. Synthetic forms of insulin have been created and may be administered to replace the insulin that is not produced by individuals with type 1 diabetes.

Insulin acts as a stimulant for the intracellular transport of glucose into tissue cells, affecting the utilization of sugar in the cell by increasing its conversion to glycogen and fat and its oxidation to carbon dioxide and water. Diminished production of insulin leads to decreased carbohydrate utilization, with consequent hyperglycemia. Without insulin, the tissue cells cannot get enough energy from food because the body's immune system begins attacking the insulin-producing beta cells in the pancreas. The beta cells become damaged, and the pancreas stops producing sufficient insulin to meet the body's needs. Diabetes is the leading cause of chronic renal failure and subsequent renal dialysis in the United States. It is also the leading cause of blindness in the United States. A report published in 2020 by the Centers for Disease Control and Prevention (CDC) estimated that 34.2 million people of all ages (10.5% of the US population) had diabetes; 34.1 million adults 18 years or older (13% of all US adults) had diabetes; the percentage of adults with diabetes increased with age, reaching 26.8% among those 65 years or older; 7.3 million adults 18 years or older (2.8% of all US adults) who met laboratory criteria for diabetes were not aware they had diabetes.*

The Greek word *diabētēs* is found in the medical writings of Galen and Aretaeus, both of the second century AD. The word *diabētēs* is from the verb *bainein* (go, walk, pass) and means "a passing through," a reference to the immoderate passage of urine affecting people who have this disease.

National Diabetes Statistics Report, 2020. Centers for Disease Control and Prevention. https://www.cdc.gov/diabetes/pdfs/data/statistics/national-diabetes-statistics-report.pdf. Accessed July 7, 2021.

VOCABULARY

Note: Latin combining forms are shown in **bold italics**.

Greek or Latin	Combining Form(s)	Meaning	Example
aktis, aktinos	**ACTIN-**	[ray] radiation	**actin**-ogenic
agra†	**-AGRA**	[hunting] (sudden) pain, gout	chir-**agra**
cortex, corticis	***CORTIC-, CORTEX***	[bark, rind] outer layer (of an organ)	adrenal **cortex**
kry(m)os‡	**CRY(M)-**	icy cold	**cry**-otherapy
glykys	**GLYC-**	sugar	hypo-**glyc**-emia
inguen, inguinis	***INGUIN-***	groin	**inguin**-al
lagneia	**-LAGNIA**	abnormal sexual excitation or gratification	algo-**lagnia**
orchis, orchios	**ORCHI(D)-,§ ORCH(E)-**	testicle	mon-**orchid**
pēnis	***PEN-***	[tail] penis	**pen**-ile
phallos	**PHALL-**	penis	**phall**-ic
pyelos	**PYEL-**	renal pelvis	**pyel**-onephritis
rhabdos	**RHABD-**	rod	**rhabd**-omyolysis
scrōtum	***SCROT-***	[bag] scrotum	**scrot**-a
sēmen, sēminis	***SEM-, SEMIN-***	seed, semen	in-**semin**-ation
sperma, spermatos	**SPERM(AT)-**	seed, sperm, semen	**sperm**-icide
ouron	**UR-**	urine, urinary tract, uric acid¶	**ur**-ine
ourētēr	**URETER-**	ureter	**ureter**-ostomy
ourēthra	**URETHR-**	urethra	**urethr**-itis
vēsīca	**VESIC-**	(urinary) bladder	**vesic**-ocele
zōon	**ZO-**	animal, organism	**zo**-ophyte

†See the Etymological Notes in this lesson.
‡There are two forms of this word in Greek: *kryos* and *krymos*, with the same meaning.
§The combining form orchid- is used as if from a genitive case *orchidos;* the -d- dropped out of this word in the Greek language, leaving the genitive case *orchios*, with an alternate form *orcheōs*.
¶Words beginning with, ending with, or containing uric- indicate the presence of uric acid, an acid that is formed as an end product of purine (protein) digestion. Uric acid is a common constituent of renal calculi and of the concretions of gout.

VESICLE

The word vesicle, as well as words beginning in vesicul-, is a modern formation (New Latin) as a diminutive of *vēsīca*; these words mean either (1) a small sac containing fluid, especially a seminal vesicle, or (2) a small, blister-like elevation on the skin containing serous fluid, as in the word vesicopustular.

ETYMOLOGICAL NOTES

The word kalium, the chemical name for the element potassium, was formed from the Arabic word *qali*, the name of the plant known in English as saltwort, from the ashes of which potash was made. Sir Humphry Davy (1778–1829) first separated potassium from potash, which previously had been considered an element, and gave it the name potassium. The Swedish chemist Jons Jacob Berzelius (1779–1848) coined the name *kalium* and applied it to the newly isolated element. Such formations are called New Latin. The word alkali is from the Arabic *al-qaliy*, the calcined ashes of the *qali* plant.

The Greek word *nitron* and the Latin *nitrum* were probably borrowed from the Arabic *natrun* (sodium carbonate). The origin of the word most likely occurred in Egypt after Alexander the Great conquered the region Nitriotes, the Greek name for the district where *nitron* was found in great quantities. Nitron is found in the Old Testament in Jeremiah 2.22 as the Hebrew word *nether*. In the King James version, the prophet says, "For though thou wash thee with nitre, and take thee much sope, yet thine iniquity is marked before me, saith the Lord God." The Hebrew word *nether* in the Old Testament is translated as *nitron* in the Septuagint and *nitrum* in the Vulgate.

The first use of the word nitrogen originated *nitrogène* in a 1790 work by French chemist Jean Chaptal (1756–1832). Antoine Lavoisier (1743–1794) recognized that this gas, which had been discovered as one of the elements of the atmosphere by the British scientist Daniel Rutherford, would not support life. For this reason, Lavoisier, in 1778, named the gas *azote* (from the Greek negative prefix *a-* and *zōē*, life). He discovered hydrogen in 1783. Lavoisier helped construct the metric system, constructed the first list of elements, and contributed to the reform of the chemical nomenclature. He also predicted the existence of silicon in 1787.

The Roman writer Pliny the Elder discourses at length about *nitrum*, soda:

In the soda-beds of Egypt, ophthalmia is unknown. Ulcers on those who visit there heal quickly, but if ulcers form on those who are already there, they are slow to heal.

Soda mixed with oil causes those who are rubbed with that mixture to sweat; it also softens the flesh. . . . Soda is good for a toothache if it is mixed with pepper in wine. If it is boiled with a leek and then cooked down to make a dentifrice, it restores the white color to blackened teeth.

[*Natural History* 31.115–117]

The Greek word *agra* meant hunting or catching game; another word, *podagra*, meant a trap for animals. This word later came to mean a disease of animals' feet, and then gout in humans, a painful, inflamed condition of a joint. Formations in English use this word as a suffix, as in **odontagra** (toothache, especially from gout), and **arthragra** (acute pain in the joints). The term **podagra** was used to mean gout. More and more, however, medical professionals simply use the term gout, especially for pain of the foot or large toe.

The word hilus, from the New Latin *hilum*, refers to "a depression or recess at the exit or entrance of a duct into a gland or nerves and vessels into an organ."* It appeared first in the mid-17th century as a Latin botanical term meaning a scar on a seed indicating a point of attachment of the ovule—for example, the "eye" of a bean. The earliest example of the word hilus in English is found in an 1840 anatomical treatise. In anatomy, hilus refers to a notch or opening in a body part, especially where blood vessels, nerves, or ducts enter or leave. Kidneys, lungs, and lymph nodes, for example, each have hilus notches. Hilus forms the base of the noun *nihil*, nothing (as used in the English word nihilism, a doctrine of destruction). According to Festus, a Roman grammarian of the second century AD, *hilum* meant "something that clings to the seed of a bean, from which we get the word *nihil*." There was no Latin form *hilus*.

Glomeruli, clusters of capillaries within the nephrons of the kidneys, take their name from the New Latin word *glomerulus*, a diminutive of Latin *glomus* (ball of yarn). The old Latin verb, *glomerāre*, meaning wind into a ball or gather together, was used by Virgil in the *Aeneid* to describe the souls of the dead gathered about the banks of the Styx, waiting to be ferried across to the realms of the dead by the boatman Charon:

quam multa in silvis autumni frigore primo
lapsa cadunt folia, aut ad terram gurgite ab alto
quam multae glomerantur aves, ubi frigidus annus
trans pontum fugat et terris immittit apricis.

As many as the leaves that fall from trees in the first frost of the autumn, and as dense as the flocks of birds that gather together in flight when the season of cold drives them across the sea, sending them to sunny lands.

[Virgil, *Aeneid* 6.309–312]

---

*Venes D, ed. *Taber's Cyclopedic Medical Dictionary*, 23rd ed. F. A. Davis, 2017, p. 1132.

Exercise 1:   Analyze and Define

Analyze and define each of the following words. In this and in succeeding exercises, analysis should consist of separating the words into prefixes (if any), combining forms, and suffixes or suffix forms (if any) and giving the meaning of each. Be certain to differentiate between nouns and adjectives in your definitions. Consult a medical dictionary for the current meanings of these words.

1. abdominovesical _____

2. actinodermatitis _____

3. actinogenic _____

4. algolagnia _____

5. anuria _____

6. aspermatogenesis _____

7. azoospermia _____

8. cerebellar cortex _____

9. chiragra _____

10. coprozoa _____

11. cortical _____

12. corticopleuritis _____

13. cryoanalgesia _____

14. cryobiology _____

15. cryptorchidectomy _____

16. dysuria _____

17. epizoon _____

18. euglycemia _____

19. genitourinary _____

20. hypoglycemia _____

21. inguinal reflex _____

22. inosuria _____

23. insemination _____

24. melanuria _____

25. monorchid _____

26. oligospermia _____

27. orchidopexy _____

28. orchioplasty _____

29. paravesical _____

30. penile _____

31. phallic _____

32. pneumaturia _____

33. protozoology _____

34. pyelogram _____

35. pyelonephritis _____

36. rhabdomyolysis _____

37. scrota _____

38. scrotal thermography _____

39. seminiferous _____

40. spermatocidal _____

41. spermicide _____

42. uremia _____

43. ureterolithiasis _____

44. urethrocele _____

45. urethrograpy _____

46. urine _____

47. urothelium _____

48. vesicouterine _____

49. vesicula _____

50. zoology _____

Exercise 2:   Word Derivation

Give the word derived from Greek and/or Latin elements that means each of the following. Verify your answer in a medical dictionary. **Note that the wording of a dictionary definition may vary from the wording used here.**

1. Surgical removal of a stone from the renal pelvis _____

2. Substance that produces low temperatures _____

3. Outer layer of the adrenal gland (2 words) _____

4. Study of the seminal fluid _____

5. Formation of a connection from one ureter to the other _____

6. Microorganism capable of causing disease of the urinary tract _____

7. Condition of having three testicles _____

8. Study of the effect of cold on biological systems _____

9. Pertaining to the groin _____

10. Excessive concentration of calcium in the urine _____

11. Hernia of the bladder (into the vagina) _____

12. Science of the diseases of animals _____

13. Inflammation of the penis _____

14. Release of urine from the body _____

15. Injection of fluid into the bladder _____

16. Surgical incision of a testicle _____

17. Resembling a rod _____

18. (Irritability or) spasm of the urethra _____

19. Inflammation of the pelvis of the kidney _____

20. (Abnormal) love of animals _____

Exercise 3: Drill and Review

Analyze and define each of the following words. Analysis should consist of separating the words into prefixes (if any), combining forms, and suffixes or suffix forms (if any) and giving the meaning of each. Be certain to differentiate between nouns and adjectives in your definitions. Using the elements in the word determine its meaning. Consult a medical dictionary for the current meanings of these words. Use a separate paper if you need more room for an answer.

1. acanthopelvis _____

2. actinotherapy _____

3. agnathia _____

4. anorchidism _____

5. antigalactic _____

6. corticoadrenal _____

7. corticosteroid _____

8. cryostat _____

9. cryotherapy _____

10. fecaluria _____

11. glycogen _____

12. hematuria _____

13. hemihyperplasia _____

14. homeopathy _____

15. hydrophilism _____

16. hyperglycemia _____

17. hyperuricemia _____

18. immunifacient _____

19. leukocoria _____

20. mastatrophia _____

21. micropenis _____

22. neophallus _____

23. neurocrine _____

24. oliguria _____

25. orchidoptosis _____

26. orchiopathy _____

27. ovicide _____

28. paraparesis _____

29. phallus _____

30. polyuria _____

31. protozoa _____

32. pubescence _____

33. pyeloplasty _____

34. rhabdovirus _____

35. seminal _____

36. sone _____

37. spermatocele _____

38. spermatorrhea _____

39. stereophotomicrograph _____

40. sternothyroid _____

41. synorchidism _____

42. thyrotroph _____

43. trophocyte _____

44. ureterosigmoidostomy _____

45. urethrotomy _____

46. urinose _____

47. ventrad _____

48. vesiculitis _____

49. zoolagnia _____

50. zoopsychology _____

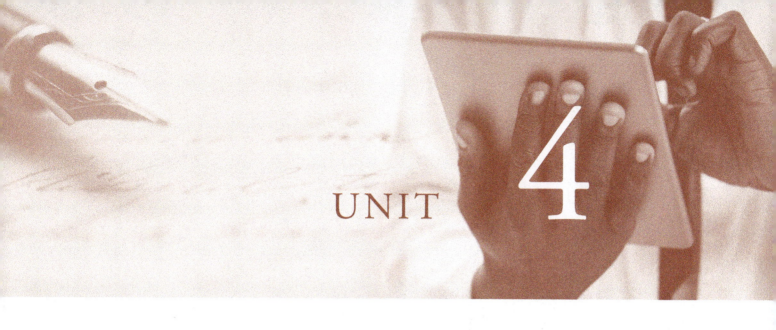

UNIT 4

ADDITIONAL STUDY

HEMATOPOIETIC AND LYMPHATIC SYSTEMS
MUSCULOSKELETAL SYSTEM
NERVOUS SYSTEM
ENDOCRINE SYSTEM

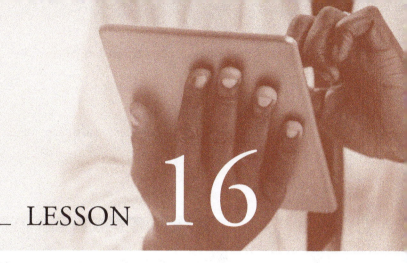

HEMATOPOIETIC AND LYMPHATIC SYSTEMS

Human blood is composed of plasma (about 52% to 62%) and cells (about 38% to 48%) (Fig. 16-1). Plasma is composed mostly of water along with ions, proteins, hormones, and lipids. The cellular components are erythrocytes, the red blood cells (RBCs); leukocytes, the white blood cells (WBCs); and thrombocytes (platelets),* the elements that play an important role in the coagulation of blood, hemostasis, and blood thrombus (clot) formation. The function of the blood is to carry nutrients, principally oxygen, to the cells and tissues of the body, and to carry away wastes, principally carbon dioxide, from the cells and tissues for disposal. In addition to these primary functions, blood plays an important part in the regulation of body temperature, and in the body's defense mechanism against infection, especially through the phagocytic action of the leukocytes (see the section on leukocytes).

ERYTHROCYTES

Erythrocytes are mature RBCs that contain hemoglobin and carry oxygen to the tissues. In adults, erythrocyte formation (called **erythropoiesis**) takes place in bone marrow, principally in the vertebrae, ribs, and sternum (breastbone); the spongy layer within the cranial bones (diploë); and the long bones of the arms and legs. During erythropoiesis, precursor cells in the bone marrow called **stem cells** go through a number of developmental stages as they mature into RBCs.† Each mature RBC is a nonnucleated biconcave

---

*Greek *platē* (flat); -let is an English diminutive suffix derived from French.
†See Venes D, ed., *Taber's Cyclopedic Medical Dictionary*, 23rd ed. F. A. Davis, 2017, pp. 843–844, s.v. erythrocyte, for further explanation of this process.

disk with a typical cell membrane and an internal stroma, or framework, made of lipids and proteins to which more than 200 million molecules of **hemoglobin** are attached. Hemoglobin is composed of **hematin,** the iron-carrying portion of the molecule, and **globin,** a simple protein.

The primary function of erythrocytes is to carry oxygen to and carbon dioxide from the cells and tissues of the body. Oxygen is carried in the hemoglobin of the blood. Hemoglobin combines with oxygen to form an unstable compound called **oxyhemoglobin,** which is carried through the arterial system to all parts of the body where the oxygen is released into the tissues. The average life span of an RBC is about 4 months. As erythrocytes age and become fragile, they are removed from circulation by macrophages in the liver, spleen, and red bone marrow. The iron in hemoglobin is reused immediately or is stored in the liver until needed for production of new RBCs in the bone marrow.

An erythrocyte from which the hemoglobin has been dissolved is called an **achromatic erythrocyte,** an RBC without color. Any excess amounts of hemoglobin in the body as a result of destruction of erythrocytes **(hemolysis)** are passed off in the urine and feces, a process that keeps the amount of hemoglobin in the body relatively stable. This principle of stability is called **homeostasis.** When it is applied to the circulating blood, it means that production and destruction of RBCs (erythrocytes) are mutually dependent on each other, and that the constituents and properties of the blood tend to remain stable. Any interference with this stability leads to hematologic disease.

When there is insufficient hemoglobin in the bloodstream to generate an adequate supply of oxygen to the

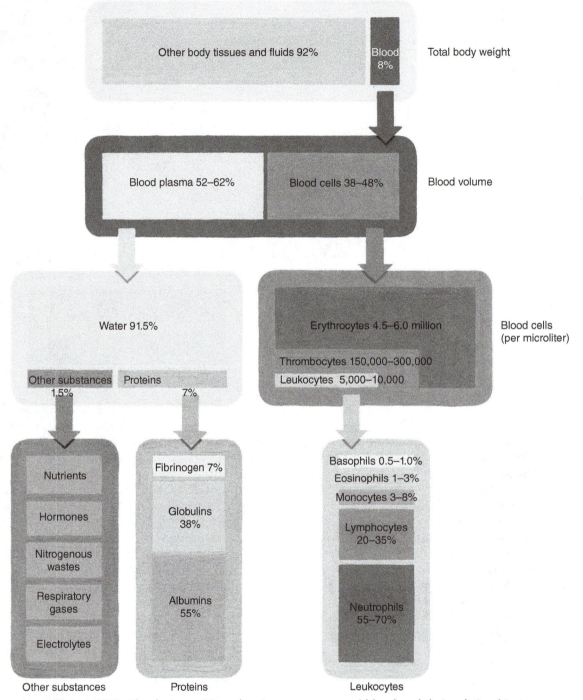

Figure 16-1. Blood composition, showing components of blood and their relationship to other body tissues. (From Scanlon, V. C., and Sanders, T., *Essentials of Anatomy and Physiology*, 7th ed. F. A. Davis, 2015, p. 285, with permission.)

cells and tissues, a substance called **erythropoietin,** which stimulates the production of erythrocytes, is released into the bloodstream. In 1906, French scientists Paul Carnot and Claude Déflandre announced their theory that the circulating blood carries a substance they called *hémopoiétin*, which stimulates the production of RBCs, but their work was largely ignored.

Subsequent investigations, especially since 1950, have confirmed the presence of this substance. Erythropoietin is a cytokine (protein) produced in the kidneys that stimulates the proliferation of RBCs. Synthetic erythropoietin is used to treat anemia, especially in patients with renal or bone marrow failure.

An insufficiency of oxygen in the body, a condition called **hypoxia,*** can result from environmental exposure, disease, or toxic substances. **Altitude hypoxia** is the

---

*Anoxia, absence of oxygen, is often used incorrectly to mean hypoxia.

result of exposure to high altitudes and can lead to headache, nausea and shortness of breath, a syndrome know as Altitude Sickness. **Anemic hypoxia** is caused by a decrease in the concentration of hemoglobin or RBCs in the blood in any process causing severe blood loss. **Anoxic hypoxia** is caused by disordered pulmonary function, respiratory obstruction, or inadequate ventilation. Exposure to toxic substances, such as snake venoms, which enter the bloodstream and cause hemolysis, can also cause hypoxia.

The normal number of erythrocytes averages about 5,500,000 per cubic millimeter (abbreviated mm³) for males and about 4,500,000 for females. The total number in an average-size person is about 35 trillion. The volume of erythrocytes packed in a given volume of blood via the process of centrifugation, which separates the solid elements from the plasma in blood, is called the **hematocrit** (Greek *kritēs*, judge). The hematocrit is expressed as the percentage of total blood volume that consists of erythrocytes, or as the volume in cubic centimeters of erythrocytes packed by centrifugation. The normal average is about 47% for men and about 42% for women. A decrease below the normal number is called **erythropenia,** and an abnormal increase in hematocrit is called **polycythemia** or **erythrocytosis.**

LEUKOCYTES

Leukocytes are the primary effector cells against infection and tissue damage. They can be classified into two groups, both of which possess nuclei. One type, called **granulocytes,** contains **granules** (Latin *grānulum*, diminutive of *grānum*, grain, seed), minute, grain like bodies located in the cytoplasm, the substance of a cell outside its nucleus. Leukocytes without granules are called **agranulocytes.**

Granular leukocytes, which readily accept certain kinds of dyes, are characterized and grouped according to the type of dye that will stain them. The granules of some leukocytes stain red. These cells are called **eosinophils,** or eosinophilic leukocytes, named for the acid dye that stains them: **eosin,** a red dye. Cells that stain blue are called **basophils** (Greek *basis*, base), or basophilic leukocytes, because the dye that stains them is a basic, or nonacidic—that is, alkaline—dye of a bluish color. Most leukocytes, however, take on a purplish color and are called **neutrophils,** or neutrophilic leukocytes, because they can be stained only by neutral dyes (dyes that are neither acidic nor alkaline), which are purple. An abnormal increase in the number of eosinophils in the blood is called **eosinophilia;** a decrease is called **eosinopenia.** An abnormal increase in the number of basophils is called **basophilia.** An abnormal increase in the number of neutrophils is called **neutrophilia,** and an abnormal decrease is called **neutropenia.**

Most leukocytes, especially granulocytes, are **phagocytes;** that is, they have the ability to engulf and neutralize or destroy microorganisms, other foreign antigens, and cell debris. When hostile bacteria invade the body, the production of leukocytes is greatly increased. An increased number of leukocytes (leukocytosis) is usually an indication of bacterial infection, inflammation, trauma, or stress. When leukocytes are destroyed by invading bacteria, the dead cells collect and form a whitish mass called pus. If the pus cannot find an outlet to the surface of the body, an abscess is formed. Normally, 1 mm³ of blood contains 5,000 to 10,000 leukocytes. A decrease in number below 5,000 is called **leukopenia,** and an increase above 10,000 is called **leukocytosis.**

PLATELETS

Platelets are microscopic flat, round or oval disks found in the blood (Fig. 16-2). They number 130,000 to 400,000 per mm³. Sometimes called **thrombocytes,** they play an important role in coagulating blood, the cessation of bleeding **(hemostasis),** and **thrombus** (blood clot) formation. When there is damage to tissue, platelets adhere to each other and to the damaged parts, forming a protective mass around the injured part, stopping the loss of blood.

An abnormal decrease in the number of platelets is called **thrombocytopenia.** The condition known as **idiopathic thrombocytopenia purpura** (ITP) (Latin *purpura*, purple) is thrombocytopenia of unknown etiology. ITP is clinically associated with the spontaneous appearance of dark blue or purple patches on the skin and/or the mucosal surfaces of the mouth caused by hemorrhages into these areas. Such discolorations, if small, are called **macules** (Latin *macula*, spot); larger patches are called **ecchymoses. Thrombocytosis,** increased platelet production, occurs after loss of blood following surgery or severe injury to tissues.

CLOTTING

When blood is exposed to air, it changes into a soft, jelly-like mass called a blood clot. This process is called blood clotting or blood **coagulation.** The physical change from liquid to a nonfluid mass is caused by **fibrinogen,** a protein substance normally present in plasma. When blood escapes from vessels that normally contain it, a substance called **thrombin** is formed from elements present in the blood. Thrombin acts on the fibrinogen and converts it to **fibrin,** a whitish filamentous protein that forms a network in which platelets are caught. These platelets cling together and form a clot. Clotting is slowed down by cold, calcium deficiency, the presence of certain mineral salts, and anticoagulants such as **heparin** or warfarin **(Coumadin),** as well as by hemolytic agents such as snake venom. Newer anticoagulants known as DOACs (direct oral anticoagulants) have made anticoagulation therapy safer for patients.

Hemophilia is a rare, hereditary blood disorder that occurs predominantly in males. It is characterized by a prolonged coagulation time; that is, blood fails to clot in the normal time because of a deficiency of blood-clotting

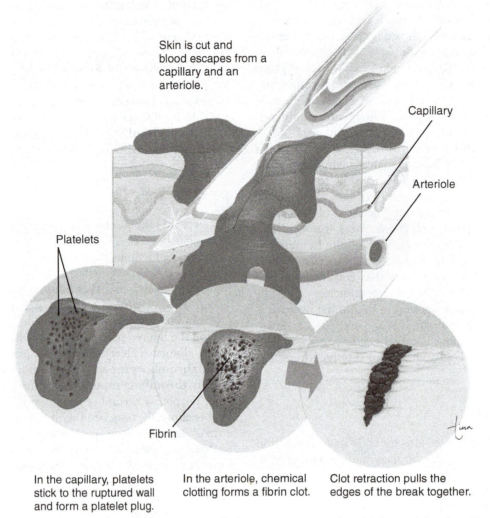

Skin is cut and blood escapes from a capillary and an arteriole.

Capillary

Arteriole

Platelets

Fibrin

In the capillary, platelets stick to the ruptured wall and form a platelet plug.

In the arteriole, chemical clotting forms a fibrin clot.

Clot retraction pulls the edges of the break together.

Figure 16-2. Platelet plug formation and clotting. (From Scanlon, V. C., and Sanders, T., *Essentials of Anatomy and Physiology*, 7th ed. F. A. Davis, 2015, p. 298, with permission.)

proteins. There are two types of hemophilia: hemophilia A, which affects 1 in 5,000 male births in the United States, and hemophilia B, which affects 1 in 30,000 male births. In hemophilia A, the blood-clotting factor VIII is either missing or defective; in hemophilia B, the blood clotting factor IX is deficient or missing. Treatment for hemophilia includes intravenous replacement of the deficient clotting factors and the addition of chemotherapeutic agents that promote clotting. Individuals with hemophilia should avoid drugs that interfere with the coagulation process (such as heparin), and must be careful to avoid trauma.

ANEMIA

Anemia is a blood disorder in which there is a reduction in the mass of circulating RBCs. This reduction occurs when the equilibrium (homeostasis) between production and destruction of erythrocytes is disturbed. Anemia is not a disease but a symptom of other illnesses or conditions. Anemia may be caused by excessive blood loss from disease or injury, vitamin or mineral deficiencies (especially vitamin B_{12}, folate, or iron

deficiency), decreased RBC production caused by the suppression of bone marrow associated with kidney failure, or excessive cell destruction **(hemolysis)** associated with sickle cell disease. Types of anemia include the following:

- **Aplastic anemia** is primarily a disease of children and young adults but can occur at any age. A form of bone marrow failure, it is caused by a severe decrease in the number of stem cells and/or white blood cell ancestors. Most patients with aplastic anemia can be treated effectively with bone marrow transplants or immunosuppressive therapy.

- **Erythroblastic anemia** (also called **Cooley anemia** after American physician Thomas Cooley, 1871–1945) is caused by an inherited trait that results in defective production of hemoglobin. This condition is also called **thalassemia major** (Greek *thalassa*, the sea) and most commonly affects people of Mediterranean, Middle Eastern, Indian, Asian, and Southeast Asian descent.

- **Iron-deficiency anemia** results from the body's demand for more iron than can normally be produced. It is caused by inadequate iron intake, malabsorption of iron, blood loss, pregnancy and lactation, intravascular hemolysis, or a combination of these factors.

- **Pernicious anemia** (Latin *perniciōsus*, destructive, from *perniciēs*, destruction) usually occurs in later adult life and is characterized by **achlorhydria** (lack of hydrochloric acid in the gastric juice) as a result of reduced absorption of vitamin B_{12}. Pernicious anemia is an autoimmune disease in which the parietal cells of the stomach lining fail to secrete enough intrinsic factor to ensure intestinal absorption of vitamin B_{12}, the extrinsic factor. There are also congenital forms of pernicious anemia caused by an inability to produce intrinsic factor.

- **Sickle cell anemia** is a hereditary, hemolytic anemia characterized by large numbers of sickle-shaped erythrocytes in the blood. Sickle cell anemia is inherited from both parents and is caused by an abnormal type of hemoglobin (hemoglobin S) in these cells (Fig. 16-3). It occurs mainly among African Americans, native Africans, and individuals of Mediterranean descent. Treatment for sickle cell anemia includes supportive therapy with supplemental iron and blood transfusions. Administration of hydroxyurea stimulates the production of hemoglobin S, decreases the need for blood transfusion and reduces the incidence of painful **sickle cell crisis,** which occurs when there is a drop in the number of blood cells as a result of abnormal cell production.

LEUKEMIA

Leukemia is a class of hematologic malignancies (cancers) of bone marrow cells in which immature blood cells multiply at the expense of normal blood cells. As normal blood cells are depleted, anemia, infection, hemorrhage, and death can result. The leukemias are categorized as acute or chronic by the type of cell from which they originate and by the genetic, chromosomal, or growth factor abnormality in the malignant cells. Treatment options include chemotherapy, bone marrow transplant, targeted therapy (drug treatments that can cause the cancer cells to die), radiation therapy, and immunotherapy. Ongoing clinical trials are testing new ways to fight hematologic cancer.

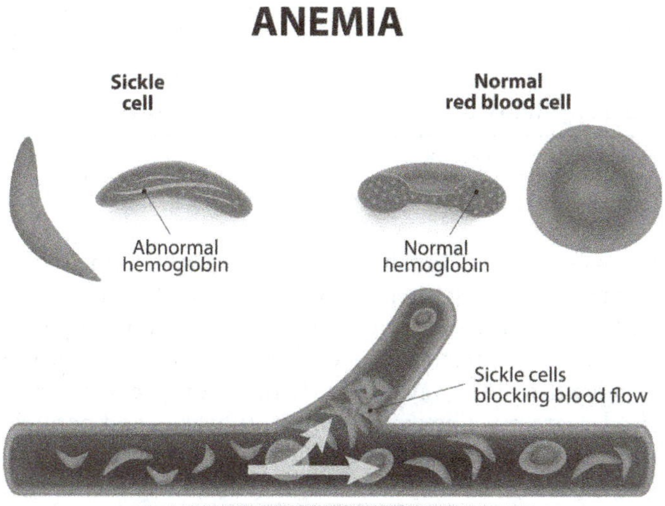

Hairy cell leukemia is a chronic, low-grade cancer in which abnormally shaped B lymphocytes, called "hairy cells" because of their fuzzy appearance, occur. This rare disease, marked by **pancytopenia** and **splenomegaly,** generally affects middle-aged people, men more often than women. Before the development of effective chemotherapeutic agents, the average survival time for patients with hairy cell leukemia was about 5 years; with chemotherapy, the survival time may be extended. Other types of leukemia include the following:

- **Acute lymphocytic leukemia,** or **ALL,** (also called acute lymphoblastic leukemia) is a hematologic cancer characterized by the unchecked multiplication of immature lymphoid cells in the bone marrow, blood, and body tissues. Although quickly fatal if left untreated, with advances in chemotherapy, about 90% of treated children achieve remission. Adult ALL is less responsive to therapy; only about one-third of adult patients are cured.

- **Acute myeloid leukemia,** or **AML,** (also called acute myelogenous leukemia and acute nonlymphocytic leukemia, ANLL), refers to a group of hematologic cancers in which neoplastic (Greek *neos*, new and *plassein*, form, develop) cells form in the blood and bone marrow, and immature cells called blasts (short for myeloblasts) circulate in the peripheral blood. Treatment with cytotoxic chemotherapy, and bone marrow and stem cell transplantation, currently results in complete remission for approximately 65% of AML patients.

- **Chronic lymphocytic leukemia,** or **CLL,** is a malignancy in which abnormal lymphocytes, usually B cells, grow and infiltrate body tissues, often resulting in enlargement of lymph nodes and immune system dysfunction. Patients with early-stage CLL are often not treated but are carefully followed. Patients in advanced stages of the disease are treated with targeted drug therapy, immunotherapy, and clinical trials of bone marrow or stem cell transplantation.*

- **Chronic myeloid leukemia,** or **CML,** (also called chronic myelogenous leukemia) is a disease marked by chronic increase in the number of granulocytes, splenomegaly, and a genetic anomaly in the bone marrow called the Philadelphia chromosome, the presence of which is used to diagnose the disease. Various chemotherapies and bone marrow transplantation are used to treat this disease.

ANEMIA

Figure 16-3. Sickle cell anemia. (Courtesy of ttsz, iStock / Getty Images Plus.)

---

*Chronic lymphocytic leukemia treatment (PDQ®)–patient version. National Cancer Institute. https://www.cancer.gov/types/leukemia/patient/cll-treatment -pdq. Accessed July 31, 2021.

THE LYMPHATIC SYSTEM

The lymphatic system is part of the circulatory and immune systems. It is a network of tissues, vessels, and organs concerned with the production and circulation of **lymph,** a colorless, alkaline fluid composed mostly of water with proteins, globulins, salts, urea, neutral fats, white blood cells, and glucose. Lymph is carried by very small, thin-walled vessels called **lymphatics** or lymphatic capillaries (Fig. 16-4). The white blood cells present in lymph are called lymphocytes; there are no erythrocytes.

Interstitial fluid is found all over the body in tissues called **interstitial spaces** (Latin *interstitium*, space between, from *inter-*, and *-stituere*, stand). When interstitial fluid enters the lymph capillaries, it is called lymph. Lymph is gathered into the lymphatics, which carry it to two central points in the body where these vessels empty into either the right lymphatic duct or the left (thoracic) duct. These two ducts empty into the venous system, returning the tissue fluid to the circulating blood. The function of the lymphatic system is twofold: (1) to return the circulating blood proteins that have leaked out of the capillaries and into the tissues, and (2) to filter foreign matter, especially bacteria, and destroy it through the phagocytic action of the lymphocytes.

All along the lymphatic vessels are small glands called lymph **nodes** (Latin *nōdus*, knot) (Fig. 16-5). Within the nodes are channels called lymph **sinuses** (Latin *sinus*, curve, hollow). Lining the walls of these sinuses are phagocytes called **reticuloendothelial cells,**** which engulf and destroy foreign material and bacteria from the lymph as these substances pass through the nodes. It is this phagocytic activity in the nodes that causes the nodes to become swollen during severe infection. Lymph nodes are particularly abundant in the axillae (Latin *axilla*, armpit) and neck because the right and left lymphatic ducts empty into the right and left jugular veins (Latin *jugulum*, throat, neck) in the neck.

The phagocytes of the lymph nodes are able to destroy some cancer cells. Many of these malignant cells may be transferred to other parts of the body through the lymphatics, creating **metastases** (singular *metastasis*, from Greek *meta-*, change, and *stasis*, position), secondary growths of malignancies spread from the site of a primary growth.

Inflammation of the lymph nodes is called **lymphadenitis.** Inflammation of the lymphatic vessels is called **lymphangitis.** Abnormal enlargement of the lymph nodes is one of the symptoms of **Hodgkin disease,** named for British physician Thomas Hodgkin (1798–1866), a form of carcinoma characterized by inflammatory infiltration of lymphocytes into the bone marrow, which results in disturbed hematopoiesis and anemia. **Lymphoma** refers to any malignancy originating from lymphocytes.

VOCABULARY

Note: Latin combining forms appear in **bold italics**.

Greek or Latin	Combining Form(s)	Meaning	Example
blastos	**BLAST-**	[bud, germ] primitive cell	myelo-**blast**
ēōs	**EOS-**	red (stain)	**eos**-in
globus	***GLOB-***	round body, globe	**glob**-ulin
grānulum	***GRANUL-***	granule	**granul**-ar
karyon	**KARY-**	[nut] nucleus	**kary**-ophage
lympha	***LYMPH-***	[clear water] lymph	**lymph**-atic
monos	**MON-**	single	**mon**-ochromatic
neuter	***NEUTR-***†	neither	**neutr**-ophil
philein	**-PHIL-**‡	having an affinity for	baso-**phil**

†In this terminology, words beginning with or containing NEUTR- refer to neutral dyes—those that are neither acid nor alkaline (basic).
‡In this terminology, words containing the combining form PHIL- refer to the capacity of a cell to accept dye. A neutrophil is a cell that stains easily with neutral dyes.

ETYMOLOGICAL NOTES

The Greek and Latin languages are called cognate, which means literally "coming into being together," because both are derived from a parent language called Indo-European. Just as there are many words in the Romance languages, which are all derived from Latin, with similar form and meaning, there are words in Greek and in Latin with these same similarities. The -penia in erythropenia, for example, is from the Greek *penia* (poverty, need), and is related in this way to the Latin noun *pēnūria* (want, need, scarcity). The words **penury** (poverty) and **penurious** (stingy) are from this Latin word. The same relationship exists between Greek *leukos* (white), and Latin *lux, lūcis* (light), as in the words **lucid** (clear) and **translucent** (transmitting light).

**Latin *rēticulum*, diminutive of *rēte*, net, Greek *endon*, within, *thēlē*, nipple. Lymph sinuses are lined with endothelial tissue.

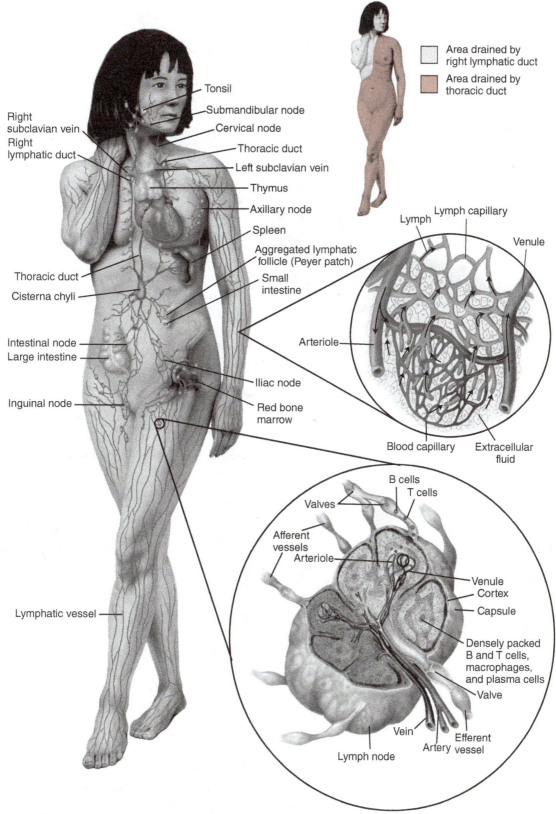

Figure 16-4. The lymphatic system. *(A)* Capillary. *(B)* Lymph node. (From Gylys, B. A., and Wedding, M. E., *Medical Terminology Systems: A Body Systems Approach*, 8th ed. F. A. Davis, with permission.)

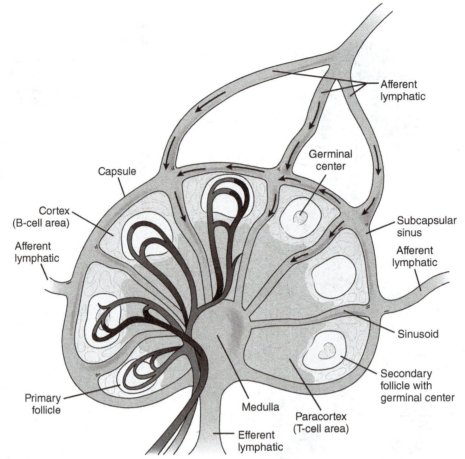

Figure 16-5. Lymph node. (From Scanlon, V. C., and Sanders, T., *Essentials of Anatomy and Physiology*, 7th ed. F. A. Davis, 2015, p. 362, with permission.)

Another group of words with this same relationship is derived from the Greek verb *histanai* (stand) and the two Latin verbs *stāre, stātus* (stand), and *statuere, statūtus, -stituere, -stitūtus* (stand, set in place). These verbs have given rise to such words as **hemostat, stasis, metastasis, homeostasis, station, statue, interstitial, constitution** and **consistent.**

Eosin, the red dye for which eosinophils have a special affinity, takes its name from the Greek word for dawn, *ēōs*. In early Greek times, Eos (Dawn), daughter of Hyperion and Theia, two of the Titans, primeval children of Sky and Earth, was thought to be a goddess. Dawn's sister Selene was the moon and her brother was Helios, the sun. In the Homeric poems, the new day was often heralded by the appearance of *rhododaktylos Eos*, rosy-fingered Dawn. On one occasion, Eos fell in love with a mortal, Tithonus, a brother of Priam, king of Troy, at the time of the Trojan War. She carried the young man away to her home in Ethiopia and secured immortality for him. But she neglected to obtain eternal youth for the unfortunate Tithonus. Although he was deathless, he continued to age. Some say that he was eventually changed into a grasshopper, a creature that renews its youth by casting off its old skin.

Tennyson recalls the sad story of this youth in his poem *Tithonus* (1860), in which the unhappy lover asks Dawn to release him from immortality:

Yet hold me not forever in thine East;
How can my nature longer mix with thine?
Coldly thy rosy shadows bathe me, cold
Are all thy lights, and cold my wrinkled feet
Upon thy glimmering thresholds, when the steam
Floats up from those dim fields about the homes
Of happy men that have the power to die,
And grassy barrows of the happier dead.
Release me, and restore me to the ground.
Thou seest all things, thou wilt see my grave;
Thou wilt renew thy beauty morn by morn,
I in earth forget these empty courts,
And thee returning on thy silver wheels.

Eos and Tithonus had two children, Emathion and Memnon. We know little about Emathion, but Memnon became king of the Ethiopians. In the closing phase of the Trojan War, Memnon came to the aid of the Trojans, leading his Ethiopian troops and wearing armor fashioned by the god Hephaestus himself. Shortly after his arrival, Memnon faced the great Greek hero Achilles in single combat and was mortally wounded in the battle. Ovid, in the *Metamorphoses*, tells us that Eos (Latin *Aurora*) appealed to Zeus to grant Memnon some special honor in death. Zeus agreed, and from the ashes that rose from Memnon's funeral pyre, countless birds came into being and were named Memnonides, daughters of Memnon. The dew on the morning grass is said to be the tears shed daily by Eos for her unfortunate son.

Lymph, the clear, alkaline fluid found in the lymphatic vessels, is named from Latin *lympha* (clear water). This Latin word is adapted from the Greek *nymphē* (or *nymphā*), young girl, maiden, nymph. Nymphs were female spirits of nature and were usually represented as living in the mountains, where they were called oreads; in the woods, where they were called dryads; or in the waters, where they were called naiads. Some nymphs were singled out in mythology for the unusual events surrounding them, and some do not appear to be oreads, dryads, or naiads. In Homer's *Odyssey*, the hero Odysseus spends 7 years on the island of Ogygia, detained by the beautiful nymph Calypso, who wants to make him immortal so that he can dwell with her forever. But his thoughts were of his home and his wife Penelope and young son Telemachus. Eventually, he was released from this unusual bondage by the order of Zeus. After almost 20 years, Odysseus returned to his home, wife, and son.

Another well-known nymph was the oread Echo. She fell in love with a handsome young man named Narcissus, the son of a naiad, Liriope, and a river god, Cephisus. Ovid tells us that when Narcissus was born, Liriope asked Tiresias, the blind prophet of Thebes, if her son would live to a ripe old age. Tiresias answered, "Only if he never knows himself."

Narcissus grew up to be a haughty young man and spurned all lovers. As the story goes, he, at last, fell in love with the image of a beautiful youth in a pool of clear water—himself (Fig. 16-6). In his frustration at this

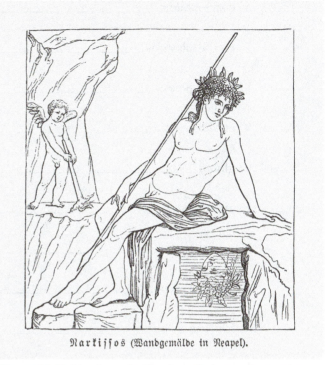

Narkissos (Wandgemälde in Neapel).

Figure 16-6. Narcissus. In Greek mythology, a hunter known for his beauty. (Courtesy Getty Images, Roman mural, Pompeii, wood engraving, published 1897.)

hopeless love, he pined away until only a flower with a yellow center surrounded by white petals remained. His last words to himself were *Heu, frustra dilecte puer. Vale* ("Alas, dear boy, loved in vain. Farewell"). Echo repeated the same words back to him. Ovid tells us that even in the Underworld, his spirit gazes eternally at its image in the waters of the river Styx. Echo, desolate, mourning for her lost love, faded away until only her voice remained, echoing through the hills and valleys, repeating whatever she heard spoken.

Exercise 1:   Analyze and Define

Analyze and define each of the following words. In this and in succeeding exercises, analysis should consist of separating the words into prefixes (if any), combining forms, and suffixes or suffix forms (if any) and giving the meaning of each. Be certain to differentiate between nouns and adjectives in your definitions. Consult a medical dictionary for the current meanings of these words.

1. agranulocyte _____

2. karyocyte _____

3. blastocyst _____

4. blastula _____

5. eosin _____

6. eosinophilous _____

7. erythroblastosis _____

8. erythropoiesis _____

9. erythropoietin _____

10. globin _____

11. granuloblast _____

12. granulocyte _____

13. granulocytopoiesis _____

14. hematin _____

15. hematophagia _____

16. hematopoiesis _____

17. hemoglobinocholia _____

18. hemoglobinolysis _____

19. hemoglobinuria _____

20. hemopathology _____

21. hypereosinophilic syndrome _____

22. karyochromatophil _____

23. karyochrome _____

24. karyophage _____

25. hemolysin _____

26. leukopoiesis _____

27. lymphadenectasis _____

28. lymphadenitis _____

29. lymphagogue _____

30. lymphangiectasis _____

31. lymphangioma _____

32. lymphangitis _____

33. lymphaticostomy* _____

34. lymphoblast _____

35. lymphocytopenia _____

36. lymphocytotoxin _____

37. lymphogranulomatosis _____

38. lymphoma _____

39. lymphopoiesis _____

40. monocyte _____

41. monocytopenia _____

42. monocytosis _____

43. myeloblast _____

44. polykaryocyte _____

45. thrombase _____

46. thrombin _____

47. thromboclasis _____

48. thrombocyte _____

49. thrombopenia _____

50. thrombophilia _____

*From New Latin *lymphaticus* (lymphatic, a lymph vessel).

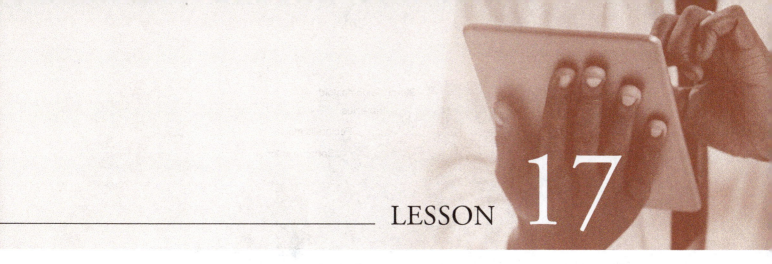

MUSCULOSKELETAL SYSTEM

The musculoskeletal system has several important functions in the body (Fig. 17-1). It supports the body, gives it shape, and protects its vital organs. The musculoskeletal system makes movement possible. Muscle (Latin *musculus*, diminutive of *mūs*, mouse; used in Latin to mean both a little mouse and a muscle) is a type of tissue composed of contractile cells or fibers. The outstanding characteristic of these cells or fibers is their elasticity, their ability to expand and contract. Muscle tissue possesses little intercellular material and, as a result, its cells or fibers lie close together.

Three types of muscle tissue are differentiated in the body: smooth, cardiac, and skeletal (Fig. 17-2). Smooth muscle tissue forms the involuntary muscles, those that are not under conscious control. These muscles are found mainly in the internal organs such as the digestive tract, the respiratory passages, the urinary and genital ducts, and the walls of blood vessels. Spindle shaped in form, smooth muscle cells each contain a central nucleus and are arranged in sheets, or layers. They are sometimes found as isolated units in connective tissue. Smooth muscle tissue contracts slowly and automatically.

Cardiac tissue is the tissue of the heart muscle. Cardiac muscle fibers branch and interconnect (**anastomose**), forming a continuous network, or **syncytium.** At intervals, the fibers are crossed by bands, or intercalated discs. Atypical muscle fibers beneath the endocardium, known as Purkinje fibers, form the impulse-conducting system of the heart. Cardiac muscle cells have one nucleus each and faint striations.

Skeletal (or striated) muscle tissue composes the voluntary muscles, those that are under conscious control. Striated muscle fibers are found in all skeletal muscles and possess alternate light and dark bands, or striations. These muscle fibers are grouped into bundles called **fasciculi,** each surrounded by a connective tissue sheath called the **perimysium.** Delicate reticular fibrils (Latin *fibrilla*, a small fiber) surround and hold together the fibers within a fasciculus forming the **endomysium.** Skeletal muscle cells are cylindrical, have several nuclei each, and appear striped (Fig. 17-3).

In anatomic terminology, body muscles are named according to the following conventions:

1. After a physical characteristic like shape or size: **bipennate muscle** (Latin *bi-*, two, *penna*, feather), so named because the muscle fibers flow down either side of a central tendon like the barbs on the two sides of a feather.

2. After the organ or part to which the muscle is attached and controls: **nasalis muscle** (Latin *nāsus*, nose). The nasalis muscle keeps the nostrils of the nose open during inspiration.

3. A combination of the preceding two: **biceps brachii muscle** (Latin *biceps*, two-headed, from *caput*, head, *brāchium*, [upper] arm; genitive case, *brāchiī*). The point of origin of a muscle is called the caput, or head. This muscle is bicipital (two headed), attached to both the scapula and the coracoid (Greek *korax*, *korakos*, crow) process, an outgrowth on the upper surface of the scapula resembling a crow's beak. The biceps brachii muscle flexes the forearm and supinates the hand, turning the hand so that the palm faces upward.

4. After the function performed by the muscle: a muscle that lifts a body part is a **levator;** one that flexes a body part is a **flexor;** one that moves a part away from

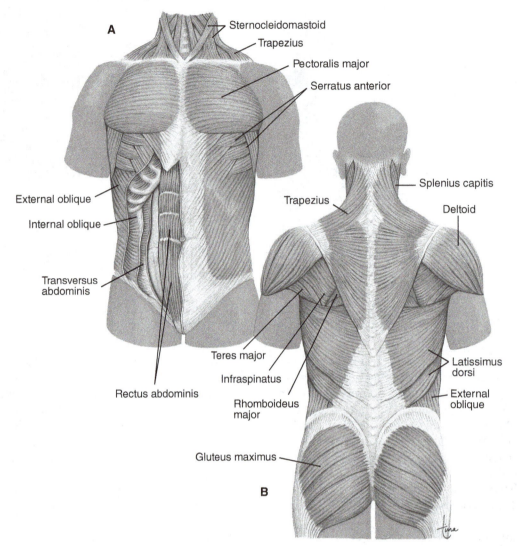

A

- Sternocleidomastoid
- Trapezius
- Pectoralis major
- Serratus anterior
- External oblique
- Internal oblique
- Transversus abdominis
- Rectus abdominis
- Splenius capitis
- Trapezius
- Deltoid
- Teres major
- Infraspinatus
- Rhomboideus major
- Latissimus dorsi
- External oblique
- Gluteus maximus

B

Figure 17-1. Muscles of the trunk. *(A)* Anterior, *(B)* posterior. (From Scanlon, V. C., and Sanders, T., *Essentials of Anatomy and Physiology*, 8th ed. F. A. Davis, 2020, with permission.)

the central plane of the body is an **abductor**; one that moves a part toward the central plane of the body is an **adductor**; and one that extends a part is an **extensor.** These terms generally, but not always, are used in combination with the part that the muscle moves. Sometimes the muscle is described as being long (Latin *longus*) or short *(brevis)*. The **abductor pollicis brevis muscle** *(pollex, pollicis,* thumb) and **abductor* pollicis longus muscle** abduct and assist in extending the thumb. The **adductor longus muscle** adducts and flexes the thigh. Note that it is not always possible to tell from the name of a muscle exactly which organ or part of the body it controls.

The names of muscles, as given in the preceding section, and other human anatomical structures are found in *Terminologia Anatomica,* usually abbreviated TA. TA is the official international terminology (nomenclature) of human anatomical structures, drafted by the Federative Committee on Anatomical Terminology (FCAT) in 1997 and accepted by the International Federation of Associations of Anatomists (IFAA) in 1999. TA replaced *Nomina Anatomica* (NA), the anatomic terminology adopted as official by the International Congress of Anatomists at various meetings after 1955. In April 2011, TA was published online by the Federative International Programme on Anatomical Terminologies (FIPAT). Latin was the standard in NA and remains the standard in TA, although in TA, Latin terms have English equivalents. For example, in TA, the Latin term **musculi intercostales interni** has an English equivalent: **internal intercostal muscles.**

---

*The noun **abductor,** as well as other agent nouns ending in -or, is in apposition to the noun muscle; it defines what kind of a muscle it is or what it does. It is easier to define these agent nouns as adjectives: the abductor muscle, which means the muscle that abducts.

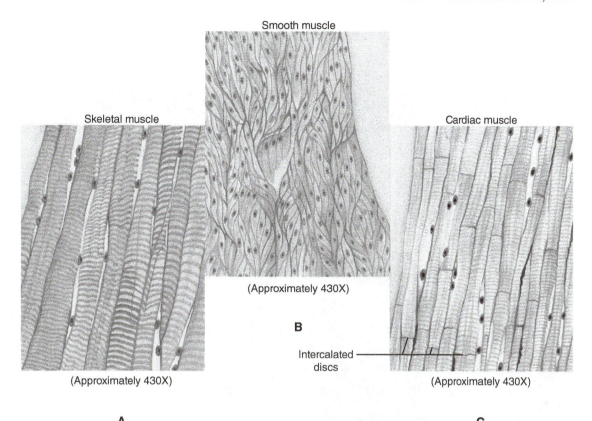

Smooth muscle

(Approximately 430X)

B

Skeletal muscle

(Approximately 430X)

A

Cardiac muscle

Intercalated discs

(Approximately 430X)

C

Figure 17-2. Comparison of properties of three types of muscle. (From Scanlon, V. C., and Sanders, T., *Essentials of Anatomy and Physiology*, 8th ed. F. A. Davis, 2020, with permission.)

NOUN DECLENSION

In naming muscles, Latin nouns and adjectives are in the forms of different grammatical cases, and in both singular and plural. The cases most commonly used are the nominative (the form found in the vocabularies) and the genitive, or possessive, case, in both singular and plural.

As presented in Lesson 8, there are five categories, called declensions, of Latin nouns and two declensions of adjectives.

First declension Latin nouns end in -*a* and are feminine; second declension nouns end in -*us* if masculine gender and -*um* if neuter gender. Third declension nouns may be masculine, feminine, or neuter, and the nominative case (the vocabulary form) is not characterized by any one ending. Nouns of the fourth and fifth declensions will not concern us here, with the exception of two fourth declension nouns: *manus* (hand) is feminine, and the genitive singular is *manūs*; *genū* (knee) is neuter, and the genitive singular is *genūs*.

A PARTIAL DECLENSION OF TYPICAL NOUNS

Singular		Plural	
Nominative	**Genitive**	**Nominative**	**Genitive**
auricula, f.,* ear	*auriculae*	*auriculae*	*auriculārum*
digitus, m., finger, toe	*digitī*	*digitī*	*digitōrum*
labium, n., lip	*labiī*	*labia*	*labiōrum*
mūs, m. and f., muscle	*mūris*	*mūrēs*	*mūrum*
manus, f., hand	*manūs*	*manūs*	*manuum*
genū, n., knee	*genūs*	*genua*	*genuum*

*The abbreviations m., f., and n. are for masculine, feminine, and neuter.

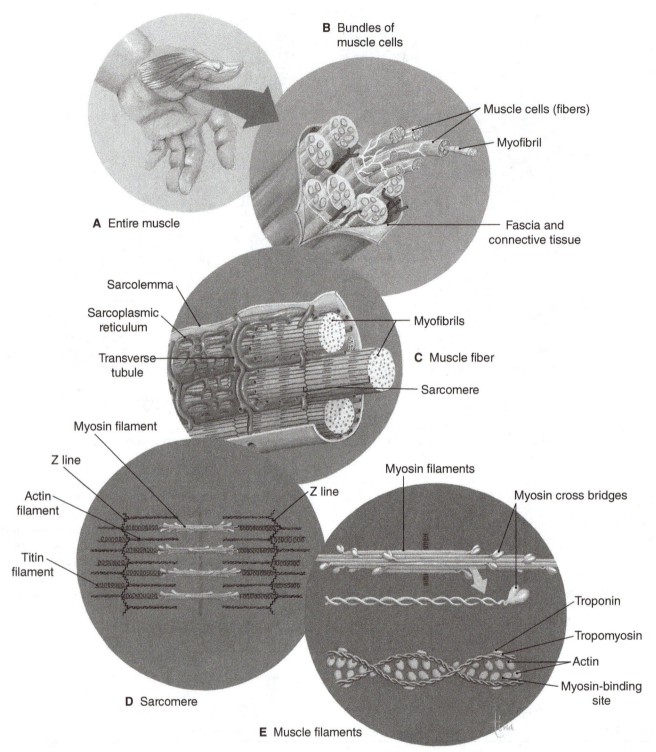

Figure 17-3. Skeletal muscle. (From Scanlon, V. C., and Sanders, T., *Essentials of Anatomy and Physiology*, 8th ed. F. A. Davis, with permission.)

LATIN ADJECTIVES

There are two categories of Latin adjectives. (1) First and second declension adjectives have the same endings as masculine, feminine, and neuter nouns of the first and second declensions. Their endings are determined by the gender of the nouns they modify. (2) Third declension adjectives usually end in *-is*. The genitive singular of third declension

adjectives also ends in *-is;* it is not always obvious whether a third declension adjective, such as *brevis*, short (genitive, *brevis*), is in the nominative or genitive case. This must be determined from the way the adjective is used in the term in which it is found.

Adjectives that end in *-ior* are in the comparative degree: *superior* (higher); *inferior* (lower). This form is used for both masculine and feminine singular. The comparative degree of neuter nouns ends in *-ius (superius, inferius)*. The genitive singular for both genders ends in *-is (superiōris, inferiōris)*, and the nominative plural for both genders ends in *-ēs (superiōrēs, inferiōrēs)*.

THE ORDER OF WORDS

In Latin, nouns in the genitive case (the possessive case) usually follow the noun on which they depend:

Nominative Singular	Genitive Singular	
rectus	**femoris**	
"the straight (muscle)	of the thigh"	The thigh muscle
extensor	**indicis**	
"the extensor (muscle)	of the index finger"	The index finger's extensor muscle

In Latin, adjectives follow the nouns they describe:

adductor longus	**adductor brevis**
"the long adductor (muscle)"	"the short adductor (muscle)"

In English, adjectives precede the nouns they describe:

flexor muscle	**adductor muscle**

SELECTED VOCABULARY FOR NAMES OF MUSCLES

Latin	Meaning
*abductor**	that which leads away, abductor
adductor	that which leads toward, adductor
āla	wing; ala nasi (wing of the nose, the lateral wall of each nostril)
angulus	angle, corner
ānus	anus, opening of the rectum
arrector	that which raises, erector
articulāris	joint (adj.), pertaining to joints
auricula	ear, the external portion of the ear
biceps	two-headed
brevis	short
buccinātor	that which has to do with the cheek (*bucca*)
corrūgātor	that which wrinkles, "wrinkle"
cubitum	elbow
dēpressor	that which lowers or depresses, depressor

*The word abductor is not found in Latin of the classical period, but had been formed on the model of other Latin words of similar construction. Such words and terms common in the terminology of anatomy and biology are called New Latin. Several other words in this vocabulary are New Latin.

Latin	Meaning
digitus	finger, toe
dīlātor	that which widens, dilator
extensor	that which extends, extensor
femur, femoris	thigh
flexor	that which flexes or bends, flexor
genū, genūs	knee
hallux, hallucis	big toe
index, indicis	index (first) finger
levātor	that which raises, levator
manus, manūs	hand
medius	middle
mentālis	of the chin (*mentum*)
minimus	smallest
nāris	nostril
nāsus	nose
oppōnēns	opposing
palpēbra	eyelid
pēs, pedis	foot
pilus	hair
pollex, pollicis	thumb
pūpilla	pupil (of the eye)
rotātor	that which turns, rotator
supercilium	eyebrow
superior, superiōris	upper, higher
sūra	calf (of the leg)
tensor	that which tenses, tensor
trīceps	three-headed
tympanum	ear drum, tympanic membrane

ETYMOLOGICAL NOTES

The abductor and adductor muscles take their name from the Latin verb *dūcere, ductus* (lead, draw). Related to this verb is the noun *dux, ducis* (leader, commander, chief). The Italian honorific title *Il Duce* (the Chief) was accorded to Benito Mussolini on his accession to the dictatorship of Italy in the years between World Wars I and II. Adherents of his party belonged to the political organization called *Fascista*, Fascists, named for the symbol of the party, the *Fasci*, from Latin *fascēs*, a bundle of rods bound around an axe and carried in procession in front of the high magistrates of Rome. A related Latin word is *fascia* (band, bandage), which gave the name to the anatomic term **fascia**, the fibrous membrane covering, supporting, and separating tissue.

The Latin word *cubitum* (elbow) is from the verb *cubāre, cubitus* (lie down). When reclining to dine, as the

Romans did, the elbow was to lean upon. The verb meaning to recline at a dining table was *recumbere* (*re-*, back, and *-cumbere*, lie down), an alternate form of *cubāre*, used with prefixes. In Roman times, the term *cubitum* also meant the distance from the elbow to the tip of the extended middle finger, a term of measurement: a cubit. The distance is variously calculated as being from 18 to 21 inches.

A number of words in current use are related to the verb *cubāre* and its alternate form—*cumbere*: cubicle, from *cubiculum*, a diminutive noun meaning a (small) place for sleeping, bedroom. Procumbent means leaning forward, and recumbent means leaning backward. The incumbent is one who is in office. The expression, "It is incumbent upon us," implies a burden "lying upon" us. The terms incubus and succubus refer to demons, or evil spirits, that visit one at night for sexual intercourse. The incubus "lies upon" women, and the succubus "lies under" men. Today, the term incubus is used to refer to anything that is oppressive, something that weighs one down. Chickens incubate their eggs. An incubator is an apparatus where eggs are artificially hatched, or a chamber used to provide a stable and healthful atmosphere for the development of premature or sick babies.

Latin *manus* (hand) has several interesting derivatives in English, among which are the words **maneuver** and **manure,** both with the same etymology: from *manus* and *opus, operis* (work). Both are disguised as a result of their transition through French before entering the English language (Fig. 17-4). Maneuver is from French *manoeuvre*, from Medieval Latin *manuopera*, meaning something done by hand, from Latin *manuoperāre* (work by hand). A maneuver is literally "something done by hand." Today, it means an evasive movement, a manipulation of affairs done for someone's advantage. (Note that the words manipulate and manipulation are from Latin *manipulus*, a handful.) Manure, barnyard refuse used as fertilizer, has the same ultimate etymology as maneuver but underwent a secondary change in form during the Middle English period, the 12th through the 15th centuries. The Middle English form is *manouren*, a verb meaning to cultivate the land (by hand), with a secondary (and modern) meaning of using manure to enrich the soil. The second component of these words, *opus, operis*, has given us such words as **operate, opera, operation,** and **inoperable.**

The modern names for the bones of the body came from the ancient Roman anatomists and their successors in the Middle Ages and Renaissance. In some instances, the bones were named after some familiar object that they resembled. In others, there seems to be no etymology to the name or any reason for it. Most of the names of bones are Latin words, but a number were borrowed from the early Greek scientists such as Hippocrates, Aristotle, and Galen.

The Latin words *digitus* (finger, toe), *ulna* (elbow, arm), *femur, femoris* (thigh), *humerus* (shoulder), *tibia* (shin), and *ilium* (flank) were originally used only to designate these parts of the body. Later, they were used to designate the

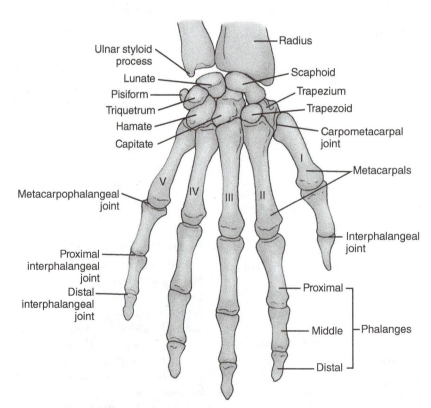

Figure 17-4. Bones of the right hand and wrist. (From Beam, J., *Orthopedic Taping, Wrapping, Bracing, and Padding*, 4th ed., F. A. Davis, 2021, with permission.)

bones underlying these parts. The following is a partial list of bones that includes some named after familiar objects:

clavicle, collar bone: "little key." Latin *clāvis* (key).

patella, kneecap: "little dish." Latin *patena* (open dish), from *patere* (lie open).

mandible, jawbone: "capable of chewing." Latin *mandere* (chew).

fibula, outer bone of leg: "safety pin." Latin *fibula* (brooch).

scaphoid, bone of the ankle and wrist: "boat-shaped." Greek *skaphē* (boat).

zygoma, bone of the cheek: "arch." Greek *zygon* (yoke).

trapezium, bone of the wrist: "little table." Greek *trapeza* (table).

cuneiform, bone of the ankle: "wedge-shaped." Latin *cuneus* (wedge).

malleus, ossicle ("little bone") of the middle ear: "hammer." Latin *malleus* (hammer).

incus, ossicle ("little bone") of the middle ear: "anvil." Latin *incūs* (anvil).

sacrum, base of the vertebral column: "sacred thing." Latin *sacer* (sacred). This part of the body of animals was burned in offerings to the gods.

lunate, bone of the wrist: "moon shaped." Latin *lūna* (moon).

hamate, bone of the wrist: "hook shaped." Latin *hāmus* (hook).

pisiform, bone of the wrist: "pea shaped." Latin *pīsum* (pea).

tarsus, ankle: "framework." Greek *tarsos* (wicker frame).

phalanges, bones of the fingers or toes: "battle line." Greek *phalanges* (plural of *phalanx,* a military unit). The Macedonian phalanx, a fighting group developed by Philip II, King of Macedonia and father of Alexander the Great, was made up of 256 men formed in a square 16 across and 16 deep and trained to maneuver with great dexterity on the field of battle.

Exercise 1: Determine the Function

Indicate, in ordinary, everyday terms, the location and function of each of the following muscles.

1. abductor* digiti minimi muscle _____

2. abductor digiti minimi pedis muscle _____

3. abductor hallucis muscle _____

4. abductor pollicis brevis muscle _____

5. abductor pollicis longus muscle _____

6. adductor brevis muscle _____

7. adductor hallucis muscle _____

8. adductor pollicis muscle _____

---

*When the first word of the names of muscles ends in -or (singular, or -ores, plural), this word is usually a noun that explains what the muscle does. All of the first five muscles in this list, for example, are abductor muscles. The part of the body that is abducted is put in the genitive case. That is, each of these muscles is the abductor of something.

9. arrectores pilorum muscles _____

10. articularis cubiti muscle _____

11. articularis genus muscle _____

12. biceps brachii muscle _____

13. femoris muscle _____

14. buccinator muscle _____

15. corrugator supercilii muscle _____

16. depressor anguli oris muscle _____

17. depressor labii inferioris muscle _____

18. dilator naris muscle _____

19. extensor digiti minimi muscle _____

20. extensor digitorum muscle _____

21. extensor hallucis brevis muscle _____

22. extensor indicis muscle _____

23. extensor pollicis brevis muscle _____

24. flexor digiti minimi brevis pedis muscle _____

25. flexor digiti minimi brevis manus muscle _____

26. flexor digitorum brevis pedis muscle _____

27. flexor hallucis brevis muscle _____

28. flexor pollicis brevis muscle _____

29. flexor pollicis longus muscle _____

30. levator anguli oris muscle _____

31. levator ani muscle _____

32. levator labii superioris muscle _____

33. levator labii superioris alaeque* nasi muscle _____

34. levator palpebrae superioris muscle _____

35. mentalis muscle _____

36. opponens digiti minimi muscle _____

37. opponens pollicis muscle _____

38. rotatores cervicis muscles _____

39. sphincter ani externus muscle _____

40. sphincter ani internus muscle _____

41. sphincter pupillae muscle _____

42. sphincter urethrae muscle _____

43. tensor tympani muscle _____

44. triceps brachii muscle _____

45. triceps surae muscle _____

---

*Latin *alaeque* "and of the wing." -*que* affixed to a noun means that this noun is to be connected with the noun that precedes it with "and." This -*que* (called an enclitic) can be affixed to any form of a noun or adjective. The initials S.P.Q.R., frequently seen on Roman inscriptions, stands for *Senatus Populusque Romanus* (the Senate and the Roman People).

THE SKELETON

The **skeleton** (Greek *skeleton*, dried up [sc. *sōma*, body]; "a dried up body") (Fig. 17-5) is the bony framework consisting of 206 bones. The distribution of these 206 bones is as follows:

cranial:	8 bones
facial:	14 bones
hyoid bone:	1 U-shaped bone lying at the base of the tongue
auditory:	6 ossicles, "little bones"
vertebrae:	26 bones

ribs:	24 bones
sternum:	1 breastbone
arms & shoulders:	10 bones
wrists:	16 bones
hands:	38 bones
legs and hips:	10 bones
ankles:	14 bones
feet:	38 bones

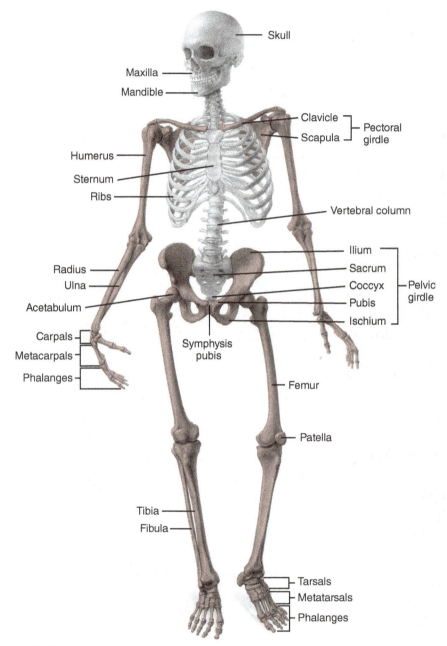

Figure 17-5. Skeleton. (From Gylys, B. A., and Wedding, M. E., *Medical Terminology Systems: A Body Systems Approach*, 8th ed., F.A. Davis, with permission.)

Exercise 2:   Identify Bones or Groups of Bones

Indicate, in ordinary, everyday terms, the location of each of the following bones or groups of bones.

1. clavicle _____

2. sternum _____

3. humerus _____

4. coccyx _____

5. metacarpals _____

6. patella _____

7. fibula _____

8. phalanges (two different sets) _____

    a. _____

    b. _____

9. scapula _____

10. sacrum _____

11. radius _____

12. femur _____

13. tibia _____

14. ilium _____

15. metatarsals _____

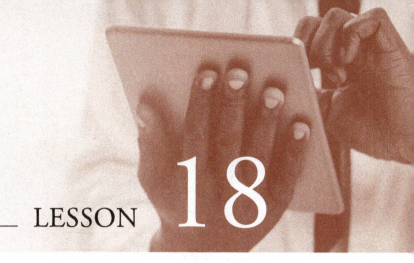

NERVOUS SYSTEM

The human body is a complex, highly organized structure composed of trillions of cells. These cells perform the many functions that keep the body in a state of dynamic equilibrium called **homeostasis.** Two systems of communication regulate body processes through electrical and chemical signals that pass between cells: the **nervous system** (discussed here), and the **endocrine system** (discussed in Lesson 19).

The nervous system has two major divisions: the **central nervous system** (CNS), and the **peripheral nervous system** (PNS), which includes the nerves of the **autonomic nervous system** (ANS) (Fig. 18-1). Both the CNS and PNS are composed of cells called **neurons,** the structural and functional units of the nervous system. Some of these neurons are short, measuring less than a millimeter in length, while others are more than 1 meter (39.37 inches) long. A nerve fiber, or axon, is a long, thin projection of a nerve cell. The terms neuron, or nerve cell, and nerve fiber are not to be confused with the term **nerve.** A nerve is an enclosed cable-like bundle of nerve fibers that connects the brain and the spinal cord to other parts of the body. A bundle of nerve fibers is called a **fasciculus** (diminutive of Latin *fascis*, bundle).* Nerves transmit electrical and chemical signals between the CNS and body tissues. Signals carried from the brain and spinal cord are called **efferent impulses;** signals carried to the brain and spinal cord are called **afferent impulses.**

SUBDIVISIONS OF THE NERVOUS SYSTEM

The **CNS** consists of the spinal cord and the brain. The spinal cord conducts sensory impulses from the PNS to the brain, and motor impulses from the brain to the various effectors, such as the skeletal muscles and glands. The brain receives sensory impulses from the spinal cord and its own nerves, and it discharges motor impulses to the muscles and glands. The brain and the spinal cord are made up of two types of tissue called gray matter **(substantia grisea)** and white matter **(substantia alba). Gray matter** is nerve tissue composed mainly of the neuronal cell bodies. **White matter** is nerve tissue composed of myelinated nerve fibers. White matter in the brain and spinal cord transmits the afferent and efferent impulses.

Bony structures protect the brain and spinal cord. The skull encloses the brain, and the vertebral column encloses the spinal cord. The **meninges** are the three membranes that lie under the bony structures of the skull and the vertebral column; they cover and protect the spinal cord and the brain (Fig. 18-2). The outermost of the three meninges is a hard membrane called the **dura mater.** The term **epidural** refers to the space around the dura. The innermost of the three is a soft membrane called the **pia mater.** Lying between the two is a weblike membrane called the **arachnoid membrane.** A blow to the head, even one that seems minor, can result in bleeding between the dura mater and arachnoid membrane. This bleeding, called **subdural hematoma,** occurs slowly; symptoms may not appear for several days or even weeks after the initial injury.†

Inflammation of any of the meninges is called **meningitis.** Inflammation of the spinal cord membranes is **spinal meningitis. Cerebral meningitis** is acute or chronic meningitis of the brain. Clinically, these two are not differentiated but are simply referred to as meningitis. Meningitis can be caused by an infection from bacteria, viruses, or fungi. It may also be caused by noninfectious

---

*See discussion in Lesson 17.

†See the Etymological Notes in this lesson for a discussion of the dura mater and pia mater.

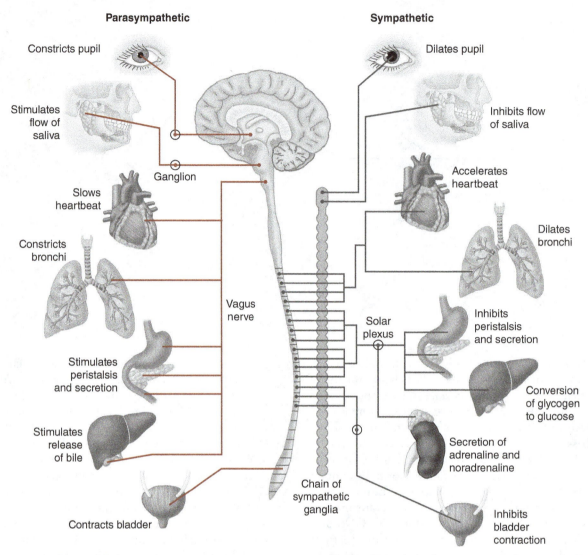

Parasympathetic

Constricts pupil

Stimulates flow of saliva

Ganglion

Slows heartbeat

Constricts bronchi

Vagus nerve

Stimulates peristalsis and secretion

Stimulates release of bile

Contracts bladder

Sympathetic

Dilates pupil

Inhibits flow of saliva

Accelerates heartbeat

Dilates bronchi

Solar plexus

Inhibits peristalsis and secretion

Conversion of glycogen to glucose

Secretion of adrenaline and noradrenaline

Chain of sympathetic ganglia

Inhibits bladder contraction

Figure 18-1. Autonomic nervous system. (From Scanlon, V. C., and Sanders, T., *Essentials of Anatomy and Physiology*, 7th ed., F. A. Davis, 2015, p. 214, with permission.)

inflammation, such as occurs with **systemic lupus erythematosus** (referred to as SLE or lupus).

Poliomyelitis (Greek *polios*, gray), usually called "polio," is a crippling inflammation of the gray matter of the spinal cord. Two important scientific advances significantly reduced the incidence of polio in the United States. In 1955, American virologist Dr. Jonas E. Salk (1914–1995) developed the first polio vaccine, the Salk vaccine, an inactivated, injectable vaccine. Six years later, Russian-born American virologist Dr. Albert B. Sabin (1906–1993) developed a live, attenuated oral polio vaccine, the Sabin vaccine. The massive public health initiative that followed resulted in the near eradication of polio in the United States, although a small number of cases continued to occur yearly.

In 1999, an advisory panel to the Centers for Disease Control and Prevention (CDC) determined that the live oral Sabin vaccine was responsible for 8 to 10 cases of polio each year. The panel recommended that routine use

of the live vaccine be discontinued, saying "the risk was too great." Only the inactivated Salk vaccine is approved for use in the United States. Polio epidemics still occur outside the United States. Recommendations for those outbreaks include the use of the live oral vaccine.*

The peripheral nervous system, or **PNS**, is made up of cranial nerves and spinal nerves. The PNS lies outside the CNS and includes nerves to and from skeletal and skin muscles. The PNS relays information to and from the CNS and includes the autonomic nervous system (ANS). Both the CNS and the PNS control the voluntary or conscious functions of the body.

The autonomic nervous system, or **ANS**, controls involuntary or unconscious bodily functions. It regulates the action of the salivary, gastric, and sweat glands, as well as the adrenal medulla, which produces epinephrine. The ANS is

---

*Venes D., ed. *Taber's Cyclopedic Medical Dictionary*. 23rd ed. F. A. Davis. 2017, p. 2458.

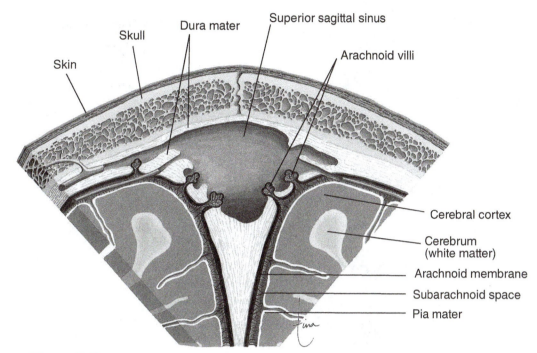

Figure 18-2. Meninges. (From Scanlon, V. C., and Sanders, T., *Essentials of Anatomy and Physiology*, 8th ed., F. A. Davis, 2020, with permission.)

divided into two parts: the **sympathetic division** and the **parasympathetic division,** each with its own functions. Often, the two divisions act in opposition to each other. Stimulation of the nerve fibers of the sympathetic division causes constriction of the vasomotor muscles, which surround the blood vessels of the body. **Vasoconstriction,** a decrease in the diameter of a blood vessel or vessels, decreases blood flow, causing a rise in blood pressure and overall heart rate. The sympathetic division is responsible for the "fight-or-flight" physiologic response.

Stimulation of the nerve fibers of the parasympathetic division produces **vasodilation,** an increase in the size of a blood vessel or vessels, which results in decreased blood pressure and heart rate. Stimulation of the nerve fibers of the sympathetic and the parasympathetic systems is brought about through the action of two **neurotransmitters: norepinephrine,** a hormone, and **acetylcholine,** an ester of choline. The endings of the nerve fibers of the sympathetic nervous system secrete norepinephrine. These fibers are said to be **adrenergic** (named after adrenaline, the name given to synthetic epinephrine). Release of this hormone causes stimulation of the sympathetic system. Norepinephrine is a **sympathetic mediator** or, sometimes, an **adrenergic mediator.**

The endings of nerve fibers of the parasympathetic nervous system secrete acetylcholine, and are said to be **cholinergic.** The action of these two substances, norepinephrine and acetylcholine, stimulates these two divisions of the ANS to produce vasoconstriction, caused by the sympathetic division, and vasodilation, caused by the parasympathetic division.

STRUCTURE OF THE NERVOUS SYSTEM

The nervous system is composed of specialized cells called nerve cells, or neurons (Fig. 18-3). Neurons are the structural and functional units of the nervous system. Each neuron consists of a cell body, an **axon,** and one or more **dendrites.** The cell bodies of neurons form the gray matter of the nervous system; myelinated axons form the white matter. Neurons make contact with each other at points called **synapses,** small spaces between the axon of one neuron and the dendrites or cell body of the next neuron. Through the synapses, the individual neurons form a complex network within the body that transmits motor and sensory information back and forth between the CNS and PNS. Dendrites, which look like tree branches when viewed under a microscope, conduct impulses to the cell body and form synaptic connections with dendrites of other neurons. Axons are structures that conduct impulses away from the cell body. "Processes" is the term used for both dendrites and axons. The axons usually are long and straight and end in synapses through which impulses are conducted to other neurons. In other words, dendrites conduct afferent impulses, and axons conduct efferent impulses.

The brain contains approximately 86 billion neurons and several hundred trillion synaptic connections. In addition to the neurons, in the gray and white matter of the nervous system are accessory cells called **glia cells,** or **neuroglia cells**. These glia cells hold the neurons in place and play an important role in brain development and function.

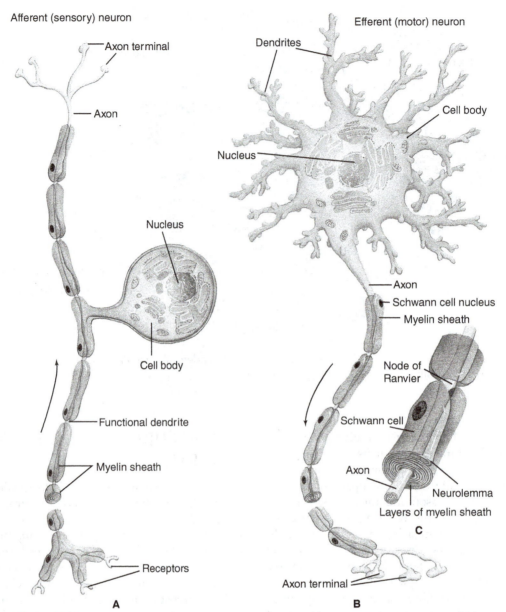

Figure 18-3. Neuron structure. *(A)* A typical sensory neuron. *(B)* A typical motor neuron. (From Scanlon, V. C., and Sanders, T., *Essentials of Anatomy and Physiology*, 8th ed., F. A. Davis, 2020, with permission.)

Tumors of the glia cells of the brain are called **gliomas** or **neurogliomas.** Gliomas, the most common type of brain tumor, account for about 25% of all tumors and 75% of malignant brain tumors.* If caught early, gliomas can often be removed with surgery.

The **spinal cord** is an ovoid column of nerve tissue about 18 inches long and about the thickness of a pencil. It extends within the vertebral column from the base of the skull to just below the ribs. Thirty-one pairs of nerves emanate from the spinal cord, and conduct impulses between the brain and the trunk and limbs of the body (Fig. 18-4). If the spinal cord is severed or damaged severely enough,

sensation and control of all muscles below the point of injury are lost. While there is no cure for spinal cord injury, laboratory research is encouraging. Depending on the injury, it may be possible to recover some degree of function.†

The **brainstem,** named for its stemlike appearance, connects the diencephalon with the spinal cord and includes the medulla oblongata, the pons, and the midbrain (Fig. 18-5). The **medulla oblongata** (from Latin *medulla*, marrow, and *oblongata*, elongated), the lower part of the brainstem, contains structures that regulate heart rate, breathing, and blood pressure. The **midbrain,** also called

*Rothman J. Brain tumors: who gets them and what is the survival rate? https://www.everydayhealth.com/brain-tumor/brain-tumor-statistics.aspx. Reviewed March 5, 2018. Accessed August 4, 2021.

†FAQs about spinal cord injury (SCI). University of Alabama at Birmingham. https://www.uab.edu/medicine/sci/faqs-about-spinal-cord-injury-sci. Accessed August 14, 2021.

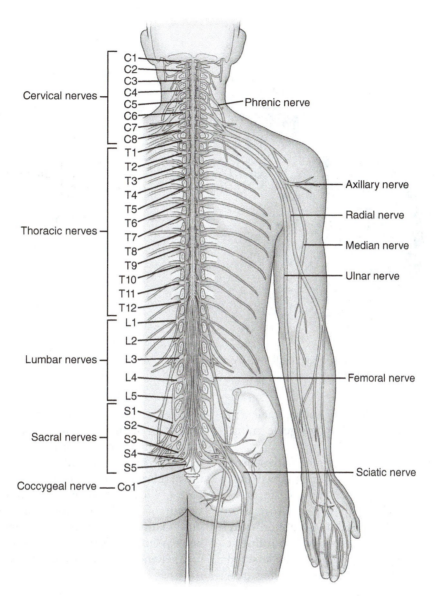

Figure 18-4. Spinal nerves (left side). (From Hoffman, J., and Sullivan, N., *Medical-Surgical Nursing: Making Connections to Practice*, 2nd Edition, F.A. Davis, 2020, with permission.)

the **mesencephalon,** is the upper part of the brainstem and contains structures that regulate respiration, touch, and hearing as well as equilibrium and posture. The **pons** lies between the medulla and the cerebrum and bridges the area between these two structures. The pons regulates transmission of impulses from the 5th, 6th, 7th, and 8th cranial nerves, which control muscles of the face and the eyes. At the upper end of the brainstem, above the midbrain, is a large mass of gray matter called the **thalamus.** The thalamus is composed of two oval-shaped structures. All sensory impulses except olfaction (the sense of smell) are processed in the thalamus, which then relays them to the cerebrum where sensations are felt.

Beneath the thalamus is a structure called the **hypothalamus,** which maintains the homeostasis of the body. It has diverse functions including regulation of body temperature and food intake as well as the production of certain hormones, such as **oxytocin.**

The largest part of the brain, the **cerebrum,** is composed of right and left hemispheres. Each hemisphere is subdivided into four lobes: frontal, parietal, occipital, and temporal. Within these two hemispheres are four paired masses of gray matter called the **basal ganglia.** These ganglia control muscle movements, such as walking or lifting, and other voluntary movements. If these ganglia become damaged, the individual loses some control over these simple muscle movements, resulting in disorders like cerebral palsy, Saint Vitus dance (Sydenham chorea), Bell palsy, Parkinson disease, and other abnormalities of voluntary muscle movement.

The **cerebral cortex** is the thin surface layer of gray matter covering each cerebral hemisphere. The word *cortex* is from Latin and meant bark (of a tree). Other organs of the body, including the adrenal gland, have outer coverings called **cortices** (singular, cortex). The cerebral cortex exerts motor control over certain muscles and controls the

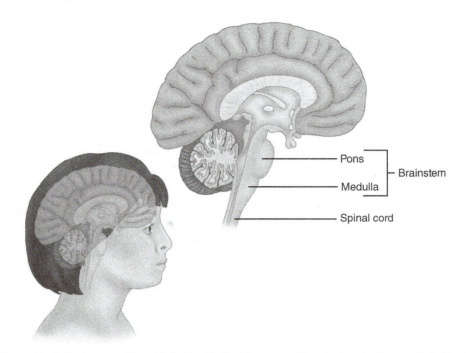

Figure 18-5. Brain stem. (From Hull, M., *Medical Language: Terminology in Context*, F. A. Davis, 2013, with permission.)

functions of the five senses: sight, hearing, touch, smell, and taste. The cerebral cortex also controls language, learning, and memory.

The area of the cerebral cortex associated with speech production and articulation is the Broca area (named after Pierre-Paul Broca, a 19th-century French physician, anatomist, and anthropologist). Damage to the Broca area causes the death of brain cells, resulting in the abnormality called **Broca aphasia,** also called **expressive** or **nonfluent aphasia.** People with this type of aphasia may understand what others are saying but they have trouble speaking, getting words out, and may omit words.*

Another area of the cerebral cortex is the Wernicke area (named for Karl Wernicke, a 19th-century German pathologist), located in the left middle section of the brain. Damage to the Wernicke area causes those affected to jumble words such that they cannot be understood by others. This condition is called **Wernicke** or **receptive aphasia**, the most common type of fluent aphasia.†

While the cerebral cortex controls memory, long-term memory is associated with another part of the brain called the **hippocampus.**‡ The hippocampus is important in memory consolidation, the process of transferring new learning to long-term memory. Damage to the hippocampus results in the loss of ability to remember anything for more than a short time—a day or even a few hours.

The **cerebellum** is a structure located above the brainstem at the back of the skull (Fig. 18-6). The word cerebellum, from the Latin word of the same name meaning "little brain," entered English in the 16th century. Like the cerebrum, the cerebellum has two hemispheres and a cortex. This portion of the brain controls the locomotor system of the body, which governs voluntary muscular movements other than those controlled by the cerebral hemispheres. This involves coordination, muscle tone, and maintenance of equilibrium and posture.

EPILEPSY

Epilepsy is defined as a chronic brain disorder marked by recurrent, abnormal electrical discharges, or seizures.§ If an individual has experienced two or more unprovoked seizures (a seizure unrelated to an underlying condition), or one seizure and an underlying condition with a high risk for more seizures, that individual is considered to have epilepsy. Between 2% and 3% of the population have epilepsy with the highest incidence in children under 10 years of age and adults age 70 or older.¶ Symptoms may vary from an almost imperceptible change in consciousness to loss of consciousness, convulsions, and amnesia of the event. Epilepsy may result from congenital or acquired brain

*Acharia AB, Wroton M. Broca Aphasia. StatPearls, NCBI Bookshelf. Updated May 4, 2022.
†Wernicke aphasia. Venes D., ed. *Taber's Cyclopedic Medical Dictionary*. 23rd ed. F. A. Davis. 2017, p. 2531.
‡Greek *hippokampos*, a mythical sea horse, a creature with the head and neck of a horse and the body and tail of a fish.

§Venes D., ed. *Taber's Cyclopedic Medical Dictionary*. 23rd ed. F. A. Davis. 2017, p. 828.
¶Sarmast ST, Abdullahi AM, Jahan N. Current classification of seizures and epilepsies: scope, limitations and recommendations for future action. *Cureus*. 2020, 12(9):e10549. https://doi.org/10.7759/cureus.10549.

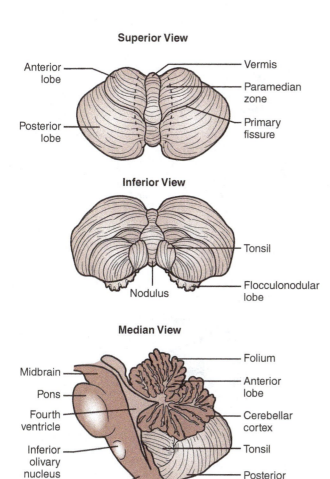

Superior View

Anterior lobe

Vermis

Paramedian zone

Primary fissure

Posterior lobe

Inferior View

Tonsil

Flocculonodular lobe

Nodulus

Median View

Midbrain

Pons

Fourth ventricle

Inferior olivary nucleus

Medulla

Folium

Anterior lobe

Cerebellar cortex

Tonsil

Posterior lobe

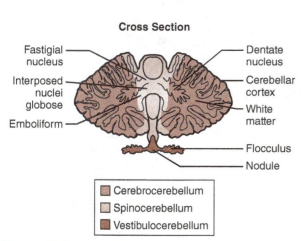

Cross Section

Fastigial nucleus

Interposed nuclei globose

Emboliform

Dentate nucleus

Cerebellar cortex

White matter

Flocculus

Nodule

☐ Cerebrocerebellum
☐ Spinocerebellum
☐ Vestibulocerebellum

Figure 18-6. Cerebellum, showing layers of the cerebellar cortex. (From Fell, D.W. Lunnen, K.Y., and Rauk R.P. *Lifespan Neurorehabilitation: A Patient-Centered Approach from Examination to Interventions and Outcomes*. Philadelphia PA: F.A. Davis, 2018.)

disease. In adulthood, epilepsy may develop as a result of strokes, tumors, brain trauma, or encephalitis. Often, the underlying cause is undetermined or idiopathic.

The International League Against Epilepsy classifies epilepsy as partial, generalized, drug-resistant, or unclassified.

Partial seizures begin with focal or local electrical discharges that occur in a small area of the brain. In generalized seizures, abnormal electrical activity occurs throughout the brain. Two common forms of generalized seizures are **absence seizures** and **tonic-clonic seizures.** Absence seizures occur mainly in children and present as a brief lapse of consciousness lasting 2 to 10 seconds. During an absence seizure, a child may appear to be staring into space. Tonic-clonic seizures (tonic means stiffening, clonic means rhythmic jerking movements) are also called convulsions. These seizures usually begin on both sides of the brain but can begin on one side and spread to the entire brain. Tonic-clonic seizures are characterized by falling, loss of consciousness, stiffening, and twitching or jerking of the extremities. Seizures may last from 1 to 3 minutes; seizures lasting 5 minutes or more require immediate medical care. In most cases, seizure disorder can be controlled and/or prevented with antiepileptic medications. If the seizures are not well controlled with medication, a condition called medically refractory epilepsy or drug-resistant epilepsy, surgical therapy may be recommended to stop seizures or limit their severity.*

NERVE PLEXUSES

Nerves from the spine and brain, from both the voluntary and the autonomic systems, connect, or anastomose (Greek *anastomōsis*, an opening), to form multiple interwoven networks of nerves, each called a **plexus** (plural plexus or plexuses). These plexuses send messages from the brain to the muscles, allowing movement to occur.

Following is a list of characteristics of some plexuses and their location in the body.

- **Brachial plexus:** Lower part of the neck to the axilla (armpit)
- **Celiac plexus:** Also called the solar plexus, behind the stomach and in front of the aorta
- **Cervical plexus:** Opposite the first four cervical vertebrae; that is, the top four of the seven vertebrae of the spinal column
- **Lumbar plexus:** Psoas muscle (lower part of the back and sides, the lumbar region)
- **Myenteric plexus:** The muscles that surround the walls of the gastrointestinal tract

CRANIAL NERVES

Twelve pairs of **cranial nerves** originate on either side of the brain, one of each pair in the left hemisphere and one in the right (Fig. 18-7). The name, function, and distribution of these 12 pairs of nerves are listed in Table 18-1.

*For more information on epilepsy and/or seizures, see *Taber's Cyclopedic Medical Dictionary*, 23rd ed. s.v. epilepsy, p. 828; s.v. seizure, p. 2120.

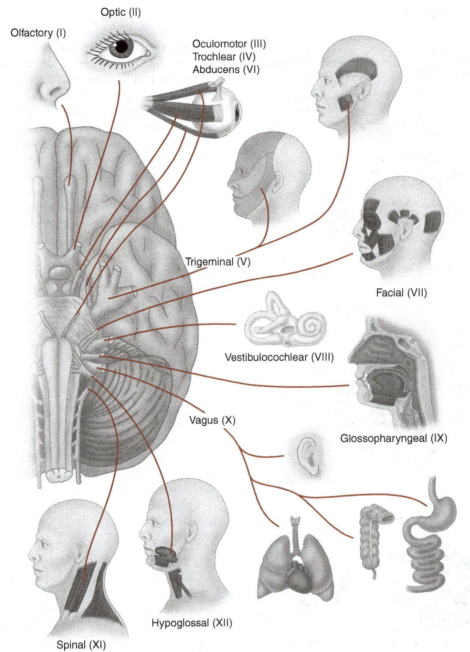

Figure 18-7. Cranial nerves and their distributions. (From Hull, M., *Medical Language: Terminology in Context*, F. A. Davis, with permission.)

Table 18-1. **Cranial Nerves**

Number	Name	Function	Distribution
1st	Olfactory	Smell	Olfactory mucosa
2nd	Optic	Sight	Retina
3rd	Oculomotor	Motor	Four of the six muscles of the eye
4th	Trochlear	Motor	Superior oblique muscles of the eye
5th	Trigeminal	Motor and chief sensory nerve of the face	Skin, mucous membranes, and sinuses of the face; muscles of mastication
6th	Abducens	Motor	Lateral rectus muscle of the eye
7th	Facial	Motor	Muscles of facial expression

Number	Name	Function	Distribution
8th	Vestibulocochlear	Hearing and equilibrium	Internal auditory meatus*
9th	Glossopharyngeal	Motor and sensory	Pharynx and posterior third of the tongue, parotid gland, ear, meninges
10th	Vagus	Motor and sensory	Pharynx, larynx, heart, lungs, esophagus, stomach, abdominal viscera
11th	Spinal Accessory	Motor	Sternomastoid and trapezius muscles
12th	Hypoglossal	Motor	Muscles of the tongue

*Latin, *meatus*, opening.

VOCABULARY

Note: Latin forms are given in ***bold italics***.

Greek or Latin	Combining Form	Meaning	Example
arachnē	**ARACHN-**	spider, web; arachnoid membrane	**arachn**-oidea
axon	**AX-, AXON-**	axis, axon	**ax**-olemma
cerebrum	***CEREBR-***	brain	**cerebr**-ospinal
cholē	**CHOL(E)-**	bile, gall	**chol**-inergic
cortex, corticis	***CORTIC-, CORTEX***	[bark, rind] outer layer (of an organ)	cerebral **cortex**
dendron	**DENDR-**	[tree] dendrite, dendron	**dendr**-oid
dendritēs	**DENDRIT-**	[pertaining to a tree] dendrite, dendron	**dendrit**-es
fasciculus†	***FASCICL-, FASCICUL-***	[little bundle] fasciculus	**fascicul**-ation
ganglion	**GANGLI-**	[knot] ganglion	**gangli**-oma
glia	**GLI-, -GLIA-**	[glue] glia, neuroglia	neuro-**glia**
medulla	***MEDULL-***	marrow, medulla oblongata	**medull**-ary
mēninx, mēningos (plural *mēninges*)	**MENING-, -MENINX**	meningeal membrane, meninges	**mening**-es
myelos	**MYEL-**	myelin, spinal cord, bone marrow	**myel**-in
neuron	**NEUR-**	[tendon] neuron, nerve, nervous system	**neur**-obiology
plexus	***PLEX-***	[braid] plexus	**plex**-opathy
pons, pontis	***PONT-, PONS***	[bridge] pons	**pont**-ine nuclei
synapsis‡	**SYNAP-, SYNAPS-**	[point of contact] synapse	**synap**-tic
thalamos	**THALAM-**	[inner chamber] thalamus	**thalam**-ic

†Diminutive of Latin, *fascis*, bundle.
‡From the Greek, *haptein*, touch.

ETYMOLOGICAL NOTES

The spinal cord and the brain are covered with three layers of protective membrane called the meninges (singular, meninx). Before the first century AD, the Greek word *mēninx* was applied to any membrane of the body. Hippocrates used it to refer to the membrane of the eye; Aristotle used it to refer to the eardrum. After the first century, the term came to be used exclusively to refer to the meninges in their modern anatomic sense. The three meninges are the **pia mater,** the delicate inner covering; the **dura mater,** the tough outer layer; and the **arachnoid,** the membrane between these two. The arachnoid (resembling a web) takes its name from Greek *arachnē* (spider, web) because of its weblike structure. The names pia mater, meaning "devout mother" in Latin, and dura mater, "hard mother," do not seem to make sense unless it is realized they are translations from Arabic.

By the fourth century AD, the Roman Empire was split into two halves, with Rome the capital of the West and Byzantium (later named Constantinople by the emperor Constantine and now called Istanbul) the capital of the East. The two halves were separated linguistically as well as geographically, with Latin used as the language of the West and Greek used in the East. The writings that survived in the West were preserved, for the most part, by the Roman church and were principally the works of Latin authors. Greek ceased to be taught in schools, and the knowledge of this language was gradually lost, along with the works of Hippocrates, Aristotle, and others. Nevertheless, these works were very much alive in the East, not only in Byzantium/Constantinople but also in other lands of the Eastern Empire.

With the rise and spread of Islam during and after the seventh century, Arabic became the common language of almost the entire East. Works of the ancient Greek writers were translated into Arabic and read in the great centers of learning all over the Islamic empire, including Spain. These Arabic translations, and Arabic literature in general, escaped the notice of most of western Europe for the simple reason that few people could read Arabic. By the early Middle Ages, practically all knowledge of ancient Greek literature, including the medical works, was lost in the West.

In the 11th and 12th centuries, monks of the Roman church began translating some of the Arabic versions of the Greek writers into Latin. In Syria, a churchman known as Stephen of Antioch produced a Latin translation of Galen from the Arabic version. At this time, only two of the three meninges were known: the dura and the pia. Galen, writing in Greek, had named the outer (the dura) the *mēninx sklēra pacheia* (the hard, thick, membrane) and the inner (the pia), the *mēninx leptē* (the thin membrane). In the Arabic translation of Galen, the Greek terms were translated as "hard mother" and "thin mother." The Arabic use of the word for mother to translate the Greek *mēninx* may have implied that the protection afforded the spinal cord by the meninges could be compared with the protection that a mother gives to her young. Stephen translated these two terms into the Latin *dura mater* and *pia mater,* "hard mother" and "devout mother." The pia (feminine of *pius,* devout, pious) should have been *tenuis* (thin), but Stephen, a monk, decided that pia was a more appropriate term, and it has remained. The arachnoid membrane was not identified until the 17th century when Dutch anatomist Frederick Ruysch realized its existence and named it.

Exercise 1

Answer each of the following questions.

1. To what part of the nervous system does each of the following refer?

   a. CNS _____

   b. PNS _____

   c. ANS _____

2. The _____ are the structural and functional units of the nervous system.

3. What is the name given to a bundle of nerve fibers? _____

4. What is the difference between an afferent and an efferent impulse?_____

   _____

5. Name the three membranes that cover and protect the spinal cord and the brain and lie under the bony structure of the skull and the vertebral column.

   a. _____

   b. _____

   c. _____

6. What is a common cause of subdural hematoma? _____

7. Immunity against the disease polio was achieved with which two vaccines?

   a. _____

   b. _____

8. What is the difference between a nerve fiber that is adrenergic and one that is cholinergic? _____

   _____

9. A/An _____ is the process that conducts impulses away from the cell body.

10. Glia cells, often called neuroglia cells, have what function? _____

11. What are gliomas and neurogliomas? _____

12. The brainstem, the continuation of the spinal cord up into the skull, contains several important structures. What are they, and where are they found? _____

    _____

13. Beneath the thalamus is a structure called the _____

14. The four lobes that subdivide each cerebral hemisphere are the:

    a. _____

    b. _____

    c. _____

    d. _____

15. Disorders such as Sydenham chorea, Parkinson disease, and Bell palsy are caused by damage to the

_____

_____

16. A person who has Broca aphasia as a result of damage to the Broca area, has difficulty doing what?

_____

_____

17. What does the term "idiopathic" mean when it is used in reference to seizures? _____

_____

18. What is a plexus? _____

19. Give five plexuses (plexus) and their location.

a. _____   _____

b. _____   _____

c. _____   _____

d. _____   _____

e. _____   _____

20. Absence seizures occur mainly in _____

ENDOCRINE SYSTEM

The state of dynamic equilibrium within the body, when all organs are functioning perfectly, is called **homeostasis.** In the body, homeostasis is controlled by two systems: the **nervous system** (discussed in Lesson 18) and the **endocrine system** (Greek *endo-*, within, and *krinein*, separate, secrete), the subject of this chapter (Fig. 19-1). The endocrine system consists of glands that produce **hormones** (Greek *horman*, set in motion), internal secretions that are discharged into the blood and then circulated throughout the body. The **endocrine glands** (Table 19-1) are ductless glands that do not transmit their secretions by way of ducts, as the sweat glands and tear glands do. Glands that release their secretions by way of ducts are called **exocrine glands,** or sometimes **eccrine glands** (in particular, the eccrine sweat glands). Hormones, which originate in a gland, an organ, or a body part, are carried to other parts of the body by the bloodstream and, through chemical action, increase or decrease functional activity of those parts. The hormones secreted by the ductless glands may have a specific effect, as in the case of estrogens, which are secreted by the ovaries and stimulate the development of female secondary sexual characteristics. Or, they may have a general effect on the entire body, as in the case of thyroid hormone, which regulates the rate of metabolism of the whole body.

THE PITUITARY GLAND

The pituitary gland, medically referred to as the **hypophysis cerebri** or **hypophysis,** is a small, round gland about the size of a pea, weighing about 0.008 ounces in humans, and located off the hypothalamus at the base of the brain (Fig. 19-2). Sometimes referred to as the "master gland" of the body, the pituitary gland controls the functions of many of the other endocrine glands. The pituitary gland is made up of three sections: the anterior lobe, the posterior lobe, and the intermediate lobe.

The **anterior lobe** of the pituitary secretes six principal hormones:

1. **Growth hormone (GH),** or **somatotropin,** regulates cell division and protein synthesis for growth. Increased production of growth hormone can cause giantism (abnormal growth) and/or **acromegaly,** abnormal enlargement of the hands, feet, jaw, and other extremities. Decreased production of growth hormone can cause dwarfism and/or **acromicria,** abnormal smallness of the extremities.
2. **Adrenocorticotropin hormone (ACTH),** also called **corticotropin,** regulates the activity of the adrenal cortex, the outer layer of the adrenal gland. The **adrenal cortex** secretes two groups of hormones that belong to the family of chemicals called **steroids.** The first group of these hormones is the **mineralocorticoids,** which regulate the retention and excretion of fluids and electrolytes. The second group, the **glucocorticoids,** is a group of chemicals that have anti-inflammatory and immunosuppressive properties. Glucocorticoids help protect the body against stress and promote the healing process. The most important glucocorticoid is cortisol (hydrocortisone). In addition to these steroids, the adrenal cortex secretes sex hormones: androgens in men and estrogens and progesterone in women.
3. **Thyroid-stimulating hormone (TSH)** manages the activity of the thyroid gland. The hormones produced regulate the rate of cellular metabolism throughout the body.
4. (Ovarian) **follicle-stimulating hormone (FSH)** is responsible for developing follicles (Latin *folliculus*, a little sac, diminutive of *follis*, sac) in the ovaries, and spermatogenesis in the testes. The ovarian follicles are spherical structures that produce an ovum every month in women of childbearing age.

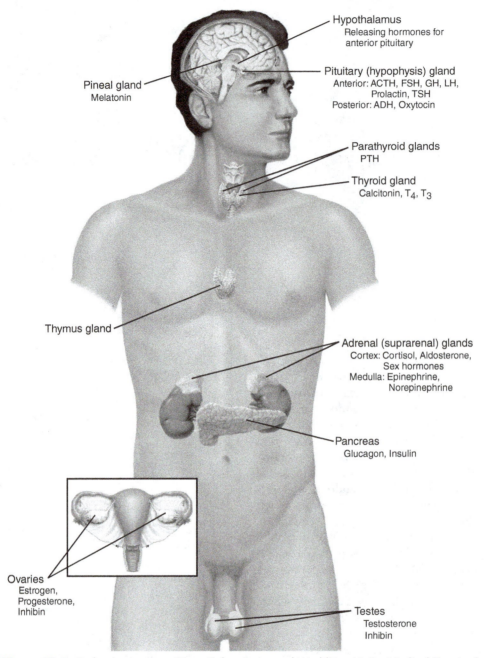

Figure 19-1. Endocrine system. (From Gylys, B. A., and Wedding, M. E., *Medical Terminology Systems: A Body Systems Approach*, 8th ed., F. A. Davis, 2017, with permission.)

5. **Luteinizing hormone (LH),** in conjunction with FSH, induces secretion of estrogens and progesterone, stimulates ovulation each month, and regulates the development of the *corpus luteum* (Latin, yellow body), a small yellow structure that develops within a ruptured ovarian follicle when the ovum is released each month in women of childbearing age. In men, LH stimulates the development of progesterone in the testes.

6. **Prolactin** or **lactogenic hormone,** in conjunction with progesterone and estrogens, stimulates breast development and induces the secretion of milk during pregnancy.

In humans, the **intermediate lobe** of the pituitary, along with the anterior lobe, produces melanocyte-stimulating hormone (MSH), which acts on cells in the skin to stimulate the production of melanin.* In cold-blooded animals, the intermediate lobe produces intermedin, also an MSH, which influences the activity of pigment cells (chromatophores) in some reptiles, fish, and amphibians.

---

*Melanocyte-stimulating hormone. Society for Endocrinology. https://www.yourhormones.info/hormones/melanocyte-stimulating-hormone/. Reviewed May 2021. Accessed August 29, 2021.

Table 19-1. Principal Endocrine Glands

Name	Position	Function	Endocrine Disorders
Adrenal cortex	Outer portion of gland on top of each kidney	Cortisol regulates carbohydrate and fat metabolism; aldosterone regulates salt and water balance	Hypofunction: Addison disease Hyperfunction: Adrenogenital syndrome; Cushing syndrome
Adrenal medulla	Inner portion of adrenal gland; surrounded by adrenal cortex	Effects of epinephrine and norepinephrine mimic those of sympathetic nervous system; increases carbohydrate use for energy	Hypofunction: Almost unknown Hyperfunction: Pheochromocytoma
Pancreas (endocrine portion)	Abdominal cavity; head adjacent to duodenum; tail close to spleen and kidney	Secretes insulin and glucagon, which regulate carbohydrate metabolism	Hypofunction: Diabetes mellitus Hyperfunction: If a tumor produces excess insulin, hypoglycemia
Parathyroid	Four or more small glands on back of thyroid	Parathyroid hormone regulates calcium and phosphorus metabolism; indirectly affects muscular irritability	Hypofunction: Hypocalcemia; tetany Hyperfunction: Hypercalcemia, resorption of bone, kidney stones, nausea, vomiting, altered mental status
Pituitary, anterior	Front portion of small gland below hypothalamus	Influences growth, sexual development, skin pigmentation, thyroid function, and adrenocortical function through effects on other endocrine glands (except for growth hormone, which acts directly on cells)	Hypofunction: Dwarfism in children; decrease in all other endocrine gland functions except parathyroids Hyperfunction: Acromegaly in adult; giantism in children
Pituitary, posterior	Back portion of small gland below hypothalamus	Oxytocin increases uterine contractions	Unknown
		Antidiuretic hormone increases absorption of water by kidney tubules	Hypofunction: Diabetes insipidus
Testes and ovaries	Testes—in the scrotum Ovaries—in the pelvic cavity	Testosterone and estrogen regulate sexual maturation and development of secondary sex characteristics; some effects on growth	Hypofunction: Lack of sex development or regression in adult Hyperfunction: Abnormal sex development
Thyroid	Two lobes in anterior portion of neck	Thyroxine and T_3 increase metabolic rate and influence growth and maturation; calcitonin regulates calcium and phosphorus metabolism	Hypofunction: Cretinism in young; myxedema in adult; goiter Hyperfunction: Goiter; thyrotoxicosis

Source: Venes, D., ed., *Taber's Cyclopedic Medical Dictionary*, 23rd ed., F. A. Davis, 2017, p. 1016, with permission.

The **posterior lobe** of the pituitary gland secretes the hormone **oxytocin** (Greek *oxys*, rapid, and *tokos*, childbirth), which increases uterine contractions during labor. **Antidiuretic hormone (ADH),** also called vasopressin, is also secreted within the posterior lobe. ADH contracts the muscles of blood vessels and elevates blood pressure. ADH acts as an antidiuretic, preventing excessive loss of fluids through the kidneys.

THE THYROID GLAND

The **thyroid gland** is situated at the base of the neck, spanning both sides of the lower part of the larynx and upper part of the trachea (Fig. 19-3). The name comes from Greek *thyreos* (shield), thyroid, "shield shaped." As noted previously, the thyroid gland is stimulated by TSH, also called **thyrotropin.** TSH is secreted within the anterior

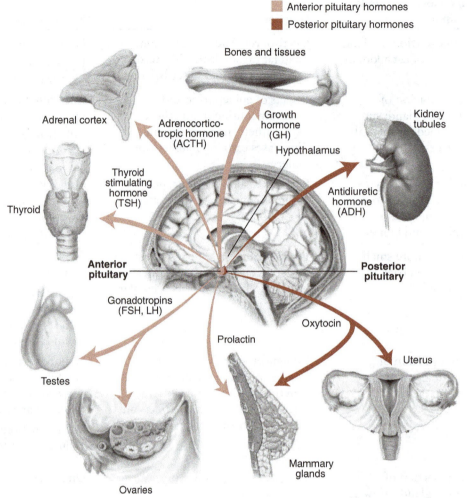

Anterior pituitary hormones
Posterior pituitary hormones

Figure 19-2. Pituitary gland. (From Eagle, S., et al., *The Professional Medical Assistant*, F. A. Davis, 2009, with permission.)

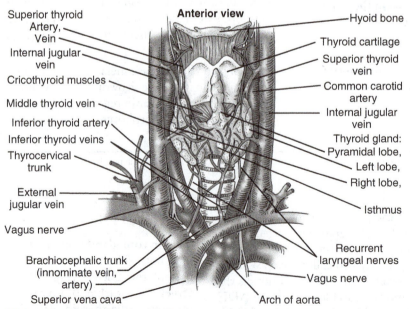

Figure 19-3. Thyroid gland and related structures. (From Venes, D., ed., *Taber's Cyclopedic Medical Dictionary*, 23rd ed., F. A. Davis, 2017, with permission.)

lobe of the pituitary gland. One of the principal hormones secreted by the thyroid gland is **thyroxine.** Oversecretion of thyroxine produces the condition called **hyperthyroidism** in which the rate of basal metabolism increases and leads to excessive stimulation of the sympathetic nervous system. Symptoms of hyperthyroidism can include increased nervousness, tremors, heat intolerance, increased heart rate, diarrhea, constipation and weight loss. About 1.5% of the U.S. population has hyperthyroidism. If overproduction of thyroxine is excessive, the condition called **thyrotoxicosis** may occur. Clinical symptoms associated with thyrotoxicosis include protruding eyes **(exophthalmos)** and, often, goiter, or enlargement of the thyroid. Treatment may involve medications, radioactive iodine ablation of the overactive gland, or surgical removal.

Insufficient production of thyroxin produces a condition called **hypothyroidism,** which results in a lowered basal metabolic rate. Symptoms of hypothyroidism are the opposite of those of hyperthyroidism and include fatigue, low blood pressure, slow pulse, increased sensitivity to cold, and decreased muscular activity. Goiter may accompany both hypothyroidism and hyperthyroidism. The underlying cause of hyperthyroidism and hypothyroidism is associated with the maintenance of proper levels of iodine in the diet. In certain regions of the world where the water is deficient in iodine salts, hypothyroidism is endemic. In recent years, however, the use of iodized salt has reduced the incidence of hypothyroidism in areas where iodine salts are at low levels in the drinking water. Treatment typically involves a daily dose of synthetic thyroid hormone (levothyroxine).

Severe lack of iodine in childhood produces the condition known as **cretinism,** characterized by lack of growth and mental development. The term cretin comes from Swiss French *creitin,* from Latin *Christiānus* (Christian). Use of this term originated in Switzerland where the water lacks iodine salts because the land is separated geologically from the sea. The Swiss are said to have used this term to indicate their realization that these cretins were children of God. Cretinism can also be a congenital condition caused by a lack of thyroid hormones and can occur as a result of antithyroid medications.

When hypothyroidism becomes severe, a condition known as **myxedema** (Greek *myxa,* mucus, and *edema,* swelling) may develop. Myxedema presents as thick, gelatinous materials called mucopolysaccharides that infiltrate the skin, giving it a waxy or coarsened appearance. Symptoms include sluggishness, cold intolerance, apathy, fatigue, and constipation that can lead to myxedema coma. Thyroid hormone replacement reverses the symptoms and reestablishes normal metabolic function.

THE PARATHYROID GLANDS

Located close to the thyroid gland are the four parathyroid glands. These glands secrete **parathyroid hormone (PTH),** which regulates the metabolism of calcium and phosphorus. **Hypoparathyroidism** results when the level of blood calcium falls and the level of blood phosphorus rises. This condition is characterized mainly by loss of calcium in the teeth and bones, with resultant tooth defects and bone lesions. Supplements to normalize calcium and phosphorous levels are used to treat this condition. The parathyroid glands are responsible for the proper maintenance of vitamin D in the body. Without normal levels of this vitamin, calcium cannot be properly utilized.

Hyperparathyroidism is the opposite of hypoparathyroidism and results when blood calcium rises and blood phosphorus falls. Symptoms of hyperparathyroidism include muscular weakness and osteoporosis, which occurs when calcium escapes from the bones into the circulating blood. The presence of abnormal amounts of calcium in the blood **(hypercalcemia)** and the inability of the kidneys to excrete this excess calcium can cause the formation of renal calculi—kidney stones—a condition known as **nephrolithiasis.** The symptoms of hyperparathyroidism are commonly referred to as stones (kidney stones), moans (gastrointestinal symptoms including constipation and abdominal pain), groans (psychological conditions including depression and dementia), and bones (bone pain).

THE ADRENAL GLANDS

There are two adrenal glands, sometimes called the **suprarenal glands,** one above each kidney (Fig. 19-4). Each adrenal gland consists of two distinct parts: the outer covering, called the **adrenal cortex,** and the inner structure, called the **adrenal medulla.** The adrenal cortex secretes three types of steroid hormones: **glucocorticoids, mineralocorticoids,** and sex hormones. Glucocorticoids regulate the metabolism of organic nutrients and have an anti-inflammatory effect. Mineralocorticoids affect metabolism

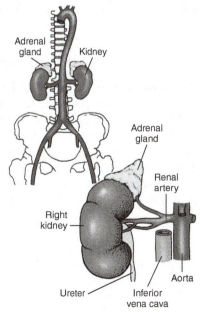

Figure 19-4. Adrenal glands. (From Venes, D., ed., *Taber's Cyclopedic Medical Dictionary,* 24th ed., F. A. Davis, 2022, with permission.)

of the electrolytes sodium and potassium. The glucocorticoid **cortisol (cortisone)** regulates the metabolism of fats, carbohydrates, sodium, potassium, and proteins. Cortisone is also manufactured synthetically and used as an anti-inflammatory agent. **Androgens,** male hormones, and **estrogens** and **progesterone,** female hormones, are also secreted in small amounts in the renal cortex. Irregularities in the production of these sex hormones can result in increased or decreased sexual development in both males and females.

The **adrenal medulla** secretes three groups of chemical substances called **catecholamines: dopamine, norepinephrine,** and **epinephrine.** The principal effects of **dopamine** on the body are dilation of the arteries and increased cardiac output, with resultant increased flow of blood to the kidneys.

The principal effect of **norepinephrine** is constriction of the arterioles and venules, the ends of the arteries and veins, where they anastomose, or join, with the capillaries. This results in increased resistance to the flow of blood through the systemic circulation, which in turn causes elevated blood pressure and slowing of the heart action **(bradycardia).**

Epinephrine increases heart activity and dilates the bronchi. Adrenalin (synthetic epinephrine) is useful in treating people with asthma. It increases the level of glucose in the blood and diminishes the activity of the gastrointestinal system.

The adrenal medulla is an extension of the sympathetic division of the autonomic nervous system.* The secretion of epinephrine and norepinephrine is closely related to emotional states. Fear, stress, and emergency situations can cause the sympathetic nervous system to "send a message" to the adrenal medulla, which can result in the immediate secretion of norepinephrine or epinephrine, giving a quick boost to the energy level of the body, the fight-or-flight response.

THE ISLETS OF LANGERHANS

The **islets of Langerhans,** named for Paul Langerhans, a 19th-century German pathologist, are clusters of cells in the pancreas. There are three types of cell clusters in the islets of Langerhans: alpha, beta, and delta cells. The beta cells, which produce insulin, occur in the greatest numbers.

Insulin (Latin *insula*, island) is essential for the proper metabolism of blood sugar (glucose) and for the proper maintenance of glucose levels in the blood. Insufficient secretion of insulin results in deficient metabolism of carbohydrates and fats and brings on the conditions called **hyperglycemia,** excessive amounts of blood sugar, and **glycosuria,** the presence of glucose in the urine. These two conditions characterize the disease called **diabetes.**

Excessive secretion of insulin brings about the condition called **hypoglycemia,** characterized by acute fatigue, irritability, and general weakness. In extreme cases, insulin shock, usually associated with excessive exogenous insulin, can bring about mental disturbances, coma, and even death.

Diabetes mellitus is a group of metabolic disorders characterized by the inability to metabolize carbohydrates.† Manifestations of the disease are hyperglycemia and glycosuria. Symptoms include **polydipsia, polyuria,** weight loss (despite **polyphagia**), and fatigue. There are two types of diabetes mellitus. Type 1 diabetes mellitus, also called insulin-dependent diabetes mellitus (IDDM), usually begins early in life and is characterized by an absolute deficiency of insulin. The isolation and eventual synthetization of insulin by the Canadian physicians Sir Frederick Banting and Charles H. Best (for which Banting won the Nobel prize in 1923) made it possible for people with type 1 diabetes to live with their disease by the injection of insulin.

Type 2 diabetes mellitus, called non-insulin-dependent diabetes mellitus (NIDDM), usually begins later in life and is characterized by resistance to the effects of insulin at the cellular level. Often, type 2 diabetes can be controlled with changes in diet and exercise. People with diabetes should test their blood sugar levels (glucose) frequently. However, if glucose concentration remains high in the blood, it may be necessary to administer medications, such as the sulfonylureas, which stimulate the pancreas to release insulin. Newer medications that work on a cellular level to increase sensitivity to insulin may also be used.

New diagnostic criteria recognize four types of diabetes: type 1, type 2, prediabetes in which blood sugar is high but not high enough to be classified as type 2, and gestational diabetes in which elevated blood sugar is related to pregnancy. Intervention at the stage of prediabetes can decrease development of type 2 diabetes. Thirty percent of those with gestational diabetes will develop type 2 diabetes later in life.

GONADS: THE TESTES AND OVARIES

The gonads are the male and female sex glands. The male gonads, the testes, secrete spermatozoa. The testes (or testicles) produce the male hormone testosterone, an androgen that stimulates and maintains secondary male sexual characteristics, including muscle strength, facial hair, and deepening of the voice.

The female gonads, the ovaries, produce an ovum each month during the parturient (childbearing) years. The ovaries produce the female hormones estrogen and progesterone, which stimulate and maintain secondary female sexual characteristics, including body fat distribution, growth of the mammary glands, and voice quality.‡

---

*See Lesson 18 for a further explanation of the autonomic nervous system.

†See Lesson 15 for a further explanation of diabetes mellitus.
‡For a more detailed discussion of ovulation, see Lesson 14.

ETYMOLOGICAL NOTES

The Greek verb *krinein* (separate), which supplies the element **-crine** in the words endocrine and exocrine, has also provided other, nontechnical words. In ancient times, the verb had additional meanings: to pick out or choose and, later, to judge. There was a noun, *krisis*, related to this verb, that meant a separating, picking out, or choosing. Extended meanings of this noun included trial, judgment, and decision. From these varied but related meanings comes the word **crisis**. Also related to the verb *krinein* was the noun *kritēs* (judge or arbiter); the adjectival form of this noun was *kritikos* (able to decide or judge, critical). This word was found in Latin as the noun *criticus* (judge or critic). Another related word was *kritērion* (a means of judging, a standard, criterion).

Estrogen, the female hormone, takes its name from Greek *oistros* (gadfly), an insect that infected cattle, plus the form **-gen**. This unusual etymology has at its root a secondary meaning of this noun: a sting, anything that excites, madness, frenzy, or vehement passion. The term estrus (or oestrus) designates the cyclic period of sexual activity in females; thus, estrogen is the name of the hormone that causes or promotes the period of estrus. The ancients were unaware of the reasons for the cyclic periods of women between menarche and menopause, and the word *oistros* (Latin *oestrus*) was used by the writers in its original sense: that which excites (something or somebody) to action; a stinging insect. Virgil writes:

> *est lucos Silari circa ilicibusque virentem*
> *plurimus Alburnum volitans, cui nomen asilo*
> *Romanum est, oestrum Grai vertere vocantes. . .*

> Around the groves of Silarus and around
> Alburnus green with oak trees
> there flies a creature which the Romans call *asilus*,
> but called *oestrus* by the Greeks. . .

> (*Georgics*, 3.146–148)

Greek legend tells us of a young girl named Io, daughter of Inachus, the river god of Argos, who had the misfortune to be desired by Zeus (Fig. 19-5). Just as Zeus

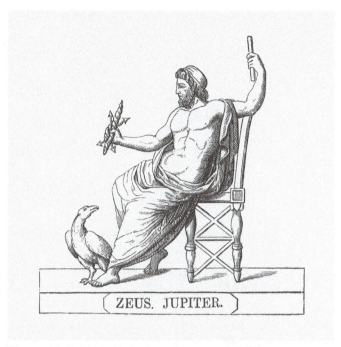

Figure 19-5. Zeus. (From Getty Images, DigitalVision, Vectors.)

was about to consummate his desires, his wife, Hera, came upon the scene; in the instant before her appearance, Zeus changed Io into a heifer, a young cow. Hera, rightfully suspicious, asked that the creature be given to her. Zeus had no choice but to comply. Hera then stationed a hundred-eyed watchman, Argus, to stand guard over the luckless Io. Zeus, unable to tolerate this state of affairs, sent his messenger, Hermes, with orders: "Kill Argus!" Hermes did as he was ordered, and Io was free, but still in bovine form. Hera took the hundred eyes of Argus and placed them in the tail of her favorite bird, the peacock. She then sent a stinging insect, the gadfly (*oistros*), to drive poor Io into flight all over the face of the earth. Eventually Zeus restored her to human form, and she settled down in the land of Egypt, where she became the mother of a son, Epaphus, sired by Zeus.

Exercise 1

Answer each of the following questions.

1. What name is given to glands that transmit their secretions through ducts? _____

2. What is the difference between the endocrine and the exocrine glands? _____

   What glands are commonly called eccrine? _____

3. What is the more common term for the gland called the hypophysis cerebri? _____

4. Which endocrine gland is often called the master gland of the body? _____

   What is the reason for this? _____

5. What are the functions of each of the following hormones, secreted in the anterior lobe of the pituitary gland?

   a. growth hormone (GH) _____

   b. adrenocorticotropic hormone (ACTH) _____

   c. lactogenic hormone _____

6. Deficient secretion of the hormone somatotropin can cause acromicria. What is the meaning of this term? _____

7. What is the main function of the hormone oxytocin, secreted in the posterior lobe of the pituitary gland? _____

8. What effect does vasopressin have on the body? _____

9. If there is excessive secretion of the hormone thyroxine by the thyroid gland, the result may be thyrotoxicosis. What is the meaning of each of the following two salient features of thyrotoxicosis?

   a. exophthalmos _____

   b. goiter _____

10. What is the cause of the condition known as cretinism? _____

11. Myxedema is a condition characterized by the accumulation of mucus in the tissues of the face and hands. What are some of the symptoms of myxedema? _____

   _____

12. Hypoparathyroidism can result in the condition known as hypercalcemia. What does this term mean? _____

   _____

13. Hypercalcemia can result in nephrolithiasis. What does this term mean? _____

14. What name is given to the outside covering of the adrenal gland? _____

15. What name is given to the inside portion of the adrenal gland? _____

16. Epinephrine, secreted in the adrenal glands, can be produced synthetically. When it is produced in this way, what is it called? _____

17. What hormones provide sudden energy to the body in emergency situations? _____

18. What hormone is secreted in the islets of Langerhans? _____

19. What is the meaning of each of the following five principal symptoms of diabetes mellitus?

    a. hyperglycemia _____

    b. glycosuria _____

    c. polyuria _____

    d. polydipsia _____

    e. polyphagia _____

20. The hormone testosterone is an androgen. What does this term mean? _____

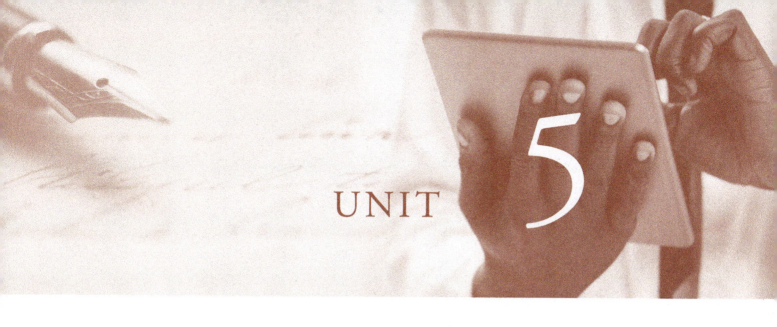

BIOLOGICAL NOMENCLATURE

BIOLOGICAL NOMENCLATURE

BIOLOGICAL NOMENCLATURE

With the advance of human knowledge of the living organisms that inhabit the world around us—plants, birds, insects, fish, and all other living things from the smallest, the virus, a minute organism not visible under ordinary light microscopy, to the largest, the honey mushroom (*Armillaria solidipes*)—it became desirable to classify these living organisms into groups. Following this classification, the next step was to name the members of each group. The term used for the classification of living organisms into groups is **taxonomy** (Greek *taxis*, arrangement, *nomos*, law). The term for the system of names used to label taxonomic groups is **nomenclature** (Latin *nōmenclātūra*, a calling by name: *nōmen*, name, *c[a]lātus*, called, and -ura, a noun-forming suffix). The Latin noun *nōmenclātūra* was first used by Pliny the Elder, a Roman scientist, in his encyclopedic *Naturalis Historia* (Natural History), completed in 77 AD. Taxonomic groups are called taxa (singular taxon); the allocation of names to these taxa is called nomenclature.

Taxonomy and nomenclature are both complementary and distinct. However, the objectives of both are the same: first, to provide a system whereby each and every living thing can be grouped according to shared characteristics and, second, to give names to these groups so that they may be referred to and discussed by all members of the scientific community in all countries, regardless of the different languages of these members. Traditionally, the language of biological and scientific nomenclature has been Latin. Included in the term "Latin" are words borrowed from other languages, mainly ancient Greek, and given the **form** of Latin words, so they look like Latin.

The reasons for the use of Latin as the language of scientific nomenclature are compelling. Latin ceased to be a spoken language centuries ago and is not subject to the changes that constantly influence living, spoken languages. Perhaps the most compelling reason for selecting Latin as a means of communication among scientists of all nations is that, in the Western world, Latin was the language of learned communities, whether the object of this learning was medicine, law, religion, philosophy, or science. The monumental work of British physician William Harvey on the circulation of the blood, published in 1628, was written in Latin: *Exercitatio Anatomica de Motu Cordis et Sanguinis* (An Anatomical Treatise Concerning the Movement of the Heart and Blood). The Polish astronomer Copernicus wrote his great work, a treatise titled *De Revolutionibus Orbium Coelestium* (Concerning the Revolutions of the Heavenly Bodies) in Latin in 1543, and the works of the Dutch theologian Erasmus (1466–1536) were written in Latin.

The Swedish botanist Carl von Linné, better known as Linnaeus (1707–1778), first formulated the principles that are still used for botanical taxonomy and nomenclature. His *Genera Plantarum* and *Classes Plantarum* (Genera of Plants and Classes of Plants), published in 1737 and 1738, are considered the beginning of systematic classification and terminology for modern botany. Following other important publications, his *Philosophia Botanica* (1751) explained fully his system for botanical nomenclature. The 10th edition of his *Systema Naturae* (1758) established the rules for zoological nomenclature. These works were written in Latin and, for the first time, laid down rules for the formulation of all subsequent biological terminology.

The system, based on Linnaeus's rules for botanical and zoological nomenclature, applies a binomial (Medieval Latin *binōmius*, having two names: Latin *bi-*, two, and *nōmen*, name) nomenclature to all living organisms. Every living organism is given two Latin names: the first identifies the **genus** (Latin *genus*, *generis*, race, stock, kind) to which it belongs. The second is a name peculiar to each member of the genus in order to differentiate it from other members of the same genus. There are many members of the cat family—the lion, the leopard, and the tiger, for

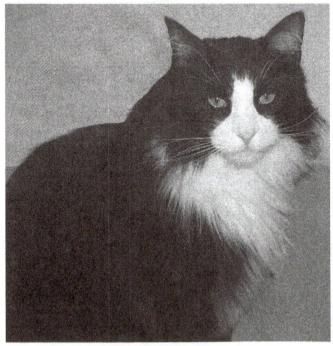

Figure 20-1. Genus *Felis* (cat). (Photograph by Laine McCarthy, 2000.)

example—obviously related to one another and, just as obviously, not related to members of the dog family—the household dog, and the coyote, for example. The genus (plural genera) of cats to which many of the great cats belong, including the lion, leopard, and tiger, is named *Panthera*. In the binomial system, the lion is *Panthera leo*; the leopard, *Panthera pardus*; and the tiger, *Panthera tigris*. The second name—the specific or **species** name–distinguishes these great cats from each other. The first, the genus or generic name, distinguishes them from the best-known member of the cat family, a member of the genus *Felis*, the domesticated feline, *Felis catus* (or *domesticus*), the common household cat (Fig. 20-1).

SPECIES AND GENERA

The binomial terms are names of **species**. The first word of the name, such as *Panthera* or *Felis*, is the genus or **generic** name. The second word, *leo*, *pardus*, or *tigris*, is the species or **specific** name that, following the generic name, indicates the species. Note that in the names of species, the generic name is capitalized but the specific name is not. Both names are customarily italicized. It takes at least two words to name a species.

A species can be defined as a group that shares similar characteristics and is usually capable of interbreeding, although not all members of each species are identical in appearance. That is, all household cats look more or less alike, although they are not identical; all leopards look more or less alike, but household cats do not look much like leopards and cannot interbreed with this species. All species of cat belong to the family Felidae, which has 18 genera, one

of which is the genus *Felis*, and another, the genus *Panthera*. All species of bears belong to the family Ursidae, which has five genera, the most diverse of which is the genus *Ursus*. The polar bear (*Ursus maritimus*), the American black bear (*Ursus americanus*), and the brown or grizzly bear (*Ursus arctos*) are species that resemble each other but none of which resembles any of the species belonging to the genus *Felis*. The household dog (*Canis familiaris*) and the coyote (*Canis latrans*) are two species of the same genus. They resemble each other, but neither resembles any members of the genus *Felis* or *Ursus*.

It should be noted that the specific name in binomial nomenclature is not used by itself. The specific names *catus*, *maritimus*, and *latrans* have no validity standing alone in this terminology.

FAMILIES

Family is the name for a group of closely related genera. The name for the cat family is Felidae and includes all its genera. The name for the bear family is Ursidae, and that for the dog family is Canidae. Names for families consist of one name only and therefore are uninomial (Latin *ūnus*, one). Family names are capitalized. Under the codes of nomenclature now in existence, the names of families of animals and protista (Latin *protista*, fr. Greek *prōtista*, the very first, "firstest")* are formed by adding **-idae** to the stem of the generic name. Names of families of plants, fungi, and prokaryotae (monera) are formed by adding **-aceae** to the stem of the generic name, with some exceptions: Compositae, Palmae, Gramineae, Leguminosae, Guttiferae, Umbelliferae, Labiatae, and Cruciferae.

These codes are drawn up in meetings of the appropriate international organizations. The naming of animals is governed by the *International Code of Zoological Nomenclature* (ICZN). The names of plants, algae, and fungi are determined by the *International Code of Nomenclature for Algae, Fungi and Plants* (ICN) and the *International Code of Nomenclature for Cultivated Plants* (ICNCP). Bacteria and archaea are governed by the *International Code of Nomenclature of Prokaryotes* (ICNP). The *International Code of Virus Classification and Nomenclature* (ICVCN) is responsible for naming viruses. In 1995, the *International Committee on Bionomenclature* (ICB) was established to expedite work toward a unified system of bionomenclature among the five codes.

TAXONOMIC HIERARCHY

The grouping of taxa into ranks or levels follows what is called the **taxonomic hierarchy** (Greek *hieros*, sacred, *archein*, rule). The smallest of the main groups within the

---

*In taxonomy, "firstest" refers to the first living organisms, the eukaryotes. These include protozoa, single-cell and multi-cell algae, and slime molds. From Venes D, ed., *Taber's Cyclopedic Medical Dictionary*, 23rd ed. F. A. Davis, 2017, p. 1942.

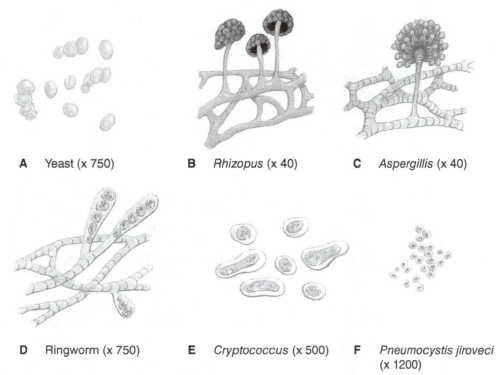

A Yeast (x 750) **B** *Rhizopus* (x 40) **C** *Aspergillis* (x 40)

D Ringworm (x 750) **E** *Cryptococcus* (x 500) **F** *Pneumocystis jiroveci* (x 1200)

Figure 20-2. Fungi. (From Scanlon, VC, and Sanders, T, *Essentials of Anatomy and Physiology*, 7th ed., F. A. Davis, 2015, p. 561, with permission.)

principal ranks is the species. Secondary ranks are generally used to subdivide large groups. Within a major group, a subgroup and supergroup may exist.

Species are grouped into genera, genera into families, families into orders, orders into classes, classes into phyla, phyla into kingdoms and kingdoms into domains.

PRINCIPAL TAXONOMIC RANKS*
Domain
Kingdom
Phylum
Class
Order
Family
Genus
Species

Domain is the largest taxon and is composed of Archaea, Bacteria, and Eukarya. Kingdom is the second highest taxonomic rank. Controversy exists concerning the actual number of kingdoms. Some taxonomies identify five kingdoms: Animalia, Plantae, Fungi (Fig. 20-2), Protista, and Prokaryotae (Monera). Others identify a six-kingdom paradigm composed of Animalia, Plantae, Fungi, Protista, Archaea, and Bacteria. Taxonomic classification continues to be an ongoing area of research and discussion as new information is discovered or old information is interpreted in new ways. The phylum (singular of phyla, from Greek *phylon*, clan, tribe) of invertebrate animals called

Arthropoda is the largest animal phylum, containing over one million species. It includes crustaceans, insects, myriapods (centipedes and millipedes), arachnids (spiders and scorpions), and other, similar forms. This phylum was well named because the term Arthropoda means "jointed feet," from Greek *arthron* (joint) and *pous, podos* (foot). All members of this group have jointed exoskeletons, segmented bodies, and jointed appendages (Fig. 20-3).

THE FORM AND ETYMOLOGICAL SIGNIFICANCE OF NAMES

Until recently all the codes of nomenclature have required that scientific names be in the form of Latin words, even if the terms used are originally from a language other than Latin (e.g., Greek, Arabic, or English). Whatever their ultimate linguistic source, these names must follow the rules of Latin grammar; that is, the names must be in the proper Latin grammatical form. An adjective that modifies a noun, for example, must agree with the noun in gender and number—feminine singular, masculine plural, neuter singular, and so forth. In the binomial nomenclature for species, the specific name—the second of the two terms—may be an adjective; thus, it must agree in gender and number with the first, or generic, name, which is always a noun.

Spirochaeta pallida (the causative organism of syphilis) is a spiral, hairlike microorganism. Its generic name is from Greek *speira* (spiral), and *chaitē* (hair). It should be noted that the Greek form for this word would be *speirochaitē* (if it

_____
*https://www.britannica.com/science/taxonomy/Ranks.

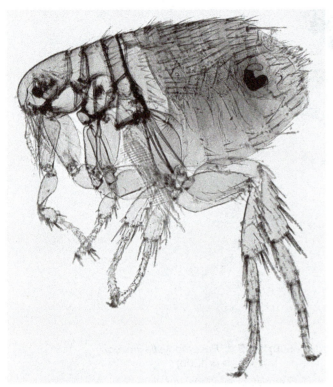

Figure 20-3. Genus *Xenopsylla* (flea). (Courtesy of the CDC, James Gathan.)

ever existed in the ancient Greek language). However, the rules of the Codes state that all of the names must be in the form of Latin. In the latinization of Greek words, the Greek diphthong *ei* usually becomes *i*, the diphthong *ai* usually becomes *ae* (often *e*), and a final -*ē* becomes -*a*. The reason for these changes is that Greek words, when borrowed by the Latin language in antiquity, were spelled in this way. The word *Spirochaeta* is a feminine noun (because the Greek noun *chaitē* was feminine) and is singular in number. The specific name, *pallida*, which identifies this particular spirochete from others of the same genus, is a Latin adjective in the form of the feminine singular, agreeing with the feminine singular noun *Spirochaeta*. The Latin adjective *pallida* means pale, pallid. Thus, *Spirochaeta pallida* means a pale, spiral, hairlike microorganism. It belongs to the family Spirochaetaceae.

Another common name for *Spirochaeta pallida* is *Treponema pallidum*. The generic name, *Treponema*, means the same etymologically as *Spirochaeta*. It is formed from the stem trep- from the Greek verb *trepein* (turn, twist) and the noun *nēma* (thread). The noun *nēma* is neuter in gender and singular in number; thus, for the Latin adjective *pallidum*, the specific name is in the form of the Latin neuter singular. *Treponema pallidum*, pale, twisted thread, is another name for *Spirochaeta pallida*, pale, spiral hair. The family name for the genus *Treponema* is Treponemataceae.

The second term, the specific name of the species, does not have to be an adjective modifying the generic name. It may be a noun in the genitive (possessive) case, or it may be a noun in the nominative singular. Examples of specific names in the form of the Latin nominative singular include *Panthera leo*, *Panthera tigris*, and *Panthera pardus*, in which the Latin nouns *leo*, *tigris*, and *pardus* meant lion, tiger, and leopard, respectively. Examples of specific names in the form of the Latin genitive singular include *Bacillus anthracis* (anthrax, *anthracis*, carbuncle), the causative agent of anthrax, a disease of animals, and *Entamoeba colī.* (colon, *colī*, colon), a species of nonpathogenic, parasitic amoeba normally found in the human intestinal tract.

It should be noted that uninomial names for genera, orders, classes, and phyla give no indication by themselves as to taxon. Thus, for example, Lepidoptera is an order of the class Insecta that includes the moths and butterflies. Annelida is the name of the phylum to which the earthworms belong. Acanthocephala is the name of a class of wormlike enterozoa related to the Platyhelminthes, a phylum of flatworms that includes the tapeworms. Anoplura is the name of the order of insects that includes the sucking lice, and *Penicillium* is a genus of fungi.

A number of genera have been named after the individual who first realized their existence. These names have been put into the form of a Latin word, usually by the addition of either the suffix -ia or the diminutive -ella: *Salmonella* (Daniel E. Salmon, American pathologist, 1850–1914); *Brucella* (Sir David Bruce, British bacteriologist, 1855–1931); *Shigella* (Kiyoshi Shiga, Japanese physician, 1870–1957); *Yersinia* (Alexandre Yersin, Swiss bacteriologist, 1863–1943); *Giardia* (Alfred Giard, French biologist, 1846–1908); *Wuchereria* (Otto Wucherer, German physician, 1820–1873).

VOCABULARY

Note: Latin combining forms are in ***bold italics***.

Greek or Latin	Combining Form	Meaning	Example
akari	**ACAR-**	mite	**Acar**-ina
amoibē	**AMOEBA**	[change] amoeba	*Ent-**amoeba***
anōphelēs*	**ANOPHELES**	useless, harmful	***Anopheles***
askos	**ASC-**	sac, bag	**Asc**-omycetes
aspergere†	***ASPERG-***	sprinkle	***Asperg**-illus*

*Greek *an-* + *ōpheleia*, help.
†Latin *ad-* + *spargere*, scatter.

Greek or Latin	Combining Form	Meaning	Example
aureus	*AURE-*	golden yellow	*Staphylococcus **aure**-us*
blatta	***BLATTA***	cockroach	***Blatta** orientalis*
botulus	***BOTUL-***	sausage	*Clostridium **botul**-inum*
bōs, bovis	***BOV-***	ox, bull, cow	*Actinomyces **bov**-is*
chaitē	**CHAET-**	hair bug	*Spiro-**chaet**-a*
cīmex	**CIMEX**	bug	***Cimex**-lectularius*
klōstēr	**CLOSTR-**	spindle	***Clostr**-idium*
culex	**CULEX**	gnat	***Culex**-pipiens*
duodēnalis	*DUODENAL-*	of the duodenum	*Ancylostoma **duodenal**-e*
*fēlineus**	*FELINEUS*	of or belonging to a cat	*Opisthorchis **felineus***
flāvus	*FLAVUS*	golden yellow	*Aspergillus **flavus***
fluere	*FLU-*	flow	in-**flu**-enza
Germānicus	*GERMANIC-*	of Germany, German	*Blatta **germanic**-a*
glaukos	**GLAUCUS**	bluish gray	*Aspergillus **glaucus***
Helvetius	*HELVET-*	Helvetian, Swiss	*Lactobacillus **helvet**-icus*
hex	**HEX-**	six	**Hex**-apoda
lectulus	*LECTUL-*	couch, bed	*Cimex **lectul**-arius*
lepis, lepidos	**LEPID-**	scale (of an animal)	**Lepid**-optera
nēma, nēmatos	**NEMA, NEMAT-**	thread	*Trepo-**nema***
opisthen	**OPISTH-**	located in the back	***Opisth**-orchis*
orchis	**ORCHIS**	testicle	*Opisth-**orchis***
orientalis	*ORIENTAL-*	of the east, oriental	*Blatta **oriental**-is*
pallidus	*PALLID-*	pale, lacking color	**pallid**-um
phtheir	**PHTHIR-**	louse	***Phthir**-us* (Fig. 20-4)
pīpīre	*PIP-*	peep, chirp	*Culex **pip**-iens*
platys	**PLATY-**	flat	**Platy**-helminthes
prōtos	**PROT-**	first	**Prot**-ozoa
pteron	**PTER-**	wing	Hemi-**pter**-a
pūbes, pūbis	*PUB-*	pubic region	*Phthirus **pub**-is*
speira	**SPIR-**	coil, spiral	***Spir**-ochaeta*
staphylē	**STAPHYL-**	bunch of grapes	***Staphyl**-ococcus*
streptos	**STREPT-**	twisted	***Strept**-ococcus*
tabānus	*TABAN-*	horsefly	Taban-idae
trepein	**TREP-**	turn, twist	*Trep-onema*

*Latin *fēlēs*, cat.

ETYMOLOGICAL NOTES

The language that was used by Linnaeus and other scientists and scholars of the Renaissance and the period following (after 1500 AD) is called New Latin. The Latin found in the writings of Cicero, Julius Caesar, and other literary figures of their time is called Classical Latin. Although the language of the Classical Period (first century BC to second century AD) was kept alive by scholars, churchmen, and literary figures in the centuries preceding the Renaissance, the spoken tongue had changed so dramatically that it resembled Classical Latin in only the vaguest outlines. This phenomenon precipitated the development of the Romance languages—Italian, Spanish, French—from the Latin spoken in the various parts of the great Roman Empire. At any age and in any place, the spoken language differs from the literary language, just as today our everyday, informal speech tends to be more idiomatic than the

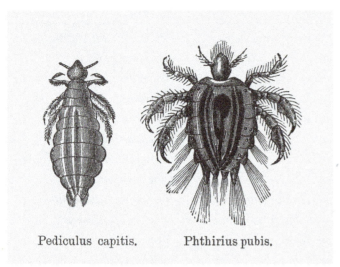

Pediculus capitis.   Phthirius pubis.

Figure 20-4. *Pediculus humanus capitis* (head louse) and *Phthirus pubis* (pubic louse). (From Getty Images, ZU_09.)

language that we use in writing. The spoken language of the ancient Romans is called Vulgar Latin, from the adjective *vulgāris* (of the people, commonplace), from the noun *vulgus* (the people, the multitude). The first great document in Vulgar Latin was the Vulgate (from *vulgata editio*, the vulgar edition), the translation of the Scriptures from Greek by Jerome (later Saint Jerome) in the early fifth century AD.

Scientists and writers of the Renaissance and the period following, schooled in Classical Latin, tried to emulate the classical writers and to revive the style of Cicero and others. They were successful to varying degrees. Although their Latin often lacks the polish of a writer such as Cicero, it is clear and straightforward and can be read with relative ease by anyone with a background in Classical Latin. Linnaeus's *Genera Plantarum, Classes Plantarum, Philosophia Botanica,* and *Systema Naturae* are good examples of this style. The language is called New Latin. Some of these New Latin writers went so far as to change their given names to the form of Latin. As noted earlier, Linnaeus's given name was Carl von Linné. Other well-known persons who Latinized their names include the composer Wolfgang Mozart, who changed his middle name, Gottlieb (God-loving), to Amadeus (Latin *amāre,* love, *deus,* god). The 15th/16th century Polish astronomer Nicolaus Koppernigk changed his name to the familiar Copernicus, and the Swiss/German physician of the same period, Aureolus Theophrastus Bombastus von Hohenheim, already given a Latin name in part, preferred to be called Paracelsus, perhaps suggesting that he was the equal of, or even superior to, the early Roman physician Celsus.

Exercise 1

Using the vocabulary from this and previous lessons, determine the etymological meaning of each of the following uninomial and binomial terms. Find the modern biological meaning of each of these terms in a medical dictionary.

1. Acarina _____

2. *Actinomyces bovis* _____

3. *Ancylostoma duodenale* _____

4. *Anopheles* _____

5. Arthropoda _____

6. Ascomycetes _____

7. *Aspergillus flavus* _____

8. *Aspergillus glaucus* _____

9. *Blatta orientalis* _____

10. *Bordetella** pertussis _____

11. *Cimex lectularius* _____

12. *Clostridium*† botulinum _____

13. *Clostridium septicum* _____

14. *Culex pipiens* _____

15. Diptera _____

16. *Entamoeba coli* _____

17. *Entamoeba gingivalis* _____

18. Hemiptera _____

19. Hexapoda _____

20. Lepidoptera _____

21. *Opisthorchis felineus* _____

22. *Phthirus pubis* _____

23. Platyhelminthes _____

24. Protozoa _____

25. Sarcophagidae _____

26. *Staphylococcus aureus* _____

27. *Streptococcus pyogenes* _____

28. Tabanidae _____

29. *Treponema pallidum* _____

30. *Trichinella spiralis* _____

---

*Named for Jules Bordet, a Belgian physician (1870–1961).
†Here, the Greek-derived suffix *-ium* (-ion) is a diminutive ending: clostridium, a little thing resembling a spindle.

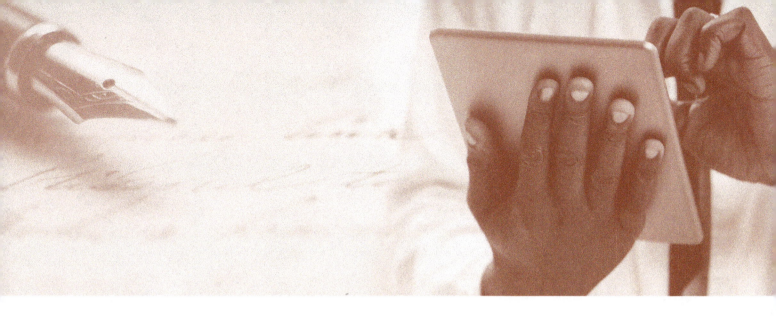

APPENDICES

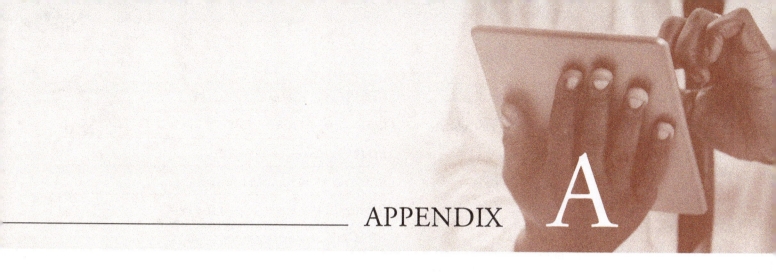

APPENDIX **A**

INDEX OF COMBINING FORMS

This index includes all of the combining forms found in this text, along with their basic meanings and the Greek or Latin term (in *italics*) from which each is formed. The combining forms are in capital letters and **bold** type; Latin combining forms are in ***bold italic*** type. The number of the lesson in which each is found is included in parentheses.

A

ABDOMIN-, *abdōmen, abdōminis,* belly, abdomen (8)

ACANTH-, *akantha,* thorn, spine (1)

ACAR-, *akari,* mite (20)

ACOU-, *akouein,* hear (5)

ACOUS-, *akouein,* hear (5)

ACR-, *akron,* [highest point] extremities (particularly the hands and feet) (2)

ACTIN-, *aktis, aktinos,* [ray] radiation (15)

ACU-, *akouein,* hear (5)

ACUS-, *akouein,* hear (5)

ADEN-, *adēn,* gland (7)

ADIP-, *adeps, adipis,* fat (8)

AER-, *aēr,* air, gas (7)

AGOG-, *agōgos,* leading, drawing forth (14)

-AGRA, *agra,* [hunting] (sudden) pain, gout (15)

ALG-, *algos,* pain (1)

ALGES-, *algēsis,* sensitivity to pain (1)

ALL-, *allos,* other, divergence, difference from (1)

ALVE-, *alveus,* hollow, cavity (11)

AMBLY-, *amblys,* dull, faint (2)

AMNI-, *amnion,* fetal membrane, amniotic sac, amnion (5)

AMOEBA, *amoibē,* [change] amoeba (20)

AMYGDAL-, *amygdalē,* [almond] tonsil (11)

AMYL-, *amylon,* starch (10)

ANCYL-, *ankylos,* fused, stiffened; hooked, crooked (6)

ANDR-, *anēr, andros,* man, male (6)

ANGI-, *angeion,* (blood) vessel, duct (1)

ANGIN-, *angina,* choking pain, angina pectoris (10)

ANKYL-, *ankylos,* fused, stiffened; hooked, crooked (6)

ANOPHELES, *anōphelēs,* useless, harmful (20)

ANTER-, *anterior,* front, in front (9)

ANTHRAC-, *anthrax, anthrakos,* coal; anthrax (11)

ANTHRAX, *anthrax, anthrakos,* coal; anthrax (11)

AORT-, *aortē,* aorta (10)

APHRODIS-, *Aphrodisios,* sexual desire (6)

APHRODISI-, *Aphrodisios,* sexual desire (6)

ARACHN-, *arachnē,* spider, web; arachnoid membrane (3, 18)

ARCH-, *archē,* beginning, origin (14)

-ARCHE, *archē,* beginning, origin (14)

ARCT-, arctāre, arctātus, compress (10)

ARCTAT-, arctāre, arctātus, compress (10)

ARTERI-, arteria, [air passage] artery (1)

ARTHR-, *arthron,* joint (1)

ASC-, *askos,* [leather bag] sac, bag, bladder (5, 20)

ASCIT-, *askos,* [leather bag] sac, bag, bladder (5)

ASPERG-, aspergere, sprinkle (20)

ATHER-, *athērē,* [soup] fatty deposit (10)

ATRI-, ātrium, [entrance hall] atrium (10)

AUR-, auris, ear (8)

AURE-, aureus, golden-yellow (20)

AUT-, autos, self (4)

AUX-, *auxein,* grow, increase (11)

-AUXE, *auxein,* grow, increase (11)

-AUXIS, *auxein,* grow, increase (11)

AX-, *axōn,* axis, axon (18)

AXON-, *axōn,* axis, axon (18)

B

BACILL-, bacillus, [rod, staff] bacillus (8)

BACTER-, *baktērion,* [small staff] bacterium (11)

BACTERI-, *baktērion,* [small staff] bacterium (11)

BAR-, *baros,* weight, pressure (5)

BI-, *bios,* life (1)

BILI-, bīlis, bile (12)

BLAST-, *blastos,* [bud, germ] primitive cell (16)

BLATTA, blatta, cockroach (20)

BLENN-, *blennos,* mucus (7)

BLEPHAR-, *blepharon,* eyelid (13)

BOL-, *bolē,* a throwing (10)

BOTUL-, botulus, sausage (20)

BOV-, bōs, bovis, ox, bull, cow (20)

BRACHI-, *bracchium,* (upper) arm (9)

BRACHY-, *brachys,* short (6)

BRADY-, *bradys,* slow (1)

BRONCH-, *bronchos,* [windpipe] bronchus (11)

BRONCHI-, *bronchos,* [windpipe] bronchus (11)

BURS-, bursa, [leather sack] bursa (8)

C

CALC-, calx, calcis, stone, calcium, lime (salts) (8)

CALOR-, calor, heat, energy (8)

CAPILL-, capillus, [hair] capillary (10)

CAPIT-, caput, capitis, head (8)

CAPN-, *kapnos,* [smoke] carbon dioxide (11)

CARCIN-, *karkinos,* [crab] carcinoma, cancer (2)

CARDI-, *kardia,* heart (1)

CARDI-, *kardia,* cardia (12)

CEC-, caecus, [blind] cecum (12)

CEL-, *koilia,* abdomen (7)

-CEL-, *kēlē,* hernia, tumor, swelling (2)

CELI-, *koilia,* abdomen (7)

CENTE-, *kentein,* pierce (5)

CEPHAL-, *kephalē,* head (1)

-CEPT-, *capere, captus,* take (9)

CEREBR-, cerebrum, brain (8, 18)

CERVIC-, cervix, cervīcis, neck (of the uterus), cervix uteri (14)

CERVIX, cervix, cervīcis, neck (of the uterus), cervix uteri (14)

CHAET-, *chaitē,* hair (20)

CHEIL-, *cheilos,* lip (7)

CHEIR-, *cheir*, hand (2)

CHIL-, *cheilos*, lip (7)

CHIR-, *cheir*, hand (2)

CHLOR-, *chlōros*, green (3)

CHOL-, *cholē*, bile, gall (2, 18)

CHOLE-, *cholē*, bile, gall (2, 18)

CHONDR-, *chondros*, cartilage (3)

CHOROID-, *chorioeidēs*, [skinlike] choroid (13)

CHROM-, *chrōma, chrōmatos*, color, pigment (5)

CHROMA-, *chrōma, chrōmatos*, color, pigment (5)

CHROMAT-, *chrōma, chrōmatos*, color, pigment (5)

CHRON-, *chronos*, time, timing (7)

-CID-, *caedere, caesus*, cut, kill (9)

CIMEX, *cīmex*, bug (20)

-CIP-, *capere, captus*, take (9)

CIRS-, *kirsos*, dilated and twisted vein, varix (10)

-CIS-, *caedere, caesus*, cut, kill (9)

CLA-, *klān*, break (up), destroy (7)

CLAS-, *klān*, break (up), destroy (7)

-CLAST, *klān*, something that breaks or destroys (7)

CLOSTR-, *klōstēr*, spindle (20)

-CLUD-, *claudere, clausus*, close (10)

-CLUS-, *claudere, clausus*, close (10)

CLY-, *klyzein*, rinse out, inject fluid (12)

CLYS-, *klyzein*, rinse out, inject fluid (12)

COCC-, *kokkos*, [berry] coccus (11)

-COCCUS, *kokkos*, [berry] coccus (11)

COL-, *kolon*, colon (2)

COLI-, *kolon, Escherichia coli* (2)

COLON-, *kolon*, colon (2)

COLP-, *kolpos*, vagina (14)

CONI-, *konis*, dust (11)

COPR-, *kopros*, excrement, fecal matter (12)

COR, *cor, cordis*, heart (10)

COR-, *korē*, [girl] pupil (of the eye) (13)

CORD-, *cor, cordis*, heart (10)

CORE-, *korē*, [girl] pupil (of the eye) (13)

CORON-, *corōna*, crown (10)

CORTEX, *cortex, corticis*, [bark, rind] outer layer (of an organ) (15, 18)

CORTIC-, *cortex, corticis*, [bark, rind] outer layer (of an organ) (15, 18)

COST-, *costa*, rib (8)

CRANI-, *kranion*, skull (1)

CREAT-, *kreas, kreatos*, flesh (12)

CRESC-, *crescere, crētus*, (begin to) grow (9)

-CRET-, *crescere, crētus*, (begin to) grow (9)

CRIN-, *krinein*, [separate] secrete, secretion (4)

CRY-, *kry(m)os*, icy cold (15)

CRYM-, *kry(m)os*, icy cold (15)

CRYPT-, *kryptos*, hidden, latent (6)

CULEX, *culex*, gnat (20)

CUSP-, *cuspis, cuspidis*, point (10)

-CUSPID, *cuspis, cuspidis*, point (10)

CYAN-, *kyanos*, blue (2)

CYCL-, *kyklos*, circle; the ciliary body (13)

CYE-, *kyein*, be pregnant (14)

CYST-, *kystis*, bladder, cyst (2)

CYSTI-, *kystis*, bladder, cyst (2)

-CYSTIS, *kystis*, bladder, cyst (2)

CYT-, *kytos*, [hollow container] cell (1)

D

DACRY-, *dakryon*, tear; lacrimal sac or duct (13)

DACTYL-, *daktylos*, finger, toe (3)

DEM-, *dēmos*, people, population (6)

DENDR-, *dendron*, [tree] dendrite, dendron (18)

DENDRIT-, *dendritēs*, [pertaining to a tree] dendrite (18)

DENT-, *dens, dentis*, tooth (8)

DERM-, *derma, dermatos*, skin (3)

-DERMA, *derma, dermatos*, skin (3)

DERMAT-, *derma, dermatos*, skin (3)

-DESIS, *desis*, binding (7)

DESM-, *desmos*, [binding] ligament, connective tissue (7)

DEXTR-, *dexter*, right (side) (10)

DIGIT-, *digitus*, finger, toe (9)

DIPLO-, *diploos*, double, twin (2)

DIPS-, *dipsa*, thirst (5)

-DOCH-, *dochos*, duct (12)

DOLICH-, *dolichos*, long, narrow, slender (6)

DORS-, *dorsum*, back (of the body) (8)

DROM-, *dromos*, a running (6)

DUC-, *dūcere, ductus*, lead, bring, conduct (9)

DUCT-, *dūcere, ductus*, lead, bring, conduct (9)

DUODEN-, *duodēnī*, [twelve] duodenum (12)

DUODENAL-, *duodēnalis*, of the duodenum (20)

DYNAM-, *dynamis*, force, power, energy (7)

E

ECHO-, *ēkhō*, reverberating sound, echo (5)

EDEMA, *oidēma, oidēmatos*, swelling (5)

EDEMAT-, *oidēma, oidēmatos*, swelling (5)

ELC-, *helkos*, ulcer (3)

-EM-, *haima, haimatos*, blood (2)

EME-, *emein*, vomit (5)

ENCEPHAL-, *enkephalon*, brain (1)

ENTER-, *enteron*, (small) intestine (2)

EOS-, *ēōs*, red (stain) (16)

ER-, *Erōs, Erōtos*, sexual desire (6)

ERG-, *ergon*, action, work (2)

EROT-, *Erōs, Erōtos*, sexual desire (6)

ERYTHR-, *erythros*, red, red blood cell (1)

ESOPHAG-, *oisophagos*, esophagus (12)

ESTHE-, *aisthēsis*, sensation, sensitivity, sense (4)

ESTHES-, *aisthēsis*, sensation, sensitivity, sense (4)

EURY-, *eurynein*, widen, dilate (14)

EURYN-, *eurynein*, widen, dilate (14)

EXTERN, *externus, -a, -um*, outer (8)

F

FAC-, *facere, factus*, make (9)

FACI-, *faciēs*, face, appearance, surface (9)

FACIES, *faciēs*, face, appearance, surface (9)

FASCICL-, *fasciculus*, [little bundle] fasciculus (18)

FASCICUL-, *fasciculus*, [little bundle] fasciculus (18)

FEBR-, *febris*, fever (9)

FEBRIS, *febris*, fever (9)

FEC-, *faex, faecis*, [sediment] excrement, fecal matter (12)

-FECT, *facere, factus*, make (9)

FELINEUS, *fēlineus*, of or belonging to a cat (20)

FER-, *ferre, lātus*, carry, bear (9)

FIBR-, *fibra*, fiber, filament (8)

-FIC-, *facere, factus*, make (9)

-FICI-, *faciēs*, face, appearance, surface (9)

FISTUL-, *fistula*, (tube, pipe) fistula, an abnormal tube like passage in the body (8)

FLAVUS, *flāvus*, golden-yellow (20)

FLECT-, *flectere, flexus*, bend (9)

FLEX-, *flectere, flexus*, bend (9)

FLU-, *fluere*, flow (20)

-FORM, *forma*, shape (10)

FRIG-, *frīgus, frīgoris*, cold (8)

FRIGOR-, *frīgus, frīgoris*, cold (8)

FUNG-, *fungus*, [mushroom] fungus (9)

FUS-, *fundere, fūsus*, pour (9)

G

GAL-, *gala, galaktos*, milk (14)

GALACT-, *gala, galaktos*, milk (14)

GANGLI-, *ganglion*, [knot] ganglion (18)

GASTR-, *gastēr, gastros*, stomach (2)

GEN-, *gignesthai*, come into being; produce (4)

GENE-, *gignesthai*, come into being; produce (4)

GENIT-, *gignere, genitus*, bring forth, give birth (9)

GER-, *gēras*, old age (7)

GER-, *gerere, gestus*, carry, bear (9)

GERMANIC-, *Germānicus*, of Germany, German (20)

GEST-, *gerere, gestus*, carry, bear (9)

GEUS-, *geuein*, taste (12)

GEUST-, *geuein*, taste (12)

GINGIV-, *gingīva*, gum (of the mouth) (12)

GLAUCUS, *glaukos*, bluish-gray (20)

GLI-, *glia*, [glue] glia, neuroglia (18)

-GLIA-, *glia*, [glue] glia, neuroglia (18)

GLOB-, *globus*, round body, globe (16)

GLOSS-, *glōssa*, tongue (12)

GLYC-, *glykys*, sugar (15)

GN-, *(g)nascī, nātus*, be born (14)

GNATH-, *gnathos*, (lower) jaw (7)

GNO-, *gignōskein*, know (5)

GNOS-, *gignōskein*, know (5)

GONAD-, *gonad*, sex glands, sex organs (14)

GRAM-, *gramma*, [something written] a record (4)

GRANUL-, *grānulum*, granule (16)

GRAPH-, *graphein*, write, record (4)

GRAVID-, *gravidus*, pregnant (14)

GURGIT-, *gurgitāre, gurgitātus*, flood, flow (10)

GURGITAT-, *gurgitāre, gurgitātus*, flood, flow (10)

GYN-, *gynē, gynaikos*, woman, female (6)

GYNEC-, *gynē, gynaikos*, woman, female (6)

H

HELC-, *helkos*, ulcer (3)

HELMINT-, *helmins, helminthos*, (intestinal) worm (6)

HELMINTH-, *helmins, helminthos*, (intestinal) worm (6)

HELVET-, *Helvetius*, Helvetian, Swiss (20)

HEM-, *haima, haimatos*, blood (2)

HEMAT-, *haima, haimatos*, blood (2)

HEPAR-, *hēpar, hēpatos*, liver (2)

HEPAT-, *hēpar, hēpatos*, liver (2)

HERPES, *herpēs, herpētos*, [shingles] herpes, a creeping skin disease (13)

HERPET-, *herpēs, herpētos*, [shingles] herpes, a creeping skin disease (13)

HEX-, *hex*, six (20)

HIDR-, *hidrōs, hidrōtos*, sweat (3)

HIDROT-, *hidrōs, hidrōtos*, sweat (3)

HIST-, *histos*, [web] tissue (3)

HISTI-, *histos*, [web] tissue (3)

HYDR-, *hydōr, hydatos*, water, fluid (3)

HYMEN-, *hymēn*, membrane; hymen (14)

HYPN-, *hypnos*, sleep (3)

HYSTER-, *hystera*, uterus (14)

I

IATR-, *iatros*, healer, physician; treatment (4)

ICTER-, *ikteros*, jaundice (3)

IDI-, *idios*, of one's self (4)

-IDR-, *hidrōs, hidrōtos*, sweat (3)

ILE-, *ileum*, ileum (12)

IMMUN-, *immūnis*, [exempt] safe, protected (9)

IN-, *is*, *inos*, fiber, muscle (3)

INFERIOR-, *inferior*, below (9)

INGUIN-, *inguen*, *inguinis*, groin (15)

INOS-, *is*, *inos*, fiber, muscle (3)

INSUL-, *insula*, island (8)

INTERN-, *internus*, *-a*, *-um*, inner (8)

IR-, *iris*, *iridos*, [rainbow] iris (13)

IRID-, *iris*, *iridos*, [rainbow] iris (13)

IS-, *isos*, equal, same, similar, alike (3)

ISCH-, *ischein*, suppress, check (7)

J

JEJUN-, *jējūnus*, [empty] jejunum (12)

JUNCT-, *jungere*, *junctus*, join (13)

K

KARY-, *karyon*, [nut] nucleus (16)

KERAT-, *keras*, *keratos*, [horn] cornea (13)

KINE-, *kinein*, move (4)

KINES-, *kinēsis*, movement, motion (4)

KINESI-, *kinēsis*, movement, motion (4)

KLEPT-, *kleptein*, steal, theft (7)

KONI-, *konis*, dust (11)

L

LAB-, *lābī*, *lapsus*, slide, slip (9)

LABI-, *labium*, lip (11)

LACRIM-, *lacrima*, tear (13)

LACHRYM-, *lacrima*, tear (13)

LACT-, *lac*, *lactis*, milk (14)

-LAGNIA, *lagneia*, abnormal sexual excitation or gratification (15)

LAL-, *lalein*, talk (5)

LAPAR-, *lapara*, abdomen, abdominal wall (5)

LAPS-, *lābī*, *lapsus*, slide, slip (9)

LARYNG-, *larynx*, *laryngos*, larynx (11)

LARYNX, *larynx*, *laryngos*, larynx (11)

LAT-, *ferre*, *lātus*, carry, bear (9)

LATER-, *latus*, *lateris*, side (9)

LECTUL-, *lectulus*, couch, bed (20)

LEI-, *leios*, smooth (7)

LEP-, *lēpsis*, attach, seizure (7)

LEPID-, *lepis*, *lepidos*, scale (of an animal) (20)

LEPT-, *leptos*, thin, fine, slight (1)

LEUK-, *leukos*, white, white blood cell (1)

LEX-, *legein*, read (5)

LIEN-, *liēn*, spleen (12)

LINGU-, *lingua*, tongue (12)

LIP-, *lipos*, fat (2)

LITH-, *lithos*, stone, calculus (1)

LOG-, *logos*, word, study (1)

LY-, *lyein*, destroy, break down (4)

LYMPH-, *lympha*, [clear water] lymph (16)

LYS-, *lyein*, destroy, break down (4)

M

MACR-, *makros*, (abnormally) large or long (2)

MALAC-, *malakos*, soft (1)

MAMM-, *mamma*, breast (14)

MAN-, *mainesthai*, be mad (7)

MAST-, *mastos*, breast (14)

MAZ-, *mastos*, breast (14)

MEAT-, *meātus*, passage, opening, meatus (8)

MEDULL-, *medulla*, marrow, medulla oblongata (18)

MEGA-, *megas*, *megalou*, (abnormally) large or long (2)

MEGAL-, *megas*, *megalou*, (abnormally) large or long (2)

MEL-, *melos*, limb (7)

MELAN-, *melas*, *melanos*, dark, black (2)

MEN-, *mēn*, [month] menstruation (14)

MENING-, *mēninx*, *mēningos*, meningeal membrane, meninges (3)

-MENINX, *mēninx*, *mēningos*, meningeal membrane, meninges (3)

MES-, *mesos*, middle, secondary, partial, mesentery (1)

-METER, *metron*, instrument for measuring (1)

METR-, *metron*, measure (1)

METR-, *mētra*, uterus (14)

-METRA, *mētra*, uterus (14)

MICR-, *mikros*, (abnormally) small (2)

MNE-, *mimnēskein*, remember (5)

MON-, *monos*, single (16)

MORPH-, *morphē*, form, shape (7)

MY-, *mys*, *myos*, [mouse] muscle (3)

MY-, *myein*, close, shut (13)

MYC-, *mykēs*, *mykētos*, [mushroom] fungus (3)

MYCET-, *mykēs*, *mykētos*, [mushroom] fungus (3)

MYEL-, *myelos*, bone marrow, spinal cord, myelin (3, 18)

MYS-, *mys*, *myos*, [mouse] muscle (3)

MYX-, *myxa*, mucus (4)

N

NARC-, *narkē*, stupor, numbness (3)

NAS-, *nāsus*, nose (8)

NAT-, (g)*nascī*, *nātus*, be born (14)

NE-, *neos*, new (5)

NECR-, *nekros*, corpse; dead (3)

NEMA, *nēma*, *nēmatos*, thread (worm) (6, 20)

NEMAT-, *nēma*, *nēmatos*, thread (worm) (6, 20)

NEPHR-, *nephros*, kidney (1)

NEUR-, *neuron*, [tendon] nerve, nervous system, neuron (1, 18)

NEUTR-, *neuter*, neither (16)

NO-, *nous*, mind, mental activity, comprehension (5)

NOM-, *nomos*, law (7)

NOS-, *nosos*, disease, illness (6)

NYCT-, *nyx*, *nyctos*, night (2)

O

OCUL-, *oculus*, eye (13)

ODONT-, *odous*, *odontos*, tooth (6)

ODYN-, *odynē*, pain (2)

OLIG-, *oligos*, few, deficient (3)

OMPHAL-, *omphalos*, navel, umbilicus (7)

ONC-, *onkos*, tumor (2)

ONYCH-, *onyx*, *onychos*, fingernail, toenail (3)

OOPHOR-, *oophoron*, ovary (14)

OP-, *ōps*, vision (13)

OPHTHALM-, *ophthalmos*, eye (13)

OPISTH-, *opisthen*, located in the back (20)

OPS-, *ōps*, vision (13)

OPT-, *optos*, [seen] vision; eye (13)

OR-, *ōs*, *ōris*, mouth, opening (9)

ORCH-, *orchis*, *orchios*, testicle (15)

ORCHE-, *orchis*, *orchios*, testicle (15)

ORCHI-, *orchis*, *orchios*, testicle (15)

ORCHID-, *orchis*, *orchios*, testicle (15)

ORCHIS, *orchis*, *orchios*, testicle (20)

OREC-, *oregein*, have an appetite (5)

OREX-, *oregein*, have an appetite (5)

ORIENTAL-, *orientalis*, of the east, oriental (20)

ORTH-, *orthos*, straight, erect; normal (4)

OS, *ōs*, *ōris*, mouth, opening (9)

OSM-, *osmē*, sense of smell; odor (12)

OSS-, *ossa*, bone (9)

OSTE-, *osteon*, bone (1)

OT-, *ous*, *ōtos*, ear (4)

OV-, *ōvum*, egg (14)

OVARI-, *ōvārium*, ovary (14)

OX-, *oxys*, acute, pointed; rapid; oxygen (5)

OXY-, *oxys*, acute, pointed; rapid; oxygen (5)

P

PACHY-, *pachys*, thick (2)

PALI-, *palin*, back, again (6)

PALIN-, *palin*, back, again (6)

PALLID-, *pallidus*, pale, lacking color (20)

PAN-, *pas*, *pantos*, all, entire, every (6)

PANT-, *pas*, *pantos*, all, entire, every (6)

-PARA, *parere*, *partus*, give birth (14)

PARESIS, *paresis*, slackening of strength, paralysis (11)

PART-, *parere*, *partus*, give birth (14)

PATH-, *pathos*, [suffering] disease (4)

PECTOR-, *pectus*, *pectoris*, breast, chest (10)

PED-, *pais*, *paidos*, child (7)

PEDICUL-, *pediculus*, louse (9)

PELV-, *pelvis*, [basin] pelvis (14)

PEN-, *penia*, decrease, deficiency (7)

PEN-, *pēnis*, [tail] penis (15)

PEPS-, *peptein*, digest (12)

PEPT-, *peptein*, digest (12)

-PEX-, *pexis*, fixing, (surgical) attachment (7)

PHA-, *phēnai*, speak, communicate (5)

PHAC-, *phakos*, [lentil] lens (13)

PHAG-, *phagein*, swallow, eat (5)

PHAK-, *phakos*, [lentil] lens (13)

PHALL-, *phallos*, penis (15)

PHARMAC-, *pharmakon*, medicine, drug (5)

PHARMACEU-, *pharmakon*, medicine, drug (5)

PHARYNG-, *pharynx*, *pharyngos*, [throat] pharynx (11)

PHARYNX, *pharynx*, *pharyngos*, [throat] pharynx (11)

PHEM-, *phēmē*, speech (5)

-PHIL-, *philein*, love; have an affinity for (4, 16)

PHLEB-, *phleps*, *phlebos*, vein (10)

PHOB-, *phobos*, (abnormal) fear (5)

PHON-, *phonē*, voice, sound (5)

PHOR-, *phoros*, bearing, carrying (6)

PHOS-, *phōs*, *phōtos*, light, daylight (6)

PHOT-, *phōs*, *phōtos*, light, daylight (6)

PHRAS-, *phrazein*, speak (5)

PHREN-, *phrēn*, mind; diaphragm (5)

PHTHIR-, *phtheir*, louse (20)

PHYLAC-, *phylattein*, protection (against disease) (5)

PHYS-, *physis*, nature, appearance (5)

PHYS-, *physa*, air, gas (11)

PHYSI-, *physis*, nature, appearance (5)

PHYT-, *phyton*, plant (organism), growth (5)

PIP-, *pīpīre*, peep, chirp (20)

PLAS-, *plassein*, form, develop (7)

PLAST-, *plassein*, form, develop (7)

PLATY-, *platys*, flat (20)

PLEC-, *plēssein*, strike, paralyze (6)

PLEG-, *plēssein*, strike, paralyze (6)

PLEUR-, *pleura*, [side] pleura (11)

PLEX-, *plēssein*, strike, paralyze (6)

PLEX-, *plexus*, [braid] plexus (18)

PNE-, *pnein*, breathe (11)

PNEUM-, *pneuma*, *pneumatos*, [breath] air, gas (11)

PNEUM-, *pneumōn*, lung (11)

PNEUMAT-, *pneuma*, *pneumatos*, [breath] air, gas (11)

PNEUMON-, *pneumōn*, lung (11)

POD-, *pous*, *podos*, foot (3)

POIE-, *poiein*, produce, make (5)

POLI-, *polios*, [gray] gray matter of the brain and spinal cord (3)

POLY-, *polys*, many, excessive (3)

PONS, *pons*, *pontis*, [bridge] pons (18)

PONT-, *pons*, *pontis*, [bridge] pons (18)

POR-, *poros*, passage, opening, duct, pore, cavity (3)

POSTER-, *posterior*, behind, in back (9)

-POSTERIOR, *posterior*, behind, in back (9)

PRAX-, *praxis*, act, action (1)

PRESBY-, *presbys*, old, old age (7)

PROCT-, *proktos*, anus (12)

PROSOP-, *prosōpon*, face (5)

PROSTAT-, *prostatēs*, [one who stands before] prostate gland (7)

PROT-, *prōtos*, first, primitive, early (1, 20)

PSEUD-, *pseudēs*, false (2)

PSYCH-, *psychē*, [soul] mind (3)

PT-, *piptein*, fall, sag, drop, prolapse (4)

PTER-, *pteron*, wing (20)

PTY-, *ptyein*, spit (7)

PTYAL-, *ptyalon*, saliva (7)

PUB-, *pūbēs*, pubic hair, pubic bone, pubic region, pubis (14, 20)

PUBER-, *pūbertās*, [manhood] puberty (14)

PUBERT-, *pūbertās*, [manhood] puberty (14)

PULM-, *pulmō*, *pulmōnis*, lung, pulmonary artery (10)

PULMON-, *pulmō*, *pulmōnis*, lung, pulmonary artery (10)

PUR-, *pus*, *puris*, pus (8)

PY-, *pyon*, pus (2)

PYEL-, *pyelos*, renal pelvis (15)

PYLE-, *pylē*, [gate] portal vein (12)

PYLOR-, *pylōrus*, [gatekeeper] pylorus (12)

PYR-, *pyr*, *pyros*, [fire] fever, burning (4)

PYRET-, *pyretos*, fever (4)

PYREX-, *pyressein*, be feverish (4)

R

RACHI-, *rhachis*, spine (6)

RAD-, *rādix*, *rādīcis*, root (8)

RADIC-, *rādix*, *rādīcis*, root (8)

RADIX, *rādix*, *rādīcis*, root (8)

RECT-, *rectus*, [straight] rectum (12)

REN-, *rēn*, *rēnis*, kidney (8)

RET-, *rēte*, *rētis*, [net] retina; network, plexus (13)

RETIN-, *rēte*, *rētis*, [net] retina; network, plexus (13)

RHABD-, *rhabdos*, rod (15)

RHACHI-, *rhachis*, spine (6)

RHAG-, *rhēgnynai*, [burst forth] flow profusely, hemorrhage (4)

RHE-, *rhein*, [run] flow, secrete (4)

RHEX-, *rhēxis*, rupture (4)

RHIN-, *rhis*, *rhīnos*, nose (4)

RHYTHM-, *rhythmos*, [steady motion] heartbeat (10)

-RRHAPH-, *rhaptein*, suture (7)

S

SALPING-, *salpinx, salpingos*, [war trumpet] fallopian tube (14)

-SALPINX, *salpinx, salpingos*, [war trumpet] fallopian tube (14)

SANGUI-, *sanguis, sanguinis*, blood (8)

SANGUIN-, *sanguis, sanguinis*, blood (8)

SAPR-, *sapros*, rotten, putrid, decaying (5)

SARC-, *sarx, sarcos*, flesh, soft tissue (2)

SCAT-, *skōr, skatos*, excrement, fecal matter (12)

-SCHE-, *ischein*, suppress, check (7)

-SCHISIS, *schizein*, split, cleft, fissure (6)

SCHIST-, *schizein*, split, cleft, fissure (6)

SCHIZ-, *schizein*, split, cleft, fissure (6)

SCLER-, *skleros*, hard (1)

SCOP-, *skopein*, look at, examine (4)

SCROT-, *scrōtum*, [bag] scrotum (15)

SECT-, *secāre, sectus*, cut (9)

SEM-, *sēmen, sēminis*, [seed] semen (15)

SEMIN-, *sēmen, sēminis*, [seed] semen (15)

SEP-, *sēpein*, [be putrid] be infected (4)

SEPT-, *saeptum*, wall, partition (10)

SIAL-, *sialon*, saliva, salivary duct (12)

SIDER-, *sidēros*, iron (11)

SIGM-, *sigma*, sigmoid colon (12)

SIN-, *sinus*, [curve, hollow] sinus (10)

SINISTR-, *sinister*, left (side) (10)

SINUS-, *sinus*, [curve, hollow] sinus (10)

SIT-, *sitos*, food (7)

SOM-, *sōma, sōmatos*, body (3)

-SOMA, *sōma, sōmatos*, body (3)

SOMAT-, *sōma, sōmatos*, body (3)

SOMN-, *somnus*, sleep (9)

SON-, *sonus*, sound (8)

SPASM-, *spasmos*, spasm, involuntary muscular contraction (2)

SPERM-, *sperma, spermatos*, seed, sperm, semen (15)

SPERMAT-, *sperma, spermatos*, seed, sperm, semen (15)

SPHINCTER-, *sphinctēr*, sphincter muscle (12)

SPHYGM-, *sphygmos*, pulse (10)

SPIR-, *spīrāre, spīrātus*, breathe (11)

SPIR-, *speira*, coil, spiral (20)

SPIRAT-, *spīrāre, spīrātus*, breathe (11)

SPLANCHN-, *splanchnon*, internal organ, viscus (12)

SPLEN-, *splēn*, spleen (2)

SPONDYL-, *spondylos*, vertebra (6)

STA-, *histanai*, stand, stop (7)

STABIL-, *stabilis*, stable, fixed (9)

STABL-, *stabilis*, stable, fixed (9)

STAL-, *stellein*, send, contraction (10)

STAPHYL-, *staphylē*, [bunch of grapes] uvula, palate; staphylococci (11, 20)

STAT-, *histanai*, stand, stop (7)

-STAT, *histanai*, device or agent for stopping the flow (of something) (7)

-STAXIA, *staxis*, dripping, oozing (of blood) (6)

-STAXIS, *staxis*, dripping, oozing (of blood) (6)

STEAR-, *stear, steatos*, fat, sebum, sebaceous glands (5)

STEAT-, *stear, steatos*, fat, sebum, sebaceous glands (5)

STEN-, *stenos*, narrow (1)

STERE-, *stereos*, solid, having three dimensions (1)

STERN-, *sternon*, chest, breast, breastbone (11)

STETH-, *stēthos*, chest, breast (11)

STHEN-, *sthenos*, strength (3)

STIGM-, *stigma, stigmatos*, point, mark, spot (13)

STIGMAT-, *stigma, stigmatos*, point, mark, spot (13)

STOL-, *stellein*, send, contraction (10)

STOM-, *stoma, stomatos*, mouth, opening (2)

STOMAT-, *stoma, stomatos*, mouth, opening (2)

STREPT-, *streptos*, [twisted] streptococci (11, 20)

SUD-, sūdor, sweat, fluid (11)

SUDOR-, sūdor, sweat, fluid (11)

SUPERIOR-, superior, above (9)

SYNAP-, *synapsis*, [point of contact] synapse (18)

SYNAPS-, *synapsis*, [point of contact] synapse (18)

SYNOV-, synovia, synovial fluid, synovial membrane or sac (8)

SYRING-, *syrinx, syringos*, [pipe] fistula, cavity, oviduct, sweat glands, syringe (14)

-SYRINX, *syrinx, syringos*, [pipe] fistula, cavity, oviduct, sweat glands, syringe (14)

T

TA-, *tasis*, stretching (4)

TABAN-, tabānus, horsefly (20)

TACHY-, *tachys*, rapid (1)

TAX-, *taxis*, (muscular) coordination (7)

TEL-, *telos*, end, completion (4)

TEN-, *tenōn, tenontos*, tendon (4)

TENON-, *tenōn, tenontos*, tendon (4)

TENONT-, *tenōn, tenontos*, tendon (4)

TENS-, tendere, tensus, stretch (10)

TENSI-, tendere, tensus, stretch (10)

THALAM-, *thalamos*, [inner chamber] thalamus (18)

THAN-, *thanatos*, death (6)

THANAT-, *thanatos*, death (6)

THE-, *tithenai*, place, put (6)

THEL-, *thēlē*, nipple (14)

THELE-, *thēlē*, nipple (14)

THERAP-, *therapeuein*, treat medically, heal (4)

THERAPEU-, *therapeuein*, treat medically, heal (4)

THERM-, *thermē*, heat, (body) temperature (7)

THORAC-, *thōrax, thōrakos*, chest cavity, pleural cavity, thorax (11)

THORAX, *thōrax, thōrakos*, chest cavity, pleural cavity, thorax (11)

THROMB-, *thrombos*, blood clot (10)

THYR-, *thyreos*, [shield] thyroid gland (7)

TOC-, *tokos*, childbirth, labor (14)

TOM-, *tomē*, a cutting, slice, incision (4)

TON-, *tonos*, [a stretching] (muscular) tone, tension (4)

TOP-, *topos*, place (10)

TOX-, *toxon*, poison (1)

TOXI-, *toxon*, poison (1)

TRACH-, *trachys*, [rough] trachea (11)

TRACHE-, *trachys*, [rough] trachea (11)

TRACHEL-, *trachēlos*, neck, cervix (3)

TRACHY-, *trachys*, [rough] trachea (11)

TREP-, *trepein*, turn, twist (20)

TRICH-, *thrix, trichos*, hair (6)

TROP-, *tropē*, turning (7)

TROPH-, *trophē*, nourishment (6)

TUB-, tuba, [trumpet] tube (8)

TUM-, tumēre, be swollen (9)

TUME-, tumēre, be swollen (9)

TUSS-, tussis, cough (8)

TYPHL-, *typhlos*, [blind] cecum (12)

U

UR-, *ouron*, urine, urinary tract, uric acid (15)

URETER-, *ourētēr*, ureter (15)

URETHR-, *ourēthra*, urethra (15)

UTER-, uterus, womb, belly, uterus (14)

V

VACC-, *vacca,* cow (8)

VAG-, *vagus,* [wandering] the vagus nerve (10)

VAGIN-, *vāgīna,* [sheath] vagina (14)

VARIC-, *varix, varicis,* dilated and twisted vein, varix (10)

VARIX, *varix, varicis,* dilated and twisted vein, varix (10)

VAS-, *vās,* (blood) vessel; vas deferens (10)

VEN-, *vēna,* vein (10)

VENTR-, *venter, ventris,* belly, abdomen, abdominal cavity (10)

VESIC-, *vēsīca,* (urinary) bladder (15)

VIR-, *vīrus,* [poison, venom] virus (8)

VIRUS-, *vīrus,* [poison, venom] virus (8)

VISCER-, *viscus, visceris,* internal organ(s) (8)

VISCUS-, *viscus, visceris,* internal organ (8)

X

XANTH-, *xanthos,* yellow (3)

XER-, *xēros,* dry (13)

Z

ZO-, *zōon,* animal, organism (15)

ZYM-, *zymē,* [leaven] ferment, enzyme, fermentation (12)

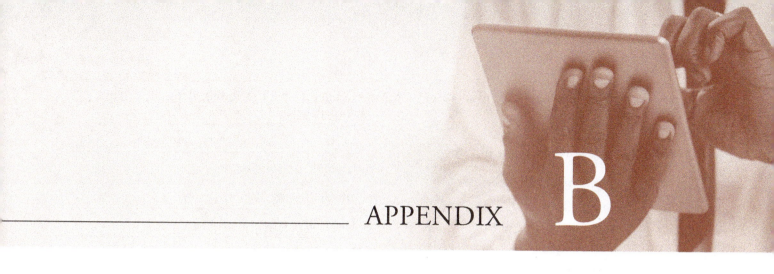

APPENDIX B

INDEX OF PREFIXES

Prefixes modify, or qualify in some way, the meaning of the word to which they are affixed. It is often difficult to assign a single specific meaning to each prefix, and it is often necessary to adapt a meaning that fits the particular use of a word. Words can have more than one prefix, and a prefix can follow a combining form.

Entries for Latin prefixes are in *italics*.

a- (an- before a vowel or *h*): not, without, lacking, deficient

ab- (a- rarely before certain consonants; *abs-* before *c* and *t*): away from

ad- (ac- before *c; af-* before *f; ag-* before *g; al-* before *l; an-* before *n; ap-* before *p; as-* before *s; a-* before *sp; at-* before *t*): to, toward

ambi-: both

amphi-, ampho-: on both sides, around, both

ana-: up, back, against

ante-: before, forward

anti- (ant- often before a vowel or *h*; hyphenated before *i*): against, opposed to, preventing, relieving

apo-: away from

bi- (bin-, bis-): two, twice, double, both

cata- (cat- before a vowel or *h*): downward; disordered

circum-: around

con- (*co-* before *h; col-* before *l; com-* before *e, m,* and *p; cor-* before *r*): together, with; thoroughly, very

contra-: against, opposite

de-: down, away from, absent

di- (rarely dis-): two, twice, double

dia- (di- before a vowel): through, across, apart

dis- (di- before *g, v,* and usually before *l; dif-* before *f*): apart, away

dys-: difficult, painful, defective, abnormal

ec- (ex- before a vowel): out of, away from

ecto- (ect- often before a vowel): outside of

en- (em- before *b, m,* and *p*): in, into, within

endo-, ento- (end-, ent- before a vowel): within

epi- (ep- before a vowel or *h*): upon, over, above

eso-: within, inner, inward

eu-: good, normal, healthy

ex- (e- before certain consonants; *ef-* before *f*): out of, away from

exo-: outside, from the outside, toward the outside

extra- (rarely extro-): on the outside, beyond

hemi-: half, partial; (often) one side of the body

heter-, hetero-: different, other, relationship to another

homo-, homeo-: same, likeness

hyper-: over, above, excessive, beyond normal

hypo- (hyp- before a vowel or *h*): under, deficient, below normal

in- (*il-* before *l*; *im-* before *b*, *m*, and *p*; *ir-* before *r*): in, into

in- (*il-* before *l*; *im-* before *b*, *m*, and *p*; *ir-* before *r*): not

in- (*il-* before *l*; *im-* before *b*, *m*, and *p*; *ir-* before *r*): very, thoroughly

infra-: beneath, below

inter-: between

intra- (rarely, *intro-*): within

meta- (met- before a vowel or *h*): change, transformation, after, behind

mono- (mon- before a vowel or *h*): one, single

mult- (often *multi-*): many, much, affecting many parts

non-: not

ob- (oc- before *c*; op- before *p*): against, toward; very, thoroughly

para- (often par- before a vowel): alongside, around, abnormal, beyond

per- (*pel-* before *l*): through; very, thoroughly

peri-: around, surrounding

post-: after, following, behind

pre-: before, in front of

pro-: before

pro-: forward, in front

pros-, prosth-: in place of

re-: back, again

retro-: backward, in back, behind

se-: apart, away from

semi-: half

sub- (*suf-* before *f*; *sup-* before *p*): under

super- (often *supra-*): over, above; excess

trans-: across, through

syn- (sym- before *b*, *p*, and *m*; *n* assimilates or is dropped before *l* and *s*): together, with, joined

ultra-: beyond, excess

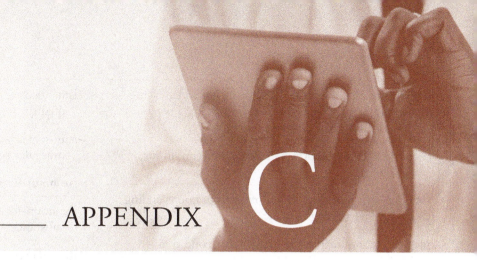

INDEX OF SUFFIXES

Suffixes form either nouns or adjectives (or, in some instances, verbs or adverbs). Most of the nouns in medical terminology are abstract, indicating a state, quality, condition, procedure, or process. Noun-forming suffixes that have special meanings, such as -itis, inflammation, will be so indicated. Adjective-forming suffixes usually have the general meaning of pertaining to, referring to, having to do with, in a condition or state of, caused by, causing, or located in. Only those meanings most commonly found are indicated here. Entries for Latin suffixes are in *italics*.

-a: abstract noun-forming suffix: state, condition

-able: adjective-forming suffix: capable of (being), able to

-ac (rare): adjective-forming suffix: pertaining to, located in

-ad: adverb-forming suffix: indicates direction toward a part of the body: toward

-al: adjective-forming suffix: pertaining to, located in

-an: adjective-forming suffix: pertaining to, located in

-ant: forms adjectives translated with -ing added to the meaning of a verb; forms nouns meaning a person who or thing that does something

-ar: adjective-forming suffix: pertaining to, located in

-arium: noun-forming suffix: denotes a place for something: place for

-ary: adjective-forming suffix: pertaining to

-ary: noun-forming suffix: denotes a place for something: place for

-ase: noun-forming suffix: forms names of enzymes

-asia, -asis (rare): abstract noun-forming suffixes: state, condition

-ate: noun-forming suffix: forms names of chemical substances

-ate: adjective-forming suffix: having the form of, possessing

-ation: noun-forming suffix indicating an action or process: the act of (being), the result of (being), something that is

-ce: noun-forming suffix: the act of (being), the state of (being)

-cle: diminutive suffix: small

-culus, -cula, -culum: diminutive suffixes: small

-cy: noun-forming suffix: the act of (being), the state of (being)

-eal: adjective-forming suffix: pertaining to, located in

-ean: adjective-forming suffix: pertaining to, located in

-ellus, -ella, -ellum: form names of biological genera

-ellus, -ella, -ellum: diminutive suffixes: small

-ema: abstract noun-forming suffix: state, condition

-ent: forms adjectives translated with -ing added to the meaning of a verb; forms nouns meaning a person who or thing that does something

-esis: abstract noun-forming suffix: state, condition, procedure

-etic: adjective forming suffix, often from nouns ending in -esis: pertaining to

-ia: abstract noun-forming suffix: state, condition

-ia: abstract noun-forming suffix: state, quality, condition

-iac (rare): noun-forming suffix: person afflicted with

-ian: noun-forming suffix: indicates an expert in a certain field

-iasis: abstract noun-forming suffix: disease, abnormal condition, abnormal presence of

-ible: adjective-forming suffix: capable of (being)

-ic: adjective-forming suffix: pertaining to, located in; noun-forming suffix: drug, agent

-ic: adjective-forming suffix: pertaining to

-ics, -tics: noun-forming suffixes indicating a particular science or study: science or study of

-id: noun- and adjective-forming suffix indicating a particular shape, form, or resemblance: resembling

-id: adjective-forming suffix: pertaining to; in a state or condition of

-ide: noun-forming suffix: forms names of chemical substances

-ient: forms adjectives translated with -ing added to the meaning of a verb; forms nouns meaning a person who or thing that does something

-il: diminutive suffix: small

-ile: adjective-forming suffix: pertaining to, capable of (being), like

-illus, -illa, -illum: diminutive suffixes: small

-in, -ine: noun-forming suffixes: form names of substances

-ine: adjective-forming suffix: pertaining to, located in

-ion: noun-forming suffix: the act of

-ism: abstract noun-forming suffix: state, condition, quality

-ismus: abstract noun-forming suffix: state, condition; muscular spasm

-ist: noun-forming suffix: a person interested in

-ite: noun-forming suffix: forms names of chemical substances

-itic: adjective-forming suffix: pertaining to; pertaining to inflammation; noun-forming suffix: drug, agent

-itides: plural of -itis: forms plural nouns: inflammation

-itis: noun-forming suffix indicating an inflamed condition: inflammation

-ium (rarely, -eum): noun-forming suffix: sometimes names a body region; membrane, connective tissue

-ive: adjective-forming suffix: pertaining to

-ize: verb-forming suffix: make, become, cause to be, subject to, engage in

-lent: adjective-forming suffix: full of

-ma: noun-forming suffix: (often) abnormal or diseased condition; sometimes forms names of substances

-ment: noun-forming suffix: agent or instrument

-oid, (rarely) -ode, -id: noun- and adjective-forming suffixes indicating a particular shape, form, or resemblance: resembling

-ole: diminutive suffix: small

-olus, -ola, -olum: diminutive suffixes: small

-oma: abstract noun-forming suffix: usually tumor; occasionally disease

-one: noun-forming suffix: forms names of chemical substances

-or: noun-forming suffix: agent or instrument

-orium: noun-forming suffix: place for (something)

-ory: adjective-forming suffix: pertaining to

-ory: noun-forming suffix: place for (something)

-ose: adjective-forming suffix: full of, resembling; noun-forming suffix: forms names of chemical substances

-osis: abstract noun-forming suffix: abnormal or diseased condition

-otic: adjective-forming suffix from nouns in -osis: pertaining to

-*ous:* adjective-forming suffix: pertaining to, characterized by, full of

-sia: abstract noun-forming suffix: state, condition

-sis: abstract noun-forming suffix: state, condition, quality, process, procedure

-ter: noun-forming suffix: instrument, device

-tic: adjective-forming suffix from nouns in -sis: pertaining to; noun-forming suffix: drug, agent; person suffering from a certain disability

-tics: noun-forming suffix indicating a particular science or study: science or study of

-*ty:* abstract noun-forming suffix: state, quality, condition

-*ule:* diminutive suffix: small

-*ulus, -ula, -ulum:* diminutive suffixes: small

-*ure, -ura:* noun-forming suffixes: result of (an action)

-*us:* noun-forming suffix: condition, person (sometimes a malformed fetus)

-y: abstract noun-forming suffix: state, condition, quality, process, procedure

-*y:* abstract noun-forming suffix: state, quality, condition

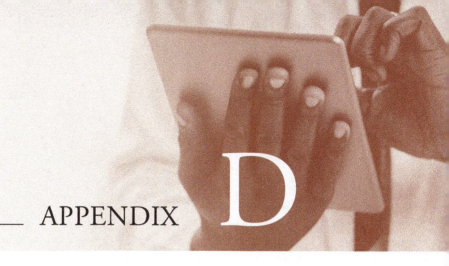
INDEX OF SUFFIX FORMS* AND COMPOUND SUFFIX FORMS

-ectasia, -ectasis: dilation, enlargement

-ectomy: surgical excision; removal of all (total excision) or part (partial excision) of an organ

-gen: substance that produces (something)

-genesis: formation, origin

-genic, -genous: causing, producing, caused by, produced by or in

-gram: a record of the activity of an organ (often an x-ray)

-graph: an instrument for recording the activity of an organ

-graphy: (1) the recording of the activity of an organ (usually by x-ray examination), (2) a descriptive treatise (on a subject)

-logy: study, science, the study or science of

-logist: one who specializes in a certain study or science

-lysis: dissolution, reduction, decomposition, disintegration

-lytic: pertaining to dissolution or decomposition, disintegration (forms adjectives from words ending in or containing -lysis)

-malacia: the softening (of tissues) of

-pathy: disease

-ptosis: dropping, sagging (of an organ or part)

-rrhagia: profuse discharge, hemorrhage

-rrhea: profuse discharge, excessive secretion

-rrhexis: bursting (of tissues), rupture

-sclerosis: the hardening (of tissues) of

-scope: an instrument for examining

-scopy: examination

-stenosis: the narrowing (of a part of the body)

-tome: a surgical instrument for cutting

-tomy: surgical incision

-toxic: poisonous (to an organ)

-toxin: a substance poisonous to (a part of the body)

---

*-logy, -logist, -malacia, -sclerosis, -stenosis, -toxic, and -toxin are suffix forms; the remaining terms are compound suffix forms.

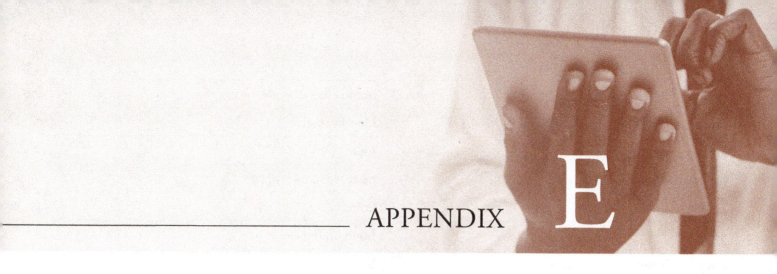

GLOSSARY OF ENGLISH-TO-GREEK/LATIN

This glossary contains the English meaning of the Greek and Latin combining forms, prefixes, suffixes, suffix forms, and compound suffix forms found in Lessons 1 to 15 of this text. It is included as an aid for your completion of Exercise 2 in each of these lessons. Verbs are given in the present infinitive form and nouns, and adjectives are given in dictionary form.

A

abdomen: abdomin-, cel(i)-, gastr-, lapar-, ventr-

abdominal cavity: ventr-

abdominal wall: lapar-

abnormal: dys-, para-, par-

above: epi-, super-, superior-

absent: de-

across: dia-, trans-

act: prax-

action: erg-, prax-

acute: ox(y)-

after: meta-, post-

again: pali(n)-, re-

against: ana-, anti-, contra-, ob-

agent that induces secretion: -agogue

agent: -e, -ment, -or

air: aer-, pneum(at)-, phys-

alike: is-

all, **entire**, **every:** pan(t)-

alongside: para-, par-

amnion: amni-

amniotic sac: amni-

angina pectoris: angin-

animal: zo-

anthrax: anthrax, anthrac-

anus: proct-

aorta: aort-

apart: dia-, dis-, se-

appearance: phys(i)-, faci-, -fici, facies

(have an) appetite: orec-, orex-

arachnoid membrane: arachn-

(upper) arm: brachi-

around: amphi-, ampho-, circum-, para-, par-, peri-

atrium: atri-

(surgical) attachment: -pex-

attack: lep-

away: dis-

away from: ab-, apo-, de-, ec-, ex-, se-

B

bacillus: bacill-

back: ana-, re-, retro-; pali(n)-

(located in the) back: opisth-, dolich-

back of the body: dors-

backward: retro-

bacterium: bacter(i)-

bear: fer-, lat-, ger-, gest-

bearing, carrying: phor-

before: ante-, pre-, pro-

beginning: arch-, -arche

behind: meta-, post-, retro-; poster-, -posterior

belly: abdomin-, ventr-, uter-

below: infra-; inferior-

below normal: hypo-

bend: flect-, flex-

beneath: infra-

between: inter-

beyond: extra-, para-, par-, ultra-

bile: chol(e)-, bili-

binding: -desis, desm-

(give) birth: genit-, part-, -para

black: melan-

bladder: cyst(i)-, -cystis, vesic-

blood: hem-, hemat-, -em-, sangui(n)-

blood clot: thromb-

blood vessel: vas-

blue: cyan-

body: som(at)-, -soma

bone: oss-

bone marrow: myel-

born: -gn-, nat-

(be) born: -gn-, nat-

both: ambi-, amphi-, ampho-, bi-

brain: cerebr-

break (up): cla(s)-

breast: pector-, mamm-, mast-, maz-, stern-, steth-

breastbone: stern-

breathe: pne-, spir(at)-

bring: duc-, duct-

bring forth: genit-

bronchus: bronch(i)-

bunch of grapes: staphyl-

burning: pyr-

bursa: burs-

bursting (of tissues): -rrhexis

C

calcium: calc-

cancer: carcin-

capillary: capill-

carbon dioxide: capn-

carcinoma: carcin-

cardia: cardi-

carry: fer-, lat-, ger-, gest-

cartilage: chondr-

caused by: -genic, -genous

causing: -genic, -genous

cavity: alve-, por-, syring-, -syrinx

cecum: cec-, typhl-

cervix uteri: cervic-, cervix, trachel-

change: meta-

check: isch-, -sche-

chemical substance: -ide, -ite, -one, -ate

chest: pector-, stern-, steth-

chest cavity: thorax, thorac-

child: ped-

childbirth: toc-

choking pain: angin-

choroid: choroid-

ciliary body: cycl-

circle: cycl-

cleft: schiz-, schist-, -schisis

close: -clud-, -clus-, my-

coal: anthrax, anthrac-

coccus: cocc-, -coccus

cold: frig-, frigor-

(icy) cold: cry(m)-

colon: col-, colon-

color: chrom-, chroma-, chromat-

come into being: gen(e)-, -gen

communicate: pha-

completion: tel-

comprehension: no-

compress: arct(at)-

conduct: duc-, duct-

connective tissue: -ium (rarely -eum); desm-

contraction: stal-, stol-

(muscular) coordination: tax-

cornea: kerat-

corpse: necr-

cough: tuss-

cow: vacc-

crown: coron-

cut: -cid-, -cis, sect-

cyst: cyst(i)-, -cystis

D

dark: melan-

daylight: phos-, phot-

dead: necr-

death: than(at)-

decaying: sapr-

decomposition: -lysis

decrease: pen-

defective: dys-

deficiency: pen-

deficient: a-, an-, hypo-; olig-

destroy: cla(s)-, -clast, ly(s)-

develop: plas(t)-

device: -ter

device or agent for stopping the flow (of something): -stat

diaphragm: phren-

different: heter-, hetero-

difficult: dys-

digest: peps-, pept-

dilate: eury(n)-

dilation: -ectasia, -ectasis

discharge: -rrhea

disease: nos-, path-, -pathy

disintegration: -lysis

disordered: cata-

double: bi-, di-, dis-, diplo-

down: de-

downward: cata-

drawing forth: agog-

dripping (of blood): -staxis, -staxia

drop: pt-

drug: -ic, -tic, -itic; pharmac(eu)-

dry: xer-

duct: -doch-, por-

dull: ambly-

duodenum: duoden-

dust: coni-, koni-

E

ear: aur-, ot-

eat: phag-

echo: echo-

egg: ov-

end: tel-

energy: calor-, dynam-

enlargement: -ectasia, -ectasis

entire: pan(t)-

enzyme: -ase; zym-

equal: is-

erect: orth-

Escherichia coli: coli-

esophagus: esophag-

every: pan(t)-

examination: -scopy

examine: scop-

excess: super-, ultra-

excessive: hyper-, poly-

(surgical) excision: -ectomy

excrement: copr-, fec-, scat-

expert (in a certain field): -ian, -ist

extremities: acr-

eye: ocul-, ophthalm-, opt-

eyelid: blephar-

F

face: faci-, -fici-, facies, prosop-

faint: ambly-

fall: pt-

falling: -ptosis

fallopian tube: salping-, -salpinx

false: pseud-

fat: adip-, lip-, stear-, steat-

fatty deposit: ather-

(abnormal) fear: phob-

fecal matter: copr-, fec-, scat-

female: gyn(ec)-

ferment: zym-

fermentation: zym-

fetal membrane: amni-

fever: febr-, febris, pyr-, pyret-

feverish: pyrex-

few: olig-

fiber: fibr-, is-, inos-

filament: fibr-

finger: dactyl-, digit-

fingernail: onych-

first: prot-

fissure: schiz-, schist-, -schisis

fistula: fistul-, syring-, -syrinx

fixed: stabil-, stabl-

fixing: -pex-

flesh: creat-, sarc-

flood: gurgit-, gurgitat-

flow: gurgit-, gurgitat-, rhe-

fluid: hydr-, sud(or)-

following: post-

food: sit-

foot: pod-

force: dynam-

form: morph-, plas(t)-

formation: -genesis

formation (of a passage): -stomy

forward: ante-, pro-

front: pro-; anter-

(in) front (of): pre-, pro-; anter-

fungus: fung-, myc(et)-

fused: ankyl-, ancyl-

G

gall: chol(e)-

gas: aer-, phys-, pneum(at)-

gland: aden-

good: eu-

gout: -agra

gray matter (of the brain and spinal cord): poli-

green: chlor-

groin: inguin-

grow: aux-, -auxe, -auxis

(begin to) grow: cresc-, -cret-

growth: phyt-

gum (of the mouth): gingiv-

H

hair: trich-

half: hemi-, semi-

hand: cheir-, chir-

hardening (of tissues) of: -sclerosis

head: capit-

heal: therap(eu)-

healer: iatr-

healthy: eu-

hear: acou(s)-, acu(s)-

heart: cor-, cord-

heartbeat: rhythm-

heat: calor-, therm-

hemorrhage: rhag-, -rrhagia

hernia: -cel-

herpes: herpes, herpet-

hidden: crypt-

hollow: alve-

hooked, crooked: ankyl-, ancyl-

hymen: hymen-

I

ileum: ile-

illness: nos-

in, into: in-, en-

in place of: pros-, prosth-

incision: tom-, -tomy

increase: aux-, -auxe, -auxis

increased: hyper-

infected: sep-

inflammation: -itis (pl. -itides)

inject fluid: cly(s)-

inner: eso-; intern-

instrument: -ment, -or, -ter

instrument (for breaking or crushing): -clast

instrument (for cutting): -tome

instrument (for examining): -scope

instrument (for recording the activity of an organ): -graph

internal organ: splanchn-, viscer-, viscus-

intestine: enter-

into: en-

inward: eso-

iris: ir(id)-

iron: sider-

island: insul-

J

jaundice: icter-

(lower) jaw: gnath-

jejunum: jejun-

join: junct-

joined: syn-

K

kidney: ren-

kill: -cid-, -cis-

know: gno(s)-

L

labor: toc-

lack: a-, an-

lacrimal sac or duct: dacry-

large: macr-, mega-, megal-

larynx: larynx, laryng-

latent: crypt-

law: nom-

lead: duc-, duct-

leading: agog-

left side: sinistr-

lens: phac-, phak-

ligament: desm-

light: phos-, phot-

limb: mel-

lip: ch(e)il-, labi-

little: use diminutive suffix

liver: hepar-, hepat-

long: macr-, mega-, megal-

louse: pedicul-

love: phil-

lung: pneum(on)-, pulm(on)-

lymph: lymph-

M

(be) mad: man-

make: fac-, -fic-, -fect, poie-

male: andr-

man: andr-

many: mult-, multi-, poly-

mark: stigm-, stigmat-

marrow: medull-

measure: metr-

meatus: meat-

medicine: pharmac(eu)-

membrane: -ium (rarely-eum); hymen-

meningeal membrane: mening-, -meninx

meninges: mening-, -meninx

menstruation: men-

mental activity: no-

mesentery: mes-

milk: gal-, galact-, lact-

mind: no-, phren-, psych-

motion: kines(i)-

mouth: or-, os, stom-, stomat-

move: kine-

movement: kines(i)-

much: mult-, multi-

mucus: blenn-, myx-

muscle: is-, inos-, my(s)-

muscular spasm: -ismus

N

narrow: dolich-

narrowing (of a part of the body): stenosis

nature: phys(i)-

navel: omphal-

neck (of the uterus): cervic-, cervix

neck: trachel-

neither: neutr-

nerve: neur-

nervous system: neur-

network: ret-, retin-

new: ne-

night: nyct-

nipple: thel(e)-

normal: eu-; orth-

nose: nas-, rhin-

not: a-, an-, in-, non-

nourishment: troph-

numbness: narc-

O

odor: osm-

of one's self: idi-

old age: ger-, presby-

on both sides: amphi-, ampho-

on the outside: extra-

one: mono-

oozing (of blood): -staxis, -staxia

opening: meat-, or-, os, por-, stom-, stomat-

opposed to: anti-

opposite: contra-

organism: zo-

origin: arch-, -arche; -genesis

out of: ec-, ex-

outer layer (of an organ): cortic-, cortex

outer: extern-

outside of: ecto-

outside: exo-

ovary: oophor-, ovari-

over: epi-, super-

oviduct: syring-, -syrinx

oxygen: ox(y)-

P

pain: odyn-

(sudden) pain: -agra

painful: dys-

palate: staphyl-

paralysis: paresis

paralyze: plec-, pleg-

partition: sept-

passage: meat-, por-

pelvis: pelv-

penis: pen-, phall-

people: dem-

pharynx: pharynx, pharyng-

physician: iatr-

pierce: cente-

pigment: chrom-, chroma-, chromat-

place for: -arium, -ary, -orium, -ory

place: the-, top-

plant organism: phyt-

plastic surgery: -plasty

pleura: pleur-

pleural cavity: thorax, thorac-

point: cusp, -cuspid

pointed: ox(y)-

poisonous (to an organ): -toxic

poisonous substance: -toxin

population: dem-

pore: por-

portal vein: pyle-

pour: fus-

power: dynam-

pregnant: gravid-, cye-

pressure: bar-

preventing: anti-

produce: gen(e)-, -gen, poie-

produced by or in: -genic, -genous

producing: -genic, -genous

prolapse: pt-

prostate gland: prostat-

protected: immun-

protection (against disease): phylac-

puberty: puber(t)-

pubic bone: pub-

pubic region: pub-

pubis: pub-

pulmonary artery: pulm(on)-

pulse: sphygm-

pupil (of the eye): cor(e)-

pus: pur-, py-

put: the-

putrid: sapr-

pylorus: pylor-

R

radiation: actin-

rapid: ox(y)-

read: lex-

record: graph-

(written) record: gram-

record of the activity of an organ (often an x-ray): -gram

rectum: rect-

reduction: -lysis

relieving: anti-

remember: mne-

renal pelvis: pyel-

resembling: -ile, -oid, -ose

retina: ret-, retin-

reverberating sound: echo-

rib: cost-

right side: dextr-

rinse out: cly(s)-

rod: rhabd-

root: radic-, rad-, radix

rotten: sapr-

rupture: rhex-, -rrhexis

S

safe: immun-

sag: pt-

sagging (of an organ or part): -ptosis

saliva: ptyal-, sial-

salivary duct: sial-

same: homo-, homeo-; is-

science, study of: -ics, -tics; -logy

scrotum: scrot-

sebaceous glands: stear-, steat-

sebum: stear-, steat-

secrete: crin-, rhe-

secretion: crin-

seed: sem-, semin-, sperm(at)-

seizure: lep-

self: aut-

semen: sem-, semin-, sperm(at)-

send: stal-, stol-

sensation: esthe(s)-

sense: esthe(s)-

sense of smell: osm-, osphr-

sensitivity: esthe(s)-

sex glands: gonad-

sex organs: gonad-

sexual desire: aphrodis(i)-, er-, erot-

(abnormal) sexual excitation or gratification: -lagnia

shape: -form, morph-

short: brachy-

shut: my-

side: later-

sigmoid colon: sigm-

similar: is-

single: mon-, mono-

sinus: sin-, sinus-

skin: derm(at)-, -derma

slackening (of strength): paresis

sleep: hypn-, somn-

slender: dolich-

slide: lab-, laps-

slip: lab-, laps-

small: micr-; use diminutive suffix

smooth: lei-

soft tissue: sarc-

softening (of tissues) of: -malacia

sound: phon-, son-

spasm: spasm-

speak: pha-, phras-

specialist: -logist

specialty: -logy

speech: phem-

sperm: sperm(at)-

sphincter muscle: sphincter-

spider: arachn-

spinal cord: myel-

spine: r(h)achi-

spit: pty-

spleen: lien-, splen-

split: schiz-, schist-, -schisis

spot: stigm-, stigmat-

stable: stabil-, stabl-

stand: sta(t)-

staphylococci: staphyl-

starch: amyl-

steal: klept-

stomach: gastr-

stone: calc-

stop: sta(t)-

straight: orth-

strength: sthen-

streptococci: strept-

stretch: tens(i)-

stretching: ta-

strike: plec-, pleg-

study: -logy

stupor: narc-

substance: -in, -ine

substance that produces (something): -gen

sugar: glyc-

suppress: isch-, -sche-

surface: faci-, -fici-, facies

surrounding: peri-

suture: -rrhaph-

swallow: phag-

sweat: hidr(ot)-, -idr-, sud(or)-

sweat glands: syring-, -syrinx

swelling: -cel-, edema, edemat-

swollen: tum(e)-

synovial fluid, synovial membrane or sac: synov(i)-

syringe: syring-, -syrinx

T

take: -cip-, -cept-

talk: lal-

taste: geus(t)-

tear: dacry-, lacrim-, lachrym-

(body) temperature: therm-

tendon: ten-, tenon(t)-

tension: ton-, tens(i)-

testicle: orchi(d)-, orch(e)-

theft: klept-

thick: pachy-

thirst: dips-

thorax: thorax, thorac-

thoroughly: con-, in-, ob-, per-

thread (worm): nemat-

through: dia-, per-, trans-

(a) throwing: bol-

thyroid gland: thyr-

time: chron-

timing: chron-

tissue: hist(i)-

to: ad-

toe: dactyl-, digit-

toenail: onych-

together: con-, syn-

tone: ton-

tongue: gloss-, lingu-

tonsil: amygdal-

tooth: dent-, odont-

toward: ad-, ob-

trachea: trach(e)-, trachy-

transformation: meta-

treatise (on a subject): -graphy

treat medically: therap(eu)-

treatment: iatr-

tube: tub-

tumor: -oma; -cel-, onc-

turning: trop-

twice: bi-, di-, dis-

twin: diplo-

twisted: strept-

two: bi-, di-, dis-

U

ulcer: (h)elc-

umbilicus: omphal-

under: sub-

up: ana-

upon: epi-

ureter: ureter-

urethra: urethr-

uric acid: ur-

urinary tract: ur-

urine: ur-

uterus: hyster-, metr-, -metra, uter-

uvula: staphyl-

V

vagina: colp-, vagin-

vagus nerve: vag-

varix: cirs-, varic-, varix

vas deferens: vas-

(dilated and twisted) vein: cirs-, varic-, varix

vein: phleb-, ven-

vertebra: spondyl-

very: con-, in-, ob-, per-

virus: vir(u)-, virus-

viscus: splanchn-

vision: op(s)-, opt-

voice: phon-

vomit: eme-

W

wall: sept-

water: hydr-

web: arachn-

weight: bar-

widen: eury(n)-

with: con-

within: en-, endo-, ento-, eso-, intra-

without: a-, an-

woman: gyn(ec)-

womb: uter-

work: erg-

(intestinal) worm: helmint(h)-

write: graph-

Y

yellow: xanth-

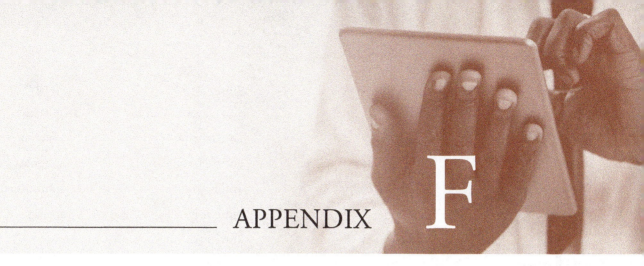

MEDICAL TERMINOLOGY USED IN LESSONS 1 TO 15

The following is a complete list of terms used in the exercises in Lessons 1 to 15, the main body of this text. Terms from the supplemental lessons (Lessons 16 to 19) and the biological nomenclature lesson (Lesson 20) are not included. This list is provided as a reference source and spelling guide.

A

abdominocentesis
abdominoplasty
abdominovesical
abduct
abenteric
abiogenesis
abiogenetic
abiosis
abiotrophy
ablation
aborad
aboral
abrachia
acanthocytosis
acanthopelvis
acephalia

achlorhydria
achondrogenesis
achromatolysis
achromatopsia
achromatosis
achromatous
acousmatamnesia
acoustic
acoustics
acroanesthesia
acrobrachycephaly
acrocephaly
acrocyanosis
acrodermatitis
acrohyperhidrosis
acromegaly
acromicria

actinodermatitis
actinogenic
actinotherapy
adduct
adenoid
adenoidectomy
adenoiditis
adenotome
adipectomy
adipocyte
adipokinesis
adipose
adiposuria
adoral
adrenal cortex
adrenalinemia
aerobe

aerometer
aerophagia
aerotitis
afebrile
afferent
ageusia
ageustia
agnathia
agnosia
agnostic
agranulocyte
agranuloplastic
akinesia
algolagnia
algometer
alloantigen
allodynia

alloplasty	androgynous	anthrax	aphakia
allostery	android	antianemic	aphasiac
alogia	andrology	antiarthritic	aphemia
alveobronchitis	anemic	antibacterial	aphonia
alveolar	anencephaly	antibiogram	aphrodisiac
alveolate	anergia	antibiosis	aplasia
alveolitis	anesthesia	antibiotic	apnea
ambidextrous	anesthesiology	anticytotoxin	apneumatosis
amblyacousia	aneurism	antiemetic	apneumia
amblyopia	angiitis	antifungal	apoplectic
amenorrhea	anginoid	antigalactic	apoplexy
amnesia	anginous	antigen	apraxia
amniocentesis	angiogram	antihemorrhagic	apraxic
amniogenesis	angiology	antihidrotic	aptyalism
amniorrhexis	anhydrous	antihypnotic	arachnodactyly
amphibious	aniridia	anti-icteric	arachnoid
amphocyte	anisocytosis	antilipemia	arachnolysin
amygdalin	ankylodactylia	antilithic	archenteron
amygdaline	ankylosis	antimicrobial	arctation
amygdaloid	ankylotia	antinarcotic	areflexia
amylogenesis	anodyne	antineuritic	arrhythmia
amyloid	anonychia	antiphagocytic	arteriosclerosis
amyloidosis	anorchidism	antipsychotic	arteriostenosis
amylolysis	anorexia	antistaphylococcic	arteriostosis
amyosthenia	anosmia	antistreptolysin	arteriovenous
amyosthenic	anosmic	antithrombin	arteritis
amyotonia	anoxia	antitoxin	arthritic
amyotrophia	antasthenic	antitussive	arthritides
anabiosis	antebrachium	anuria	arthritis
analgesic	antenatal	aortarctia	arthrocentesis
analogy	antepartum	aortocoronary	arthroclasia
anamnesis	antepyretic	aortoiliac	arthrodesis
anamniotic	anterolateral	aortopathy	arthrology
anaphylaxis	anteroposterior	aortostenosis	arthropyosis
anastomosis	anthelmintic	aphacia	arthrosclerosis
anatoxin	anthracosis	aphagia	arthrosis

ascus

aspermatogenesis

aspiration

aspirator

asternia

asthenia

astigmatism

astigmia

astigmometer

asynergy

asystolia

ataxia

ataxiaphasia

atelencephalia

atelia

atherogenesis

atheroma

atheromatosis

atrial

atrichia

atrioventricular

atrophy

aural

auricula

auriculotherapy

auris interna

autism

autoantitoxin

autoerotism

autohemolysis

autosepticemia

auxin

auxology

auxotrophic

aviremia

azoospermia

B

bacillar

bacillary

bacillemia

bacteriolysin

bacteriophage

bacteriotherapy

bacteriotoxin

bacteroid

baresthesia

bariatrics

barognosis

biceps

bicuspid

biliary

bilious

biloma

binauricular

binocular

binotic

biocide

biodynamics

biokinetics

biologic

biologist

biometry

biotoxin

bisection

blastocyst

blastocyte

blastoderm

blastogenesis

blennorrhagia

blennorrhea

blepharodiastasis

blepharoplasty

blepharoptosis

blepharostat

blepharotomy

brachia

brachial

brachialgia

brachiocephalic

brachycephalic

brachycephalous

brachytherapy

bradyarrhythmia

bradycardia

bradykinesia

bradyphrenia

bradypnea

bradytachycardia

bronchiolectasis

bronchiolitis

bronchomycosis

bursae

bursolith

bursotomy

C

calcemia

calciferous

calcification

calcipexy

calculogenesis

calculus

califerous

calorific

calorigenic

calorimeter

calorimetry

capillarectasia

capillariasis

capillaropathy

capillaroscopy

capillary

capitate

capitulum

capnography

capnometry

carcinogen

carcinogenesis

carcinogenic

carcinoma

cardia

cardiac

cardialgia

cardioangiology

cardioesophageal

cardiomalacia

cardionephric

cardioptosis

cardiopyloric

cardiospasm

cardiotomy

cardiovascular

catagenesis

cataphoresis

cataplexia

cataplexy

cecopexy

cecoptosis

cecostomy

celiac

celiocentesis

celiohysterectomy

celiomyositis

celiopathy

celiorrhaphy

centesis

cephalalgia

cephalocele

cephalothoracic

cerebellar ataxia

cerebellar cortex

cerebellum

cerebral

cerebropathy

cervicitis

cervicovaginitis

cheilectomy

cheilitis

cheiloschisis

cheirognostic

chiragra

chiromegaly

chirospasm

chloroleukemia

chloronychia

chloropia

chlorosis

cholagogue

cholangioma

cholangiotomy

cholecystectomy

cholecystic

cholecystogastrostomy

cholecystolithiasis

cholecystopexy

choledochal

choledochoenterostomy

choledochorrhaphy

cholelithiasis

cholemesis

cholestasia

chondralgia

chondrectomy

chondritis

chondrocostal

chondrocranium

chondrocyte

chondrodystrophy

chondrolipoma

chondromyxosarcoma

chondroplasty

choroid

choroiditis

choroidocyclitis

choroidoiritis

chromatogram

chromatophore

chromatoptometry

chromidrosis

chromophobia

chromophore

chromotherapy

chronobiology

chronograph

chronological

chronophobia

cirsectomy

cirsoid

cirsotomy

clysis

coarctate

coccobacilli

coccobacteria

coccoid

colicolitis

colicystitis

coliform

colinephritis

colitis

collapsotherapy

coloenteritis

colonic

colonitis

colonocyte

colorectostomy

colostomy

colpocystocele

colpocystotomy

colpomicroscope

concrescence

coniofibrosis

coniology

coniosis

conjunctiva

conjunctivitis

conjunctivoma

conjunctivoplasty

contralateral

copremesis

coprolalia

coprolith

coprophilic

coproscopy

coprozoa

cordate

corectopia

corelysis

coremorphosis

coreoplasty

corestenoma

corona dentis

coronary

coronavirus

coronoid

coronoidectomy

cortical

corticoadrenal

corticopleuritis

corticotherapy

costalgia

costochondral

costochondritis

costopneumopexy

costotome

craniology

craniomalacia

craniorhachischisis

craniosclerosis

creatorrhea

cryoanalgesia

cryobiology

cryogen

cryostat

cryotherapy

cryptic

cryptogenic

cryptography

cryptolith

cryptomnesia

cryptorchidectomy

cusp

cuspid

cyanopia

cyanosis

cyanotic

cyclectomy

cyclochoroiditis

cyclokeratitis

cycloplegia

cyesis

cystalgia

cystic

cystigerous

cystocele

cystoid

cystolith

cystoma

cystopexy

cystorrhexis

cystoscopy

cytobiology

cytocide

cytoclasis

cytometer

cytotoxic

cytotoxin

D

dacryocystitis

dacryocystorhinostomy

decalcification

decalcify

decimeter

defecation

deferent

demographics

demography

denticle

dentigerous

dentilabial

dentin

dentist

dentofacial

dentolabial

dermatitis

dermatocyst

dermatology

dermatomycosis

dermatomyoma

dermatomyositis

dermatopathology

dermatophyte

dermatoscopy

dermatotherapy

dermic

desmoplasia

desmoplastic

detoxification

detoxify

dextral

dextrocardia

diagnosis

diaphoresis

diaphoretic

diastole

diencephalon

digestion

digitate

digitation

digiti

diglossia

diplegia

diplegic

diplocephaly

diplococcus

diploid

diplopia

dipsophobia

dissection

dolichocephalic

dolichoectasia

dolichomorphic

dolichosigmoid

dorsad

dorsal

dorsiflection

dorsiflexion

dorsolateral

dorsoventral

dromotropic

ductile

ductogram

ductule

duodenoenterostomy

duodenojejunostomy

duodenorrhaphy

dynamic

dynamometer

dynamometry

dysarthrosis

dyscephaly

dyschiria

dyschromatopsia

dysentery

dysgeusia

dysgraphia

dyshidrosis

dyskinesia

dyslexia

dysmenorrhea

dysmnesia

dysodontiasis

dysopsia

dysostosis

dyspepsia

dyspeptic

dysphagia

dysphasia

dysphonia

dysphoria

dyspnea

dyspraxia

dysrhythmia

dysstasia

dysthyroidism

dystrophoneurosis

dystrophy

dysuria

E

echoendoscope

echogenic

echogram

echolalia

echopathy

ectasis

ectocardia

ectophyte

ectopia

ectopotomy

ectostosis

edema

edematogenic

efferent

embolism

emesis

emetic

emphysema

emphysematous

encephalalgia

encephalic

encephalolith

encephalomalacia

encephalomyelopathy

endangiitis

endaortitis

endarteritis

endemic

endemoepidemic

endocardium

endocranium

endocrinology

endocrinopathy

endocrinotherapy

endocystitis

endodontics

endodontitis

endogastritis

endomastoiditis

endometriosis

endometrium

endoneurium

endoparasite

endoscope

endosteum

endostoma

endotoscope

endotoxin

enophthalmos

enteralgia

enterocentesis

enterocholecystostomy

enteroclysis

enterocystocele

enterodynia

enteromegaly

enteromycosis

enterorrhaphy

enterosepsis

enterostenosis

entopic

eosin

eosinopenia

eosinophilia

epicardium

epicranium

epidemic

epidemiologist

epidermitis

epidermoid

epidermomycosis

epigastrium

epileptic

epinephrine

epiotic

epipharynx

episcleritis

epistaxis

episternum

epizoon

ergometer

ergonomics

erogenous

erotic

eroticism

erotogenic

erotomania

erythralgia

erythrism

erythroblastosis

erythrocyte

erythrocytometer

erythrocytopenia

erythrocytorrhexis

erythrocytosis

erythroleukemia

erythromelalgia

erythromelia

erythropenia

erythrophage

erythropia

erythropoiesis

erythropoietin

erythropsia

erythrosis

esogastritis

esophagismus

esophagocele

esophagodynia

esthesiometer

eubiotics

eucapnia

euglycemia

euphonia

euphoria

euthanasia

excise

excision

exclusion

excrescence

exencephalia

exocardia

exocrine

exocytosis

exodontia

exoerythrocytic

exogastritis

exogenous

exomphalos

exotoxin

expectorant

expectoration

expiration

expiratory

exsanguination

external

externalize

extrauterine

extravasation

F

facial

facial
   hemiplegia

faciobrachial

febrifacient

febrile

fecaloid

fecaluria

feculent

fibromyalgia

fibromyoma

fibroplasia

fibrosis

fistula

fistuloenterostomy

flexile

flexor

formation

frigid

frigolabile

frigostabile

fungi

fungicide

fungistasis

fungistatic

fungoid

G

galactic

galactopoiesis

galactorrhea

gastrectomy

gastroenteralgia

gastroenteric

gastroenteritis

gastrohepatic

gastropexy

gastrorrhagia

gastroschisis

gastroscope

genetics

genitalia

genitourinary

geriatric

geriatrician

geriatrics

gestosis

gingivitis

gingivostomatitis

globin

glossectomy

glossoptosis

glycogen

gonadal dysgenesis

gonadarche

gonadotropin

granulocyte

granulocytopenia

granulocytopoiesis

granuloma

graphology

gynecoid pelvis

gynecologist

gynecology

gynecomastia

H

helcoid

helminthiasis

helminthic

helminthology

hemangiectasis

hemangioma

hemangiosarcoma

hemarthrosis

hematin

hematoma

hematomyelia

hematopathology

hematophagous

hematopoiesis

hematosalpinx

hematuria

hemianalgesia

hemiangiosarcoma

hemiataxia

hemiatrophy

hemic

hemicephalic

hemicrania

hemifacial

hemihyperplasia

hemilaryngectomy

hemiparesis

hemiplegia

hemithorax

hemocyte

hemocytoblast

hemocytology

hemocytometer

hemodynamics

hemoglobin

hemoglobinemia

hemoglobinolysis

hemoglobinopathy

hemoglobinuria

hemopericardium

hemopexin

hemophiliac

hemoptysis

hemosiderin

hemosiderosis

hemostasis

hemotrophic

heparin

heparinoid

hepaticotomy

hepatocarcinogen

hepatogastric

hepatogenous

hepatologist

hepatolytic

hepatomegaly

hepatomelanosis

hepatorrhaphy

hepatosplenomegaly

herpes facialis

herpes labialis

herpes ocular

herpesvirus

herpetic

herpetiform

heterocephalus

heterochromia iridis

heterotaxia

hidradenitis

hidrosis

histiocyte

histiocytoma

histiocytosis

histolysis

histoma

histopathology

histophysiology

homeopathy

homeostasis

homeotherm

homoerotic

homogenize

homolateral

homology

homophobe

hydrocephalus

hydrocolpos

hydrometra

hydronephrosis

hydropenia

hydrophilism

hydropneumothorax

hymen

hymenal

hypacousia

hypalgesia

hyperacusis

hyperalgesia

hyperalgia

hypercalcemia

hypercalciuria

hypercapnia

hyperchlorhydria

hyperchromatic

hyperemesis

hyperemesis
    gravidarum

hyperemia

hypereosinophilia

hyperesthesia

hyperglycemia

hyperhidrosis

hyperinsulinemia

hyperinsulinism

hyperleukocytosis

hyperlipemia

hypermetropia

hyperopia

hyperostosis

hypertension

hypertonus

hypertrichosis

hypertrophy

hyperuricemia

hypnogenic

hypnoidal

hypnotic

hypnotize

hypocapnia

hypochloremia

hypodermoclysis

hypogastrium

hypogenitalism

hypoglossal

hypoglycemia

hypokinesia

hypologia

hypomelanosis

hypophonia

hypoplasia

hypostosis

hypotensive

hypotrichosis

hypoxemia

hypoxia

hysterectomy

hysteromyoma

hysterosalpingography

hysteroscope

hysterotrachelorrhaphy

I

iatrogenesis

iatrogenic

iatrology

icterohepatitis

icteroid

idiogram

idioisolysin

idiolysin

idiopathic

idiotropic

ileocolic

ileocolostomy

ileocystoplasty

ileoproctostomy

ileotomy

iliocecal sphincter

immunifacient

immunochromatography

immunogenic

immunology

immunotherapy

immunotoxin

inception

incipient

incise

incisor

indigestible

inframammary

infrarenal

infusion

ingestant

ingestion

inguinal

inguinal reflex

inosemia

inositis

inosuria

insemination

insomnia

insomniac

inspiration

insulin

insulinase

insulinemia

interatrial

intercostal

internal

internalize

interventricular

intra-atrial

intracranial

intraduodenal

intrapulmonary

intrauterine

introflexion

intubation

intumesce

intumescent

ipsilateral

iridadenosis

iridalgia

iridectropium

iridemia

iridocele

iridocystectomy

iridopathy

ischemia

ischemic

ischidrosis

isochromatic

isocoria

isocytosis

isocytotoxin

isodactylism

isodiametric

isomorphism

isotonia

J

jaundice

jejunojejunostomy

jejunostomy

K

karyochrome

karyokinesis

karyophage

karyostasis

keratectasia

keratectomy

keratocele

keratomalacia

keratomycosis

keratoprosthesis

keratorrhexis

kinesiatrics

kinesimeter

kleptomaniac

L

labial

labile

labiodental

labiogingival

labioplasty

lachrymal

lachrymation

lacrimal

lacrimation

lactation

lactiferous

lactobacillus

lactogen

lalorrhea

laparocele

laparocholecystotomy

laparoileotomy

laparorrhaphy

laparoscope

laparoscopy

laparotomy

laryngismus

laryngomalacia

laryngopharyngeal

laryngoscopist

lateral

leiomyofibroma

leiomyoma

leiomyomata

leiomyosarcoma

leptocephalus

leptochromatic

leptomeninges

leukocidin

leukocoria

leukocyte

leukocytic

leukoedema

leukoencephalitis

leukopenia

leukopoiesis

leukopoietic

leukorrhea

leukotoxin

lienal

lienomyelomalacia

lingual

lingula

lingulae

lipemia

lipocyte

lipodermatosclerosis

lipoid

liposarcoma

lithiasis

lithoclast

lithogenesis

lithology

logopenia

lymphadenitis

lymphadenopathy

lymphangiectasis

lymphangioma

lymphangiosarcoma

lymphangitis

lymphedema

lymphoblast

lymphocytopenia

lymphogranulomatosis

lymphoma

lymphopoiesis

lymphogenous

M

macrocephalous

macrocephaly

macrocheilia

macrocranial

macrocythemia

macropsia

macrosomia

macrostoma

macrotia

mammogram

mammography

maniacal

mastalgia

mastatrophia

mastectomy

mastitis

mastodynia

meatometer

meatotomy

megacolon

megalocephaly

melalgia

melanin

melanoderma

melanoma

melanomatosis

melanonychia

melanophore

melanuria

menarche

meningitis

meningocele

meningococcemia

mesencephalic

mesentery

mesocardia

mesocephalic

mesoderm

mesogastrium

mesojejunum

mesonephric

metabiosis

metachromasia

metakinesis

metamyelocyte

metrectasia

metritis

metrology

microbe

microbicide

microcephaly

microdontism

microgastria

micrognathia

microlithiasis

micropenis

microphakia

microphotograph

micropsia

micropsychotic

microstomia

monoblast

monobrachius

monochromatic

monochromatism

monocular

monocyte

monocytopenia

mononeuritis

monophasia

monorchid

monosomy

morphogen

morphography

morphometry

multigravida

myasthenia

myatonia

mycethemia

mycetoma

mycobacterium

mycology

mycosis

myectomy

myeloblast

myelocystocele

myelodysplasia

myelofibrosis

myeloid

myeloma

myelopoiesis

myeloradiculopathy

myocyte

myofibril

myofibroma

myolipoma

myoneural

myopathy

myope

myopia

myospasm

myotasis

myotome

myotonia

myxoid

myxolipoma

myxoma

N

narcohypnia

narcolepsy

narcosis

narcotism

narcotize

nasal

nasogastric

nasolacrimal

nasoscope

nasosinusitis

natal

necrobiosis

necrogenous

necrophagous

necrosis

nematocide

nematocyst

nematoid

nematology

neogenesis

neologism

neonate

neonatology

neophallus

neophobia

neostomy

nephrectomy

nephritis

nephrocystitis

nephrolithiasis

nephrolithotomy

nephroscope

nephrotoxin

neuralgia

neurasthenia

neuritis

neurocrine

neurodermatitis

neuroectoderm

neurohistology

neurosclerosis

neurotoxin

neurotropic virus

neutrophil

nomogram

nomography

nonose

nonseptate

nontoxic

nosode

nosology

nosophyte

nyctalopia

nyctamblyopia

O

occipital

occiput

occlude

ocular herpes

ocularist

oculofacial

oculonasal

oculoplastics

odontalgia

odontectomy

odontocele

odontoclasis

odontogenesis

odontogenic

odontography

odontonecrosis

odontoschism

odynometer

odynophagia

oligoarthritis

oligodontia

oligogenic

oligohydramnios

oligomenorrhea

oligospermia

oliguria

omphalitis

omphalocele

omphalotomy

oncology

oncotherapy

onychodystrophy

onychoid

onychomycosis

oophorectomy

oophoritis

ophthalmia neonatorum

ophthalmologist

ophthalmomycosis

ophthalmoplegia

ophthalmorrhea

ophthalmoscope

optogram

optometrist

optometry

orad

oral

orchidopexy

orchidoptosis

orchiopathy

orchioplasty

orchiotomy

orexigen

orifice

oropharynx

orotracheal

orthokinetics

orthopsychiatry

orthoptic

orthosis

orthotics

osmesthesia

ossicle

ossific

ossification

ossify

ostalgia

osteitis

osteoarthropathy

osteocarcinoma

osteochondroma

osteoclast

osteocyte

osteogen

osteogenesis

osteogeny

osteomalacia

osteometry

osteomyelitis

osteophlebitis

osteophyte

osteoporosis

osteosclerosis

osteosynthesis

ostosis

otitis

otolaryngologist

otomycosis

otoncus

otorhinolaryngology

otorhinology

ototoxic

ovariotomy

ovariotubal

ovicide

oviduct

oviform

ovocyte

ovogenesis

ovoid

oxygenase

oxygenic

oxytocic

oxytocin

P

pachyderma

pachymeter

pachymetry

pachyonychia

palindromic

panarteritis

pancarditis

pancreatic

pancreatitis

pancreatoduodenectomy

pancytopenia

pandemic

panencephalitis

panendoscope

panhysterectomy

pansinusitis

parabiosis

paracentesis

parahepatic

paraneural

paranoia

paranoid

paraparesis

paraphasia

paraplegia

pararenal

parasitemia

parasitize

parasitologist

parasternal

paravesical

parenteral

paresis

paronychia

parotic

partogram

pathogenetic

pathogenic

pathologist

pathology

pectoral

pedagogy

pediatrician

pediatrics

pedicular

pediculosis

pediculus

pelves

pelvic

pelvimetry

penile

penitis

pepsin

peptic

perfusion

periarterial

periarteritis

periarthritis

peribronchiolar

pericarditis

pericardium

pericholangitis

perichondrium

pericoronitis

pericyte

perihepatic

perinephric

perinephritis

perinephrium

periodontal

perioral

periosteitis

periostitis

periostosis

peripharyngeal

periradicular

peristalsis

peritrichous

perivaginitis

pertussis

phacoscope

phage

phagocyte

phagocytize

phagocytosis

phallic

phallus

pharmaceutics

pharmacology

pharmacotherapy

pharyngoplasty

phlebography

phlebolith

phlebolithiasis

phlebosclerosis

phlebotomy

phonasthenia

phoniatrics

phonocardiogram

phonophobia

phosphorolysis

photobiology

photogenic

photolysis

photometer

photosynthesis

phototherapy

phototropism

phrenic

physical

physiologist

phytotherapy

phytotoxin

pleurectomy

pleurodesis

pleurodynia

pleuropneumonia

pleuropulmonary

pneumatics

pneumatocele

pneumatosis

pneumaturia

pneumocephalus

pneumocyte

pneumohypoderma

pneumolysin

pneumonectomy

pneumonolysis

pneumonorrhaphy

podalgia

podiatrist

podocyte

polioencephalitis

polioencephalomyelitis

poliomyelitis

poliovirus

polyarthritis

polycythemia

polydactyly

polydipsia

polymorphism

polymyositis

polyneuritis

polyostotic

polyotia

polyp

polyphagia

polyradiculitis

polyuria

porous

posterosuperior

postlingual

postnasal

postnatal

postpartum

postpuberty

postvaccinal

predentin

preformation

pregnant

prenatal

prepuberal

prepubescent

presbycardia

presbyopia

proctalgia

proctocolitis

proctologist

proctopexia

proctopexy

proctosigmoiditis

prodromal

prognathic

prognathous

prognosis

prolactin

prolapse

prophylactic

prosopagnosia

prostatectomy

prostatodynia

prosthesis

prosthodontics

protopathic

protozoa

protozoology

pseudoanemia

pseudoaneurysm

pseudoarthrosis

pseudobacteremia

pseudocyesis

pseudocyst

pseudoicterus

pseudophakia

psychodiagnosis

psychodiagnostics

psychokinesis

psychometry

psychoneurotic

psychopharmacology

psychophysical

psychosis

psychosomatic

ptosis

ptyalism

pubarche

puberty

pubescence

pulmonary

pulmonic

pulmonologist

puriform

purulent

purulent conjunctivitis

purulent synovitis

pyelitis

pyelogram

pyelolithotomy

pyelonephritis

pyeloplasty

pyemia

pyemic

pylethrombophlebitis

pylethrombosis

pyloristenosis

pyloromyotomy

pyloroplasty

pylorospasm

pyocephalus

pyoid

pyonephrosis

pyosalpinx

pyrexia

pyrogen

pyrogenic

Q

quadriceps

quadriplegia

R

rachiometer

rachischisis

rachitis

rachitome

radiculalgia

radiculoneuritis

radix

receptor

rectocele

rectoclysis

rectocolitis

rectocystotomy

rectopexy

rectostenosis

reflex

reflexogenic

reflexology

regurgitant

regurgitation

relapse

renal calculus

renogram

resectable

resectoscope

respiration

retinochoroid

retinodialysis

retinopathy

retinopexy

retrocecal

retrocervical

retroesophageal

retrolingual

retronasal

retropubic

retrouterine

retrovirus

rhabdoid

rhabdomyolysis

rhabdovirus

rhachialgia

rhinocephaly

rhinodacryolith

rhinogenous

rhinolith

rhinomycosis

rhinopharyngeal

rhinopharyngocele

rhinoplasty

rhinorrhagia

rhinorrhea

rhinoscleroma

rhinoscope

S

salpingo-oophoritis

salpingoscopy

sanguine

sanguineous

sanguinopurulent

saprobes

saprophyte

sarcocele

sarcoma

sarcomatoid

scatology

schistocyte

schistocytosis

schistoprosopia

schizencephaly

schizophrenia

scleroderma

scleromalacia

scleronychia

sclero-oophoritis

sclerosis

sclerotic

sclerotome

scrota

scrotal thermography

section

seminal

seminiferous

semisynthetic

sepsis

septicemia

septorhinoplasty

sialadenosis

sialagogue

sialocele

sialolith

sialolithiasis

sialorrhea

sialosyrinx

sideropenia

siderophore

sigmoiditis

sigmoidoscope

sigmoidoscopy

sincipital

sinistrad

sinistrality

sinogram

sinonasal

sinusitis

sinusoid

somatic

somatogenic

somatoparaphrenia

somatotropic

somnipathy

somnogen

somnolent

somnology

sone

sonic

sonogram

sonography

spasm

spasmolytic

spermatocele

spermatocidal

spermatology

spermatorrhea

spermicide

spermology

sphincterectomy

sphincteroplasty

sphincterotome

sphincterotomy

sphygmogram

sphygmograph

sphygmometer

spirogram

spirometry

splanchna

splanchnic

splanchnicectomy

splanchnocranium

splanchnology

splanchnoptosis

splenicterus

splenocele

splenocolic

splenocyte

splenohepatomegaly

splenomegaly

spondylarthritis

spondylopathy

spondyloptosis

spondylosis

stabile

stabilize

staphylococcemia

staphylococci

staphylococcus

staphylolysin

staphyloma

stasis

stearin

steatohepatitis

steatoma

steatonecrosis

steatorrhea

steatosis

stenosis

stenotic

stereognosis

stereogram

stereology

stereometry

stereophotomicrograph

stereopsis

stereotropism

sternad

sternocostal

sternomastoid

sternothyroid

sternotomy

stethoscope

sthenia

stigmatic

stomatitis

stomatocyte

stomatogastric

streptococcal

streptococcus

streptolysin

subcostal

sublingual

sudor

sudorific

superficial

supervirulent

supradiaphragmatic

suprarenal

symbiosis

symbiotic

symbiotics

symblepharon

symmetry

sympodia

synbiotic

synchondrosis

syndactyly

syndesis

syndesmopexy

synergy

synopsis

synoptophore

synoptoscope

synorchidism

synosteology

synostosis

synovectomy

synoviocyte

synovioma

synthetic

syringectomy

syringocarcinoma

syringoencephalomyelia

syringoma

systole

systolic

T

tachyarrhythmia

tachycardia

tachycardiac

tachygastria

tachyphylaxis

telangiectasis

telogen

tenocyte

tenodesis

tenolysis

tenorrhaphy

tenosynovitis

tenotomy

tensiometer

tension

tensor

thanatology

thelarche

thelium

therapeutics

therapist

therapy

thermodynamics

thermogenesis

thermolabile

thermometry

thermostabile

thoracic

thoracoplasty

thoracoscope

thoracostomy

thrombasthenia

thrombectomy

thrombocyte

thrombocytopoiesis

thrombogenic

thrombophilia

thyroplasty

thyrotome

thyrotoxicosis

thyrotroph

thyrotropin

thyrotropism

tocodynamometer

tocolytic

tomography

tomosynthesis

tonometer

topical

topographical

topography

topology

topophobic

toxemia
toxic
toxicoderma
toxicologist
toxicology
toxicosis
toxigenic
toxin
trachelismus
trachelitis
trachelocele
trachelodynia
trachelology
tracheocele
tracheomalacia
tracheopathy
tracheostomy
tracheotome
trachychromatic
transabdominal
translation
transthoracic
transtracheal
transudate
transudation
trichomycosis
trichonosis
trichophobia
trichotoxin
tricuspid
triorchidism
trophedema
trophic
trophocyte
tubectomy
tuboabdominal

tuboplasty
tuborrhea
tumefacient
tumefaction
tumescence
tussive
typhlectasis
typhlenteritis
typhlitis

U

ultrasonogram
uremia
ureterolithiasis
ureterosigmoidostomy
ureteroureterostomy
urethrismus
urethrocele
urethrography
urethrotomy
urination
urine
urinose
uropathogen
urothelium
uterine
uterocervical
uteropexy
uterotubal

V

vaccine
vaccinology
vaccinotherapeutics
vaginismus
vaginodynia

vaginogenic
vaginolabial
vaginomycosis
vagolysis
vagolytic
vagotonia
vagovagal
varices
varicoblepharon
varicomphalus
varicophlebitis
varicula
vascular
vascularization
vascularize
vasculitis
vasectomy
vasitis
vasohypertonic
vasorrhaphy
vasotomy
vasovagal
venectasia
venoclysis
venospasm
ventrad
ventricle
ventricular
ventroscopy
vesicocele
vesicoclysis
vesicoureteral
vesicouterine
vesicula
vesiculitis
viremia

virucide
virulent
virusemia
virustatic
visceromegaly
viscerosomatic
viscerotropic
viscus

X

xanthine
xanthochromia
xanthoma
xanthomatosis
xanthomatous
xanthophose
xanthous
xerocheilia
xeroderma
xerography
xeropthalmia
xerosis
xerostomia

Z

zoolagnia
zoology
zoopathology
zoophilism
zoophyte
zoopsychology
zymase
zymogen
zymolysis
zymolytic

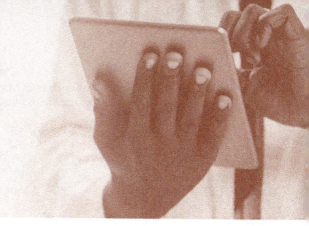

Bibliography

Definitions in this manual have been taken from the following sources:

Latin Words: Lewis CT, Short C, eds. *Harper's Latin Dictionary*. New York, NY: American Book Company, 1907.

Greek Words: Liddell HG, Scott R. *A Greek-English Lexicon*. London, England: Oxford University Press, 1953.

Medical Terms: Venes D, ed. *Taber's Cyclopedic Medical Dictionary*, 23rd ed. Philadelphia, PA: FA Davis, 2017.

Acharia AB, Wroton M. Broca Aphasia. StatPearls, NCBI Bookshelf. Updated May 4, 2022.

Age-related macular degeneration. Centers for Disease Control and Prevention. https://www.cdc.gov/visionhealth/basics/ced/index.html#a3. Accessed February 6, 2021.

Aminoff MJ, Greenberg DA, Simon RP. *Clinical Neurology*. Stamford, CT: Appleton & Lange, 1996.

Ayers DM. *English Words from Latin and Greek Elements*. Tucson, AZ: University of Arizona Press, 1965.

Bauer J. *Differential Diagnosis of Internal Disease*. New York, NY: Grune & Stratton, 1967.

Benson RC. *Handbook of Obstetrics and Gynecology*. Los Altos, CA: Lange Medical Publications, 1980.

Boggs DR, Winkelstein A. *White Cell Manual*. Philadelphia, PA: FA Davis, 1975.

Burriss EE, Casson L. *Latin and Greek in Current Use*. Englewood Cliffs, NJ: Prentice-Hall, 1949.

Carmichael AG, Razan RM, eds. *Medicine: A Treasury of Art and Literature*. New York, NY: Harkavy Publishing Service, 1991.

Chronic lymphocytic leukemia treatment (PDQ®)–patient version. National Cancer Institute. https://www.cancer.gov/types/leukemia/patient/cll-treatment-pdq. Accessed July 31, 2021.

Corpus luteum and the menstrual cycle. *MedicalNewsToday*. https://www.medicalnewstoday.com/articles/320433#corpus-luteum-and-the-menstrual-cycle. Accessed May 5, 2021.

Couch M. *Greek and Roman Mythology*. New York, NY: Metrobooks, 1997.

Daviel's method was explained in an article in the Annals of the Royal Academy of Surgery (Paris), *Sur une nouvelle méthode de guérir la cataracte par l'extraction du cristallin*, in 1753.

Dunmore CW, Fleischer RM. *Medical Terminology: Lessons in Etymology*, 3rd ed. Philadelphia, PA: FA Davis, 2004.

Episcleritis. Healthline. https://www.healthline.com/health/episcleritis. Accessed February 6, 2021.

FAQs about spinal cord injury (SCI). University of Alabama at Birmingham. https://www.uab.edu/medicine/sci/faqs-about-spinal-cord-injury-sci. Accessed August 14, 2021

Federative Committee on Anatomical Terminology. *Terminologia Anatomica*. Stuttgart, Germany: Georg Thieme Verlag, 1998.

Feldman M. *Sleisenger and Fordtran's Gastrointestinal and Liver Disease*, 7th ed. Philadelphia, PA: WB Saunders, 2002.

Fell DW, Lunnen KY, Rauk RP. Lifespan Neurorehabilitation: A Patient-Centered Approach from Examination to Interventions and Outcomes. Philadelphia, PA: FA Davis, 2018.

Flynn CA, D'Amico F, Smith G. Should we patch corneal abrasions? A meta-analysis. J Fam Pract. 1998, 47:264-270.

Garrison FH. *An Introduction to the History of Medicine*, 3rd ed. Philadelphia, PA: WB Saunders, 1927.

Goldman L, Bennett JC, eds. *Cecil Textbook of Medicine*, 21st ed. Philadelphia, PA: WB Saunders, 2000.

Grendell JH, McQuaid KR, Friedman SL. *Current Diagnosis and Treatment in Gastroenterology*. Stamford, CT: Appleton & Lange, 1996.

Gylys B, Masters R. *Medical Terminology Simplified: A Programmed Learning Approach by Body System*, 6th ed. Philadelphia, PA: FA Davis, 2019.

Gylys, BA, Wedding ME. *Medical Terminology Systems: A Body Systems Approach*, 8th ed. Philadelphia, PA: FA Davis, 2017.

Harker LA. *Hemostasis Manual*. Philadelphia, PA: FA Davis, 1974.

Harvey AM. *The Principles and Practice of Medicine*, 17th ed. New York, NY: Appleton-Century-Crofts, 1968.

Healthy contact lens wear and care. Centers for Disease Control and Prevention. https://www.cdc.gov/contactlenses/fast-facts.html. Accessed February 6, 2021.

Henry RK, Goldie MP. *Dental Hygiene: Applications to Clinical Practice*. Philadelphia, PA: FA Davis, 2016.

Herness J, Buttolph A, Hammer NC. Acute pyelonephritis in adults: rapid evidence review. Am Fam Physician. 2020;102(3):173-180. https://www.aafp.org/afp/2020/0801/p173.html. Accessed July 5, 2021.

Hillman RS, Finch CA. *Red Cell Manual*. Philadelphia, PA: FA Davis, 1974.

Hoffman J, Sullivan N. *Medical-Surgical Nursing: Making Connections to Practice*, 2nd ed. Philadelphia, PA: FA Davis, 2020.

Holvey DN, ed. *The Merck Manual of Diagnosis and Therapy*, 12th ed. Rahway, NJ: Sharp & Dohme Research Laboratories, 1972.

Houston JC, Joiner CL, Trounce JR. *A Short Textbook of Medicine*. London, England: English Universities Press, 1972.

Journal of the American Medical Association. Chicago, IL: 1974, 1975, 1976.

Keefer CS, Wilkins RW. *Medicine, Essentials of Clinical Practice*. Boston, MA: Little, Brown, 1970.

Kidney stones. Mayo Clinic. https://www.mayoclinic.org/diseases -conditions/kidney-stones/diagnosis-treatment/drc-20355759. Accessed June 17, 2021.

Lewis AE. *The Principles of Hematology*. New York, NY: Appleton-Century-Crofts, 1970.

Lewis CT, Short C, eds. *Harper's Latin Dictionary*. New York, NY: American Book Company, 1907.

Liddell HG, Robert S. *A Greek-English Lexicon*. London, England: Oxford University Press, 1953.

Lippert L. *Clinical Kinesiology and Anatomy*, 6th ed. Philadelphia, PA: FA Davis, 2017.

Male infertility. Mayo Clinic. https://www.mayoclinic.org /diseases-conditions/male-infertility/symptoms-causes /syc-20374773. Updated April 13, 2021. Accessed June 12, 2021.

McCrum R, Cran W, MacNeil R. *The Story of English*. New York, NY: Viking, 1986.

Melanocyte-stimulating hormone. Society for Endocrinology. https://www.yourhormones.info/hormones/melanocyte -stimulating-hormone/. Reviewed May 2021. Accessed August 29, 2021.

Morbidity & Mortality Weekly Report, Centers for Disease Control and Prevention, January 16, 2015.

National Diabetes Statistics Report, 2020. Centers for Disease Control and Prevention. https://www.cdc.gov/diabetes /pdfs/data/statistics/national-diabetes-statistics-report.pdf. Accessed July 7, 2021.

National Library of Medicine. *MedlinePlus Medical Encyclopedia*. https://medlineplus.gov/encyclopedia.html. Accessed September 18, 2022.

New York Heart Association. *Nomenclature and Criteria for Diagnosis of Diseases of the Heart and Great Vessels*, 7th ed. Boston, MA: Little, Brown, 1973.

Nybakken OE. *Greek and Latin in Scientific Terminology*. Ames, IA: Iowa State University Press, 1959.

Orchitis. Mayo Clinic. https://www.mayoclinic.org/diseases -conditions/orchitis/symptoms-causes/syc-20375860. Published November 6, 2020. Accessed June 6, 2021.

Rothman J. Brain tumors: who gets them and what is the survival rate? https://www.everydayhealth.com/brain -tumor/brain-tumor-statistics.aspx. Reviewed March 5, 2018. Accessed August 4, 2021.

Ryan KJ, Berkowitz RS, Barbieri RL, eds. *Kistner's Gynecology and Women's Health*, 7th ed. St. Louis, MO: Mosby, 2000.

Sarmast ST, Abdullahi AM, Jahan N. Current classification of seizures and epilepsies: scope, limitations and recommendations for future action. *Cureus*. 2020, 12(9): e10549. https://doi.org/10.7759/cureus.10549.

Scanlon VC, Sanders T. *Essentials of Anatomy and Physiology*, 8th ed. Philadelphia, PA: FA Davis, 2020.

Shaw I, ed. *The Oxford History of Ancient Egypt*. New York, NY: Oxford University Press, 2000.

Seminiferous tubule. Science Direct. https://www.sciencedirect .com/topics/neuro science/seminiferous-tubule. Accessed June 6, 2021.

Tanagho EA, McAninch JW. *Smith's General Urology*, 14th ed. Norwalk, CT: Appleton & Lange, 1995.

The LASIK Institute (http://www.lasikinstitute.org). Accessed February 6, 2021.

Treatment for fungal eye infections. Centers for Disease Control and Prevention. https://www.cdc.gov/fungal/diseases/fungal -eye-infections/treatment.html. Accessed February 6, 2021.

Undescended testicle (cryptorchidism). Harvard Health Publishing. https://www.health.harvard.edu/a_to_z/undescended-testicle -a-to-z. Published July 1, 2019. Accessed June 11, 2021.

Undescended testicle. Mayo Clinic. https://www.mayoclinic.org /diseases-conditions/undescended-testicle/diagnosis-treatment /drc-20352000. Accessed June 11, 2021.

Vaughan D, Asbury T, Cook R. *General Ophthalmology*. Los Altos, CA: Lange Medical Publications, 1971.

Vaughan D, Asbury T, Riordan-Eva P. *General Ophthalmology*. Stamford, CT: Appleton & Lange, 1995.

Venes D, ed. *Taber's Cyclopedic Medical Dictionary*, 19th ed. Philadelphia, PA: FA Davis, 2001.

Venes D, ed. *Taber's Cyclopedic Medical Dictionary*, 23rd ed. Philadelphia, PA: FA Davis, 2017.

Vitamin A and carotenoids. National Institutes of Health. http:// ods.od.nih.gov/factsheets/VitaminA-HealthProfessional/#h2. Accessed February 6, 2021.

Walsh PC, Retik AB, Darracott Vaughan E, et al. *Campbell's Urology*, 8th ed., 4 vols. Philadelphia, PA: WB Saunders, 2002.

Wernicke aphasia. Venes D, ed. *Taber's Cyclopedic Medical Dictionary*, 23rd ed. FA Davis, 2017, p. 2531.

What to know about acute renal failure. *MedicalNewsToday*. https://www.medicalnewstoday.com/articles/324627#causes. Reviewed March 5, 2019. Accessed June 15, 2021.

Wilson RH. *Williams Textbook of Endocrinology*, 9th ed. Philadelphia, PA: WB Saunders, 1998.

World Health Organization, Measles Fact Sheet, December 2019, https://www.who.int/news-room.fact-sheets/detail/measles

World Health Organization, Poliomyelitis, July 22, 2019, https:// www.who.int/news-room/fact-sheets/detail/poliomyelitis

Yanoff M, Duker JW, eds. *Ophthalmology*. London, England: CV Mosby, 1999.

Zagaria MAE. HSV Keratitis: An Important Infectious Cause of Blindness. *US Pharm*. 2015;40(4):16-18.